BASIC
MEDICAL
LABORATORY
TECHNIQUES

Second Edition

BASIC MEDICAL LABORATORY TECHNIQUES

Second Edition

NORMA J. WALTERS, R.N., PH.D.
ASSOCIATE PROFESSOR, TEACHER EDUCATOR, AND COORDINATOR
HEALTH OCCUPATIONS EDUCATION
COLLEGE OF EDUCATION
AUBURN UNIVERSITY
AUBURN, ALABAMA 36849

BARBARA H. ESTRIDGE, B.S., MT(ASCP)
RESEARCH ASSOCIATE
COLLEGE OF SCIENCES AND MATHEMATICS
(FORMERLY INSTRUCTOR, MEDICAL TECHNOLOGY)
AUBURN UNIVERSITY
AUBURN, ALABAMA 36849

ANNA P. REYNOLDS, B.S., MT(ASCP)
CHIEF MEDICAL TECHNOLOGIST
DRAKE STUDENT HEALTH CENTER
(FORMERLY INSTRUCTOR, MEDICAL TECHNOLOGY)
AUBURN UNIVERSITY
AUBURN, ALABAMA 36849

 DELMAR PUBLISHERS INC.®

NOTICE TO THE READER

Front cover photographs courtesy of Joseph Schuyler Photography.
Back cover photograph courtesy of Becton Dickinson Vacutainer Systems.

Delmar Staff:

Executive Editor: Leslie F. Boyer

Managing Editor: Gerry East

Project Editor: Marlene McHugh Pratt

Senior Production Supervisor: Karen Seebald

Design Coordinator: Susan Mathews

For information, address Delmar Publishers Inc.
3 Columbia Circle
Albany, New York 12212

10 9 8 7 6 5

Printed in the United States of America
Published simultaneously in Canada
by Nelson Canada,
a Division of The Thomson Corporation

Library of Congress Cataloging-in-Publication Data

Walters, Norma J.
    Basic medical laboratory techniques / Norma J. Walters, Barbara H.
    Estridge, Anna P. Reynolds. — 2nd ed.
        p. cm.
    Includes bibliographical references.
    ISBN 0-8273-3948-8 (pbk.)
    1. Diagnosis, Laboratory. 2. Medical laboratory technology.
I. Estridge, Barbara H. II. Reynolds, Anna P. III. Title.
    [DNLM: 1. Diagnosis, Laboratory. 2. Technology, Medical. QY 25
W235b]
RB37.W25   1990
616.07′5—dc20
DNLM/DLC   89–17168
for Library of Congress   CIP

Contents

List of Color Plates   ix
List of Figures and Tables   xi
Preface   xvii
About the Book   xix

UNIT 1: INTRODUCTION TO THE MEDICAL LABORATORY   1

LESSON 1-1   The Medical Laboratory   3
LESSON 1-2   The Medical Laboratory Professional   8
LESSON 1-3   Laboratory Safety   14
LESSON 1-4   Laboratory Glassware and Equipment   23
LESSON 1-5   The Microscope   33
LESSON 1-6   Introduction to Medical Terminology   44
LESSON 1-7   The Metric System   50
LESSON 1-8   Laboratory Math   58
LESSON 1-9   Isolation Techniques for the Laboratory Worker   66

UNIT 2: BASIC HEMATOLOGY   77

LESSON 2-1   Capillary Puncture   79
LESSON 2-2   Microhematocrit   85
LESSON 2-3   Blood Diluting Pipets   94
LESSON 2-4   The Hemacytometer   107
LESSON 2-5   The Red Blood Cell Count   119
LESSON 2-6   The White Blood Cell Count   134
LESSON 2-7   Hemoglobin Determination   146
LESSON 2-8   Preparation of a Blood Smear   156
LESSON 2-9   Staining a Blood Smear   163
LESSON 2-10   Identification of Normal Blood Cells   171
LESSON 2-11   Differential Leukocyte Count   178

UNIT 3: ADVANCED HEMATOLOGY 187

LESSON 3-1   Venipuncture 189
LESSON 3-2   Erythrocyte Sedimentation Rate 202
LESSON 3-3   Reticulocyte Count 209
LESSON 3-4   Platelet Count 215
LESSON 3-5   Prothrombin Time 228
LESSON 3-6   Erythrocyte Indices 236
LESSON 3-7   Bleeding Time 243
LESSON 3-8   Capillary Coagulation 249

UNIT 4: INTRODUCTION TO SEROLOGY 255

LESSON 4-1   ABO Slide Typing 257
LESSON 4-2   ABO Tube Typing 264
LESSON 4-3   Rh Slide Typing 270
LESSON 4-4   Urine Pregnancy Test 277
LESSON 4-5   Slide Test for Infectious Mononucleosis 283
LESSON 4-6   Slide Test for Rheumatoid Factors 290

UNIT 5: URINALYSIS 297

LESSON 5-1   Collection and Preservation of Urine 299
LESSON 5-2   Physical Examination of Urine 307
LESSON 5-3   Chemical Examination of Urine 315
LESSON 5-4   Identification of Urine Sediment 324
LESSON 5-5   Microscopic Examination of Urine Sediment 336

UNIT 6: INTRODUCTION TO BACTERIOLOGY 343

LESSON 6-1   Identification of Stained Bacteria 345
LESSON 6-2   Preparation of a Bacteriological Smear 350
LESSON 6-3   The Gram Stain 361
LESSON 6-4   Inoculation of Media 368
LESSON 6-5   Collection and Handling of Bacteriological Specimens 377
LESSON 6-6   Performing a Throat Culture and a Rapid Test for Group A *Streptococcus* 382
LESSON 6-7   Performing a Urine Culture 390

UNIT 7: BASIC CLINICAL CHEMISTRY 397

LESSON 7-1   Introduction to Clinical Chemistry 399
LESSON 7-2   Quality Control 410
LESSON 7-3   The Spectrophotometer 422
LESSON 7-4   Instrumentation in the Small Laboratory 432
LESSON 7-5   Measurement of Blood Cholesterol 441
LESSON 7-6   Measurement of Blood Glucose 450

REFERENCES AND SUGGESTED READINGS   469

GLOSSARY   471

APPENDICES   479

Appendix A: Safety Agreement Form   479
Appendix B: Abbreviations, Prefixes, Suffixes, and Stems   481
Appendix C: Metric Conversions   488
Appendix D: Temperature Conversions   490
Appendix E: Examples of Preparing Solutions and Dilutions   491
Appendix F: Table of Normal Hematological Values   493
Appendix G: Hematology—CBC Report Form   495
Appendix H: Table of Normal Clinical Chemistry Values   497
Appendix I: Percent Transmittance—Absorbance Conversion Chart   498
Appendix J: Table of Normal Urine Values   500
Appendix K: Routine Urinalysis Report Form   501
Appendix L: Guide for Selection of Vacuum Tubes   503
Appendix M: Examples of Laboratory Requisition Forms   504
Appendix N: Preparation of Reagents   505
Appendix O: Sources of Laboratory Supplies   507

INDEX   509

List of Color Plates

HEMATOLOGY

PLATE 1:   Segmented neutrophils
PLATE 2:   Neutrophilic bands
PLATE 3:   Eosinophils
PLATE 4:   Basophils
PLATE 5:   Lymphocytes
PLATE 6:   Monocytes
PLATE 7:   Normal erythrocytes in peripheral blood (Wright's stain)
PLATE 8:   Platelets in peripheral blood (1000X)
PLATE 9:   Photomicrograph of Wright's stained erythrocytes and platelets in peripheral blood (1000X)
PLATE 10:   Examples of blood cells seen in peripheral blood smear from a normal individual
PLATE 11:   Photomicrograph of lymphocyte and segmented neutrophil (1000X)
PLATE 12:   Photomicrograph of reticulocytes stained with New Methylene Blue (1000X)
PLATE 13:   Photomicrograph of erythroctyes as they appear in an RBC count (400X)
PLATE 14:   Photomicrograph of leukocytes as they appear in a hemacytometer (100X)
PLATE 15:   Photomicrograph of platelets (arrows) as they appear in a platelet count (400X)
PLATE 16:   Normal peripheral blood.   A. basophil B. monocyte

URINALYSIS

PLATE 17:   Reagent strips used for chemical analysis of urine (positive reactions, left)
PLATE 18:   Squamous epithelial cells, red blood cells, leukocyte
PLATE 19:   Renal epithelial cell and erythrocytes
PLATE 20:   Hyaline casts
PLATE 21:   Granular casts and a leukocyte
PLATE 22:   Two uric acid crystals
PLATE 23:   Two ammonium magnesium phosphate crystals (triple phosphate) with amorphous phosphate granules
PLATE 24:   Fibers in urine

BACTERIOLOGY

PLATE 25:   Gram positive coccus from a pure culture
PLATE 26:   Gram negative rod from a pure culture
PLATE 27:   Gram positive bacillus from a pure culture
PLATE 28:   A blood agar plate showing isolated colonies of bacteria
PLATE 29:   Antibiotic susceptibility test plate
PLATE 30:   Biochemical strip tests for bacterial identification

Color Plates 1-7 and 10. Courtesy of John Estridge

Color Plate 20. Coutresy of Ames Division of Miles Laboratories, Inc., Elkhart, IN. From *Modern Urine Chemistry*, 1982.

Color Plates 21, 22, 23. Courtesy of W.B. Saunders Co., Philadelphia, PA. From *Clinical Diagnosis by Laboratory Methods*, 17th Ed., 1984.

List of Figures and Tables

UNIT 1: INTRODUCTION TO THE MEDICAL LABORATORY

Figures

1-1   Organizational chart of a typical medical laboratory   5
1-2   Physical hazards   15
1-3   Chemical hazards   16
1-4   Examples of biohazard containers   18
1-5   Biological hazards   18
1-6   A safe laboratory   19
1-7   Beakers with markings   24
1-8   Flasks   25
1-9   Meniscus   25
1-10   Test tubes   26
1-11   Volumetric pipet   26
1-12   Serological pipet   26
1-13   Micropipets   27
1-14   Graduated cylinder with markings   28
1-15   Examples of mechanical automatic pipetters   29
1-16   Example of electrical automatic pipetter   29
1-17   The Micro-Pipex pipet filler   29
1-18   Monocular microscope   35
1-19   Parts of a microscope   36
1-20   Transporting the microscope   38
1-21   Example of Fahrenheit temperature converted to Celsius   59
1-22   Example of Celsius temperature converted to Fahrenheit   59
1-23   Preparing a solution using proportions   60
1-24   Using the formula: $C_1 \times V_1 = C_2 \times V_2$ to prepare a solution   60
1-25   Preparation of a weight to volume (w/v) percentage solution   61
1-26   Preparation of a volume to volume (v/v) percentage solution   61
1-27   Preparation of a 1:10 dilution   61
1-28   Handwashing technique   68
1-29   Putting on a clean mask and cover gown before entering the patient's room   69
1-30   Removing the contaminated gown   70
1-31   Donning sterile gloves   71
1-32   A clean cover gown is put on before entering the patient's room   72
1-33   Double-bagging technique   72

Tables

1-1   Selected prefixes commonly used in medical terminology   45–46
1-2   Selected stems commonly used in medical terminology   47
1-3   Selected suffixes commonly used in medical terminology   48
1-4   Abbreviations commonly used in a medical laboratory   48–49
1-5   Commonly used prefixes in the metric system   52
1-6   Conversion of English units to metric units   52
1-7   Conversion of metric units to English units   53
1-8   Common metric equivalents   53
1-9   International System of Units   54

UNIT 2: BASIC HEMATOLOGY

Figures

2-1	Capillary puncture	80
2-2	Massaging the finger gently to increase blood flow	81
2-3	Collecting capillary blood into a capillary tube	81
2-4	Diagram of packed cell column	86
2-5	Filling the capillary tube from a tube of blood	87
2-6	Sealing the capillary tube with sealing clay	87
2-7	Microhematocrit centrifuge with built-in reader	88
2-8	Microhematocrit centrifuge without reader	89
2-9	Microhematocrit reader	90
2-10	Red and white cell diluting pipets	95
2-11	Parts of a red cell diluting pipet	96
2-12	Aspirating a sample using the RBC pipet	97
2-13	Diluting a sample using the RBC pipet	98
2-14	Manual rotation of blood diluting pipet using figure-eight motion	99
2-15	Automatic pipet shaker	100
2-16	Dispensing four to five drops from blood diluting pipet onto a gauze pad	101
2-17	Cleaning a blood diluting pipet using suction apparatus	102
2-18	Parts of a disposable blood diluting unit such as Unopette®	103
2-19	Hemacytometer with coverglass in place	108
2-20	Side view of hemacytometer with coverglass in place	108
2-21	Ruled area of hemacytometer showing dimensions	109
2-22	WBC counting area	110
2-23	RBC counting area	111
2-24	Filling the hemacytometer	112
2-25	Left-to-right, right-to-left counting pattern	112
2-26	Boundaries and dimensions of ruled area	113
2-27	RBC counting area	121
2-28	Sample count in square ''a'' on one side of chamber	122
2-29	Sample calculation of an RBC count	123
2-30	Automated cell counters	124
2-31	WBC counting area	135
2-32	Sample count in square one of WBC counting area	136
2-33	Sample calculation of a WBC count	137
2-34	Sahli pipet	148
2-35	Sample calculation of hemoglobin using the absorbance formula	149
2-36	The Hb-Direct™ system	149
2-37	Positioning the spreader slide in front of the drop of blood	157
2-38	Spreading the blood with a spreader slide	157
2-39	Properly prepared smear vs improper smears	158
2-40	Applying Wright's stain to a blood smear	164
2-41	Applying buffer to Wright's stain	164
2-42	Mixing buffer and stain	165
2-43	Parts of a stained erythrocyte, segmented neutrophil, and lymphocyte	166
2-44	Proper area of slide to view	174
2-45	Proper area of slide to be viewed for differential count	179
2-46	Differential counter	180

Tables

2-1	Normal microhematocrit values	87
2-2	Normal RBC counts in adult males and adult females	120
2-3	Normal leukocyte counts	135
2-4	Normal hemoglobin values	147
2-5	Leukocyte identification guide	173
2-6	Normal values for differential count	180

UNIT 3: ADVANCED HEMATOLOGY

Figures

3-1   Materials for venipuncture   190
3-2   Tying a tourniquet   192
3-3   Releasing the tourniquet   193
3-4   Veins most commonly used for venipuncture   193
3-5   Palpating a vein with fingertip   194
3-6   Performing the puncture   195
3-7   Withdrawing needle from puncture   196
3-8   Vacuum tube blood collecting system   197
3-9   Materials for erythrocyte sedimentation rate   203
3-10   Erythrocyte sedimentation rate   203
3-11   Sedimentation tube showing settling of cells   204
3-12   Erythrocytes forming rouleau   205
3-13   Reticulocytes showing stained reticulum   210
3-14   Sample calculation of reticulocyte percentage   211
3-15   Hemacytometer in moist chamber   216
3-16   Platelet counting area   217
3-17   Sample calculation of platelet count   218
3-18   Unopette® microcollection system   219
3-19   Illustrating manual tilt-tube method of determining prothrombin time   230
3-20   Using the Fibrometer® to perform a prothrombin time test   231
3-21   Calculation of mean corpuscular volume   237
3-22   Calculation of mean corpuscular hemoglobin   237
3-23   Calculation of mean corpuscular hemoglobin concentration   237
3-24   Puncture site in Ivy bleeding time   244
3-25   Simplate® device used in performing bleeding time test   244
3-26   Performing a bleeding time test using a Simplate®   245
3-27   Puncture site for Duke bleeding time   245
3-28   Capillary coagulation: breaking the capillary tube   250
3-29   Capillary coagulation: appearance of the fibrin thread   251

Tables

3-1   Guide for selection of vacuum tubes   197
3-2   Normal values for Wintrobe method of erythrocyte sedimentation rate   204
3-3   Normal reticulocyte percentages   211
3-4   Normal values for erythrocyte indices   238

UNIT 4: INTRODUCTION TO SEROLOGY

Figures

4-1   ABO slide typing: microscope slide with antisera and blood added   259
4-2   ABO slide typing: mixing antisera and blood   259
4-3   Agglutination of blood cells by anti-A in ABO typing   259
4-4   Rh slide typing using viewbox   272
4-5   Principle of agglutination inhibition test for pregnancy   278
4-6   Monospot® slide with reagents added   284
4-7   Mixing reagents on Monospot® slide using wooden applicator   285
4-8   Principle of agglutination test for rheumatoid factors   291
4-9   Example of latex agglutination   292

Tables

4-1   Table of ABO antigens and antibodies   258
4-2   Reactions of ABO groups with anti-A and anti-B   260
4-3   Forward and reverse typing results for ABO blood groups   265
4-4   Fisher-Race and Wiener nomenclature for Rh system   271
4-5   Interpretation of results of Rh slide typing   273
4-6   Interpretation of results of Monospot® test   285

UNIT 5: URINALYSIS

Figures
5-1   Refractometer   309
5-2   Urinometer   310
5-3   Various types of reagent strips used for urine testing   316
5-4   Erythrocytes in urine sediment   325
5-5   Leukocytes in urine sediment   325
5-6   Squamous epithelial cells   325
5-7   Bladder and renal tubular epithelial cells   326
5-8   Bacteria in urine sediment   326
5-9   Yeasts in urine sediment   327
5-10   Protozoa in urine sediment   327
5-11   Spermatozoa in urine sediment   327
5-12   Casts in urine sediment   328
5-13   Amorphous urates in urine sediment   329
5-14   Uric acid crystals in urine sediment   329
5-15   Calcium oxalate crystals in urine sediment   329
5-16   Amorphous phosphates in urine sediment   330
5-17   Triple phosphate crystals in urine sediment   330
5-18   Calcium carbonate crystals in urine sediment   330
5-19   Cystine crystals in urine sediment   331
5-20   Tyrosine crystals in urine sediment   331
5-21   Leucine crystals in urine sediment   331
5-22   Cholesterol crystals in urine sediment   332
5-23   Sulfonamide crystals in urine sediment   332
5-24   Mucus threads in urine sediment   333
5-25   Examples of artifacts which may be seen in urine sediment   333

Tables
5-1   Normal 24-hour urine volumes   301
5-2   Table of urine colors and their causes   308
5-3   Physical characteristics of normal urine   310
5-4   Normal values for urine chemical tests   318
5-5   Normal values for components of urine sediment   337

UNIT 6: INTRODUCTION TO BACTERIOLOGY

Figures
6-1   Microscopic appearance of round bacteria   346
6-2   Microscopic appearance of rod-shaped bacteria   347
6-3   Microscopic appearance of spiral bacteria   347
6-4   Preparation of a direct smear from a swab   351
6-5   Heat-fixing a bacteriological smear   352
6-6   Sterilizing the inoculating loop   352
6-7   Flaming a culture tube   353
6-8   Transferring bacteria from a culture tube to a slide   353
6-9   Making a bacterial smear using the inoculating loop   354
6-10   Removing bacteria from an agar plate using the inoculating loop   355
6-11   Slide staining rack   362
6-12   Transferring organisms from agar slant to broth   369
6-13   Inoculation of broth   370
6-14   Streaking an agar plate in four quadrants   370
6-15   Inoculation of an agar slant   372
6-16   Examples of supplies for collection and transport of bacteriological specimens   378
6-17   Culturette® system for collection and transport of bacteriological specimens   379
6-18   Transferring throat culture swab to an agar plate   384
6-19   EIA test for strep   385
6-20   Results of a rapid strep test   386
6-21   Streaking a urine plate   391

6-22   Isolated colonies on a blood agar plate   391
6-23   Antibiotic susceptibility test plate   392

Table
6-1   Steps of Gram stain procedure   363

UNIT 7: BASIC CLINICAL CHEMISTRY

Figures
7-1   Relative intracellular and extracellular electrolyte concentration   404
7-2   Accuracy versus precision   412
7-3   Normal distribution curves   414
7-4   Levey-Jennings charts   416
7-5   An example of a spectrophotometer   423
7-6   Diagram of internal parts of a spectrophotometer   424
7-7   Illustration of a standard curve showing absorbance versus concentration   425
7-8   Determining the concentration of an unknown using a standard curve   426
7-9   Illustration of a solid-phase reagent strip   434
7-10   Illustration of the insertion of the sample card into the Kodak Ektachem DT60   435
7-11   The VISION™ System clinical chemistry analyzer   436
7-12   The NOVA 12 clinical chemistry analyzer   436
7-13   Glucometer® II with parts labeled   454

Table
7-1   Normal levels of blood cholesterol   443
7-2   Normal ranges for HDL and LDL cholesterol   443

Preface

Basic Medical Laboratory Techniques, 2nd edition, was written in response to a need to provide students, prospective teachers and teachers with a text which combines both theory and techniques of basic medical laboratory procedures. This second edition incorporates suggestions from reviewers and has been expanded to meet the needs requested.

Educational Challenges

Individuals interested in pursuing careers in health fields such as clinical laboratory medicine, nursing, pharmacy, dental assisting, respiratory therapy, medical assisting, or medical records can no longer acquire mastery of the chosen field by learning only on the job. Even though on-the-job training remains important, training in the various health care skills must also be taught in the classroom and laboratory. There is a need for well-trained personnel prepared to teach these skills.

Educators have encountered many challenges in trying to provide well-designed materials for training personnel for the various health careers and have been handicapped by a lack of appropri-

ate textbooks. Students being introduced to health careers in laboratory medicine have found it very difficult to obtain fundamental information in one text written in a concise, sequential, and clear manner to meet their needs. In addition, personnel already employed in a health career have not been able to obtain educational materials concerning clinical laboratory procedures which provide a basic review or supplement their knowledge and experience.

In order to respond to the needs of teacher educators, classroom teachers and students, the authors conducted workshops for health occupations teachers in which basic medical laboratory procedures were taught. As a result of the positive response to these workshops, the idea of a textbook of *Basic Medical Laboratory Techniques* and the *Basic Medical Laboratory Techniques Instructor's Guide* was conceived. *Basic Medical Laboratory Techniques* incorporates the workshop materials and evaluations from workshop participants as well as reviewers. The performance-based text and guide have been carefully designed to promote learning and to aid teaching in group sessions as well as individualized study.

ACKNOWLEDGMENTS

The authors wish to express their appreciation to all who gave freely of their time, despite busy schedules, in the development of the book including:

John A. Estridge
   Illustrations and photographs

David A. Estridge
   Illustrations

Student assistants
   Johnny deGuzman   Howard Scott
   Donda Huett   Carol Stewart
   Kathy Kirby   Pamela White
   Susan McDonald   Dottie Whitehead
   Kelley Patterson

Health Occupations teachers and students
Participants in workshops

   The authors also wish to thank the following companies and institutions for providing some of the information and photographs:

   Abbott Laboratories
   Ames Company, Division of Miles Laboratories, Inc.
   Becton-Dickinson Labware
   Boehringer-Mannheim Diagnostics
   Clay-Adams Division, Becton-Dickinson and Company
   Drake Student Health Center, Auburn University, AL
   East Alabama Medical Center, Opelika, AL
   Eastman Kodak Company
   Fisher Scientific Company
   General Diagnostics, Division of Warner Lambert Company
   Hybritech
   International Equipment Company, Division of Damon Corporation
   ISOLAB, Inc.
   Marion Laboratories, Inc., Marion Scientific Division
   NOVA biomedical
   Ortho Diagnostics Systems, Inc.
   Reichert Scientific Instruments
   Sigma Chemical Company
   TIP Industries, Inc.
   W. B. Saunders Company

About the Book

Basic Medical Laboratory Techniques, 2nd edition, has been specifically designed for maximum use by the health occupations teacher educators in training prospective student teachers for teaching in a cluster or a specific program. The book may also be used by classroom teachers and students in other allied health training programs, such as the medical laboratory technician programs, medical assistant programs, and the medical laboratory assistant programs. In addition, persons already employed in the medical field may use the book as a reference to augment or supplement their knowledge base and experience.

The content and organization of the book provides for unlimited flexibility in the teaching and learning processes. The book has been written emphasizing many basic manual laboratory procedures which illustrate fundamental principles and are taught in most training programs, even though larger hospitals and laboratories use automation for most procedures.

The topics of the seven units in the text include: Introduction to the Medical Laboratory, Basic Hematology, Advanced Hematology, Introduction to Serology, Urinalysis, Introduction to Bacteriology, and Basic Clinical Chemistry. New additions in this second edition include: a new lesson on safety and a new lesson on isolation techniques in Unit 1; a new unit on basic clinical chemistry which includes glucose and cholesterol; a rapid strep test in the unit on bacteriology; a prothrombin time (PT) in the unit on advanced hematology; the rheumatoid factor in the unit on serology; additional illustrations and photographs throughout the textbook; and use of vacuum tubes and examples of laboratory requisition forms in the appendices. An overview precedes each unit and includes a list of unit objectives. Each lesson in the units contains objectives, glossary terms, and basic information. Precautions, student activities, lesson reviews, worksheets, and student performance guides are included where appropriate. Figures, tables, and photographs are incorporated to aid in understanding and interpreting the information and procedures. Color plates are also included to assist the student to identify blood cells, components of urine sediment, and bacteria. In addition, a glossary and list of references have been provided to supplement the text.

The appendices contain important information which is easily located. These include abbreviations; prefixes; suffixes and stems; tables of normal values; metric and temperature conversion charts; %T-A conversion chart; samples of hematology and urinalysis report forms; use of vacuum tubes; and examples of laboratory requisition forms. Helpful information on preparation of reagents, examples of preparing solutions and dilutions, and sources of laboratory supplies is also included. In addition, a safety agreement form has been included which should be read and completed by each student and filed before any laboratory procedure is performed.

An instructor's guide is also available to assist the teacher in teaching various procedures. The guide includes self-contained lesson plans for each lesson in the student text. These contain objectives, glossary terms, introduction, lesson content, method of teaching, resources, student learning activities, equipment and materials, a method of evaluation, summary of lesson, test/test key, and a final performance check sheet and worksheets, as appropriate. After Unit 1 has been completed, Units 2, 4, 5, 6, or 7 may be studied in the order of preference of the instructor, depending on the availability of time, laboratory space, and equipment. Unit 3 should be used as a sequel to Unit 2.

Educators and students should find this book an essential aid in understanding and teaching basic laboratory techniques. The book can be used as a methodology text and as a valuable reference book.

TO THE STUDENT

Basic Medical Laboratory Techniques was written primarily to introduce the prospective teacher or student to the basic principles and techniques of some commonly performed medical laboratory procedures. The information is presented in a brief and interesting manner to facilitate learning.

New additions in this second edition include: a new lesson on safety and a new lesson on isolation techniques in Unit 1; a new unit on basic clinical chemistry which includes glucose and cholesterol; a rapid strep test in the unit on bacteriology; a prothrombin time (PT) in the unit on advanced hematology; the rheumatoid factor in the unit on serology; additional illustrations and photographs throughout the textbook; and use of vacuum tubes and examples of laboratory requisition forms in the appendices.

The book is divided into seven units, each containing a list of objectives of the unit and an introduction to the unit. The units are divided into lessons with each procedure in the unit represented by a lesson.

Each lesson begins with the objectives followed by a list of glossary terms, words which may be unfamiliar or need further explanation. Basic theoretical concepts are briefly presented along with clinical information. Figures, tables, photographs, and color plates are included where appropriate to clarify points and expand your understanding. Precautions which should be observed, both for safety and for technical reasons, are emphasized in each procedure and restated in the "Precautions" sections. Review questions and learning activities have been included to test and reinforce understanding of the material.

Basic Medical Laboratory Techniques is performance-based and includes Student Performance Guides which allow you to practice a procedure to become proficient before evaluation. Where appropriate, worksheets have been included for calculations and the recording of results. Care must be taken in each procedure to read and follow the instructions given in the text and any additional ones the instructor may add. All parts of the lesson must be completed before attempting to practice the procedure. If there are any questions regarding content or procedure, the instructor should be consulted.

The performance guide has been designed to allow you to practice a procedure and judge individual performance. The Student Performance Guide includes instructions, a materials and equipment list, a step-by-step procedure with a satisfactory and unsatisfactory check column and a comment section for you and the instructor to note errors or positive comments, and the date and the signature of the instructor to verify practice performance. Once you feel a specific procedure has been mastered, the instructor can observe your performance and complete the final performance evaluation.

The final evaluation is basd on two components: 1) results of a written examination, and 2) completion of a final performance of the procedure using the instructor's Performance Check Sheet. The format of the final Performance Check Sheet includes the same step-by-step procedure as the Performance Guide.

By using the Student Performance Guide and the instructor's Performance Check Sheet, you will be able to achieve higher standards of performance and learn to master all steps of the procedures. Repetition of the procedures is an important requirement in the development of technique. Thus, the more you practice the methods and procedures, the more proficient you will become in terms of speed and accuracy. This also provides an opportunity for you to develop confidence in performance capabilities. You must always remember that all laboratory tests must be performed in an exacting manner and with the highest accuracy since the results submitted are relied upon by the physician in the diagnosis and prognosis of disease and in charting a course of treatment for a patient.

The authors hope that through the performance of the procedures and the completion of the lessons you will obtain much self-satisfaction in becoming knowledgeable and proficient in laboratory procedures. It is also hoped that you will come to realize the special qualities that are required of the person who works in the medical laboratory.

Norma J. Walters
Barbara H. Estridge
Anna P. Reynolds

UNIT 1

Introduction to the Medical Laboratory

UNIT OBJECTIVES

After studying this unit, you should be able to:
- Discuss the organization and function of the medical laboratory.
- Discuss the qualifications and functions of medical laboratory personnel.
- Discuss laboratory safety rules which must be followed to guard against chemical, physical, and biological hazards.
- Identify and use laboratory glassware and equipment.
- Use the compound microscope.
- Identify prefixes, stems, and suffixes in selected medical terms.
- Perform measurements and conversions using the metric system.
- Perform common laboratory mathematical calculations.

OVERVIEW

The medical laboratory is a place where blood, body fluids, and other biological specimens are tested, analyzed, or evaluated. Precise measurements are made and the results are calculated and interpreted. The observations may be macroscopic or microscopic. The tests may be performed manually or by using specialized instruments. Because of this, laboratory workers must have the skills necessary to perform a variety of tasks.

This unit is an introduction to the laboratory environment as a work place. Key procedures or concepts that a laboratory worker needs to know are described. This unit discusses the organization and function of the laboratory. Qualifications and job functions of laboratory personnel are also reviewed. A lesson on laboratory safety is included because everyone working in the laboratory must be thoroughly aware of potential hazards. The worker must also be familiar with all safety practices before any laboratory exercises can be conducted.

The care, use, and cleaning of frequently used laboratory glassware is also explained. This includes pipets, beakers, test tubes, and flasks. Basic laboratory equipment such as centrifuges, automatic pipets, pH meters, autoclaves, and laboratory balances are described. The proper care and use of the microscope is included since it is required in the bacteriology, hematology, and urinalysis units.

Since most laboratory analyses use the metric system and require some calculations, there is a brief introduction to the metric system. Simple calculations such as percentages and ratios are also presented. The principles of the metric system and laboratory mathematics which are covered in this unit will be expanded upon in Units 2 and 3. To learn the structure of medical terms, medical terminology is included in one lesson. As other units are studied, additional vocabulary terms will be introduced and defined.

Unit 1 is an introduction to the techniques, rules, and skills that are needed to perform the exercises in Units 2–7. Unit 1 may also be used alone as an introduction to the laboratory. After Unit 1 has been completed, Units 2, 4, 5, 6 or 7 may be studied in the order of the instructor's preference. This usually depends on the availability of time, laboratory space, and equipment. Unit 3 should be studied only after finishing Unit 2.

LESSON 1–1
The Medical Laboratory

LESSON OBJECTIVES

After studying this lesson, you should be able to:
- Draw an organizational chart of a typical medical laboratory.
- List the major departments of a medical laboratory and name a test which might be performed in each department.
- List locations of non-hospital medical laboratories.
- Define the glossary terms.

GLOSSARY

hematology / the science concerned with the study of blood and blood-forming tissues

immunohematology / blood banking; the study of blood group antigens and antibodies

microbiology / the scientific study of microorganisms such as bacteria

pathologist / a physician specially trained in the nature and cause of disease

phlebotomist / one trained to draw blood; venipuncturist

reference laboratory / an independent regional laboratory which offers routine as well as specialized testing for hospitals and physicians

serum / the liquid portion of blood which has been allowed to clot

stat test / a test that should be performed immediately

INTRODUCTION

Many medical (clinical) laboratories are located in a hospital. Others are found in clinics, group practices, public health departments, physicians' offices, and reference laboratories.

The type of laboratory facility found in a hospital depends on the hospital's size. A small hospital, under 100 beds, may have the ability to perform only very routine test procedures. More complicated or seldomly requested tests are

3

usually sent to reference laboratories. In a medium-size hospital, up to 300 beds, routine tests and some of the more complicated test procedures may be performed. Only the most recently developed tests or ones with complicated procedures need to be sent to a reference laboratory. The laboratories in most larger hospitals, over 300 beds, can handle large volumes of work and perform most test procedures.

ORGANIZATION OF THE LABORATORY

Although the details may vary, the organization of most hospital laboratories follows a general outline (Figure 1–1). Usually the head of the laboratory is a **pathologist,** a physician who is specially trained in the nature and cause of disease. Directly under the pathologist's authority is the laboratory manager. This is usually someone with an education in the medical laboratory sciences and a business or management degree. In addition, some laboratories have a chief or head technologist. The heads of the various departments report to this person. The department heads are responsible for the quality and quantity of work performed. The number of major departments in laboratories varies. Chemistry, hematology, microbiology, and the blood bank usually operate as independent units, each with its own department head. The subdivisions within each department may differ from one laboratory to another.

Chemistry

In the chemistry department, test procedures are usually performed on **serum,** the liquid part of blood left after a clot has formed. Tests may also be performed on urine. Although urine and serum are the most frequently used specimens, spinal fluid, joint fluid and other body fluids are tested also. The more commonly performed procedures in this department include blood glucose content, assays of enzymes to determine if heart damage has occurred, and the electrolytes—a set of tests which determine the chloride, bicarbonate, potassium, and sodium levels in the blood. The chemistry department usually has one or more subdivisions. One common subdivision is special chemistry. In this department, a patient's blood may be analyzed to discover what drug is involved in an overdose. The blood level of prescribed drugs may also be monitored.

The number of instruments available for chemistry analysis has grown rapidly in the last 20 years. Thus, it is possible for almost every laboratory to have instruments capable of performing most routine test procedures.

Microbiology

The **microbiology** department is responsible for growing and identifying the organisms obtained from a patient's blood, urine or other body fluid, sputum, or wound. After the organism is grown out, susceptibility testing can be performed. Susceptibility testing involves exposing the organism to different antibiotics. This helps to determine which antibiotic is most effective against the organism.

The parasitology laboratory is often included as a part of the microbiology department. This department examines patient specimens for parasites. The patient's blood may be examined for evidence of the blood parasite which causes malaria. Or, the stools may be examined for evidence of intestinal parasites such as tapeworms or hookworms.

Traditionally, the microbiology department has been less automated than other departments; however, this is rapidly changing. Automated systems are available which can detect growth of an organism, identify an organism, and determine the most effective antibiotic for treatment.

Hematology

In the **hematology** department, whole blood is used for the majority of test procedures. Hematology procedures can be qualitative or quantitative. The quantitative procedures include actual counts of the various blood components. For example,

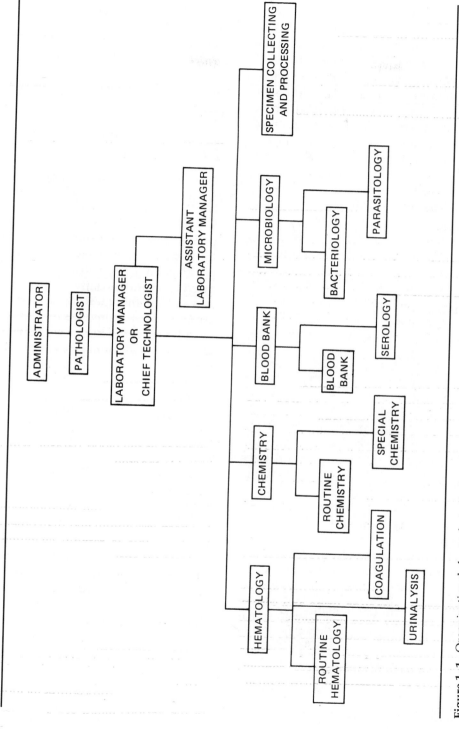

Figure 1–1. Organizational chart of a typical medical laboratory

the number of leukocytes (white blood cells), erythrocytes (red blood cells), and platelets in a blood sample can be determined. All of these counts can be performed using automated systems. The qualitative procedures are ones in which the various blood components are observed for qualities such as cell size, shape, and maturity level. Using a microscope, a laboratory worker can view a blood smear to determine the types of leukocytes present or to estimate the size, shape, and hemoglobin content of erythrocytes. The number of platelets can also be estimated. The presence of any abnormalities can also be noted during the microscopic examination of the blood smear. This may include identifying immature leukocytes or erythrocytes. The microhematocrit, the blood indices, and the blood hemoglobin content are additional tests commonly performed. The results of these three tests can be used to diagnose anemias. Many companies have developed sophisticated instruments capable of performing the routine hematology procedures.

Coagulation and Urinalysis. In some laboratories, coagulation tests and urinalyses are also performed in the hematology department. Coagulation tests help to diagnose and monitor patients who have defects in their blood clotting mechanism. Automated systems for coagulation tests have been in use for several years. Urinalysis includes physical, chemical, and microscopic examinations of urine specimens. Several methods of automation are now being used for the physical and chemical examination of urine.

Blood Bank

The blood bank department is also known as transfusion services or **immunohematology.** Here, several procedures can be performed, depending on the needs of the patient. If a transfusion is required, the patient's ABO blood type and Rh type are determined by blood bank technologists. The technologists then test the blood units in storage to determine which are correct for the patient.

The blood bank department may also have the capability to process the units of whole blood into specialized components such as concentrated red blood cells.

Serology may be a part of the blood bank or microbiology department. In serology, specimens are tested using antigen-antibody methods. Tests such as pregnancy tests and tests for rheumatoid arthritis and infectious mononucleosis are performed in this section.

SPECIMEN COLLECTING AND PROCESSING

Some hospitals have a separate phlebotomy department which is responsible for specimen collecting and processing. **Phlebotomists** are the personnel who collect the necessary blood specimen. They are specially trained to efficiently obtain a blood specimen with as little discomfort to the patient as possible. In other laboratories, some or all of the regular staff share this responsibility. In some instances, nursing personnel also may be responsible for all or partial blood collecting.

REQUESTING A LABORATORY TEST

Only the physician may request laboratory testing on a patient. Usually the physician writes the request in the patient's chart. Sometimes, however, the order may be given to the registered nurse to record. The laboratory personnel can collect a blood specimen and perform a particular test procedure only after the proper request has been received. Examples of Laboratory Requisition Forms can be found in Appendix M, p. 504.

COMMUNICATIONS

Communication problems may arise between laboratory personnel and other hospital personnel. These problems usually involve the test request procedure and/or the delivery of the test results to the physicians. Following the health agency's procedure manual will eliminate many of these problems. All laboratory personnel must strive to perform the test procedures as efficiently and accurately as possible. They must insure that emergency requests are treated as such and that the test results are reported as soon as possible. Likewise, other employees in the hospital must realize that only a physician can request a **stat test.** A stat test is one that must be performed immediately because of an emergency. Other hospital personnel must carry out their responsibilities to see that test requests and specimens are transported to the laboratory as quickly as possible. A breakdown in communication causes stress and bad feelings among all personnel involved. Health care employees must remember that the welfare of the patient is of uppermost importance.

NON-HOSPITAL MEDICAL LABORATORIES

Non-hospital medical laboratories may be associated with a group practice, such as internal medicine specialists. These laboratories may also be located in the office of a physician who has a specialty such as hematology. A physician with a general practice may have laboratory facilities to perform some of the more routine procedures. These laboratories are called physician's office laboratories (POLs). State Public Health Departments may have medical laboratory facilities; these laboratories perform a variety of medical tests such as those for tuberculosis and venereal and viral diseases. Additional procedures can include tests for water and milk purity.

Reference laboratories are regional laboratories which do high volume testing and offer a wide variety of procedures. Large hospitals use reference laboratories primarily to perform complicated or rarely ordered tests. Small hospitals or doctors' offices may use them for a wide range of tests.

A recent development is the walk-in medical facility, usually located near shopping centers. Routine laboratory procedures such as blood counts, throat cultures, and urine tests are performed in these offices. As a greater number of patients use these facilities, the laboratories in the facilities will grow and new or additional tests will be added as necessary.

LESSON REVIEW

1. Draw an organizational chart of a typical medical laboratory.
2. Name five major departments a hospital medical laboratory might have.
3. Name two procedures which are performed in a hematology department.
4. Name one procedure performed in the chemistry department.
5. Why is cooperation between laboratory personnel and other hospital personnel so important?
6. List three locations of medical laboratory facilities other than in a hospital.
7. Define hematology, immunohematology, microbiology, pathologist, phlebotomist, reference laboratory, serum, and stat test.

STUDENT ACTIVITIES

1. Re-read the information on the medical laboratory.
2. Review the glossary terms.
3. Interview an employee of a medical laboratory in a health agency. Inquire about the organization of the laboratory and the types of tests which are performed. Obtain various laboratory test report forms and note the types of tests performed in each department.
4. Tour a medical laboratory in your community.

LESSON 1–2
The Medical Laboratory Professional

LESSON OBJECTIVES

After studying this lesson, you should be able to:
- Give a brief history of medical technology.
- List five qualities which are desirable in a medical laboratory professional.
- Describe the educational requirements for medical technologists and medical laboratory technicians.
- Discuss the relationship between laboratory personnel and the patient.
- Discuss rules of ethical conduct for laboratory workers.
- Name five areas of employment for laboratory personnel other than in a hospital laboratory.
- Define the glossary terms.

GLOSSARY

certified medical laboratory technician / a professional who has completed a minimum of two years of specific training in an accredited program, consisting of one year of college and one year of clinical training, and has passed a national certifying examination

certified medical technologist / a professional who has a bachelor's degree from an accredited college or university, has completed one year of clinical training, and has passed a national certifying examination

ethics / a system of conduct or behavior; professional rules of right and wrong

medical technology / the health profession concerned with the performance of laboratory analyses used in the diagnosis and treatment of disease as well as in health maintenance

MEDICAL TECHNOLOGY

Medical technology is the health profession concerned with performing laboratory analyses. The analyses are used to diagnose and treat disease as well as maintain good health. The tests are performed by trained, skilled medical technologists and technicians, or by other medical laboratory or allied health personnel. The laboratory tests are standardized and controlled. This insures reliable and accurate results.

History of Medical Technology

Medical technology can be traced back several centuries. Papyrus writings dated before 1000 B.C. record descriptions of intestinal parasites, an early example of parasitology. Before medieval times, Hindu doctors performed crude urinalyses when they observed that some urines had a sweet taste and attracted ants. With the invention and improvement of the microscope in the seventeenth century, the study of biological specimens progressed from simple visual examination to microscopic examination.

The first clinical laboratories in the United States appeared in the late nineteenth century and were very crude. Some consisted of only a table and a microscope. They were staffed mostly by doctors who showed special interest in "laboratory medicine." The U.S. census of 1900 listed only one hundred laboratory technicians, all male.

After World War I, laboratories grew in size and in number. This is when schools to train laboratory workers were organized. Since World War II, the technology for laboratory testing has become more complex. At that time, laboratory tests began to play an important role in medicine. Today's technology allows us to provide a level of health care which was only imagined a few years ago.

Presently, there are thousands of medical laboratories, both large and small. Laboratories are highly sophisticated and offer many complex tests. The technologists and technicians staffing these laboratories are highly skilled professionals who perform complicated analyses. They may also serve as laboratory managers, teachers, supervisors, and administrators. Laboratories may also employ laboratory assistants and phlebotomists to collect blood, process specimens, and perform routine laboratory duties, both technical and clerical.

Educational Requirements for Medical Laboratory Professionals

Soon after the emergence of medical laboratories, it was clear that there was a need for (1) educating laboratory workers, (2) defining educational requirements, and (3) identifying adequately trained persons. By the 1930s, schools of medical technology were training laboratory workers and basic educational requirements were established. At that time, certifying examinations were being given to measure the knowledge and ability of workers. Trained workers now comprise most of the work force in the medical laboratory. The two most common levels of professionals in the medical laboratory are the technician and the technologist.

Medical Laboratory Technician. The **medical laboratory technician** is a worker who has two years of training after high school—one year of college and one year of clinical training. After the clinical training has been completed satisfactorily, the worker takes a national certifying examination. Upon receiving satisfactory scores on the exam, the medical laboratory technician is certified.

Medical Technologist. The **medical technologist** is a laboratory worker who has a bachelor's degree from a college or university and one year of clinical training. To become a certified medical technologist, the individual must also pass a national certifying exam for medical technologists. These examinations are administered by agencies such as the American Society of Clinical Pathologists (ASCP), the National Certification Agency for Medical Laboratory Personnel (NCAMLP), the American Medical Technologists (AMT) and the International Society for Clinical Laboratory Technology (ISCLT). Certified medical technologists are qualified to perform analyses in all departments of the laboratory. These individuals may be supervisors or department heads. They may also work in other leadership positions in the laboratory.

Areas of Specialization

Some laboratory workers may specialize in one area of laboratory work such as chemistry or microbiology. Usually, these workers have a four-year degree in the area of specialization and are certified by examination in the specialty area.

Laboratory managers oversee the day-to-day management of the laboratory. They are usually medical technologists who have some additional educational training in business, management, or other health-related field. With the increasing cost of health care and the emphasis on cost containment, efficient medical laboratory management is becoming more important.

Qualities of Laboratory Workers

Dedication, cooperation, neatness, and a caring attitude are essential qualities of the health care professional. In addition, there are special characteristics needed in persons performing laboratory analyses. The workers in each department need to be knowledgeable of the procedures performed in that department. They should be willing to attend continuing education programs to keep up with new developments in their field. Laboratory workers must be able to perform accurate, precise manipulations and calculations. Communication skills, reliability, honesty, and the ability to relate well to fellow workers are important qualities for laboratory workers. Organizational skills must also be developed. To function professionally in any laboratory, the personnel must learn how to prioritize laboratory requests and schedules.

Ethics and Professionalism

Laboratory workers should consider themselves health care professionals. They should observe professional **ethics,** which is a code of conduct and behavior. Patient information is confidential. It should only be discussed with health care workers who are directly related to the case and who have a need to know. Test results should not be discussed with the patients, their relatives, or other inappropriate persons. The results should be reported only to the physician or other appropriate designated employee.

The Patient and the Laboratory Professional

The field of medical technology exists for the patient, as do all other fields of health care. In order for a patient to receive the best possible care, a physician must make the proper diagnosis. To make this diagnosis, the physicians rely on laboratory analyses along with information gained from the medical history, physical examination and clinical symptoms. For this reason, it is important that the laboratory analyses are performed carefully and accurately, using the best techniques available.

The only contact patients may have with the laboratory is through the lab assistant, technologist, or phlebotomist who collects a blood sample from them for testing. At best, it is not pleasant to have blood taken from a vein or finger. At all times, the technologist needs to be aware of the stress the patient is feeling when hospitalized. The technologist must be professional, courteous, and considerate when obtaining the specimen.

Responsibilities of Laboratory Workers

Set rules and regulations govern health care in all states. Most health care agencies have very specific standards, rules, and regulations governing the responsibilities of various health care employees. Each health care worker must assume the responsibility of learning exactly what activities are allowed in their position. They should understand their job responsibilities fully for their protection, the protection of their employer, and the safety of the patient.

Licensing

Although certification is usually sufficient to meet most employment requirements, some states regulate laboratory personnel by requiring state licensure. Licensing laws vary from state to state and are nonexistent in some. The state may require a fee to obtain a license, or it may require that a test be taken before the license is issued; some states require both.

Professional Organizations

Laboratory personnel usually have a choice of membership in one or more professional societies. These societies provide opportunities for professional growth and continuing education by offering workshops and seminars, and by publishing journals. Membership in a national society usually also includes membership in the state affiliate. It is important for all laboratory professionals to be active in one or more of these organizations.

Employment Opportunities

There are many employment opportunities for medical laboratory workers. Most of the nation's laboratory workers are employed in hospitals. However, some are employed in physician's offices or clinics, public health agencies, reference laboratories, the military, research, education, veterinary medicine, and in sales or product development for medical suppliers.

LESSON REVIEW

1. What is medical technology?
2. Describe the beginnings of medical technology.
3. What are the educational requirements for medical technologists—for medical technicians?
4. List five qualities that a laboratory worker should possess.
5. What is the obligation of the medical laboratory professional to the patient?
6. List five places of employment for laboratory personnel other than in hospitals.
7. Define certified medical laboratory technician, certified medical technologist, ethics, and medical technology.

STUDENT ACTIVITIES

1. Re-read the information on the medical laboratory professional.
2. Review the glossary terms.
3. Complete a Career Information Fact Sheet on the medical laboratory technician and the medical laboratory technologist. This should include the educational training, cost of program, nature of job, advantages and disadvantages, employment opportunities, and salary range of occupation.
4. Interview a laboratory worker using the fact sheet format provided by the instructor. Be sure to consider the following areas: his or her job functions, relationships with co-workers and patients, advantages and disadvantages, satisfactions, dissatisfactions, salary range, and opportunities for advancement with appropriate educational training. Describe the benefits of talking to the laboratory worker in person rather than reading the information in a book.

Career Information Fact Sheet

NAME_____   DATE _____

LESSON 1–2 THE MEDICAL LABORATORY PROFESSIONAL

Title:

Legal Requirement:

Length of Program:

Educational Institution:

Cost of Program:

Admission Requirements:

Nature of the Job:

Earnings:

Advancement:

Related Occupation(s):

Advantages:

Disadvantages:

Interview Fact Sheet

NAME_____ DATE _____

LESSON 1–2 THE MEDICAL LABORATORY PROFESSIONAL

Title:

Educational Preparation:

Approximate Cost of Education Program:

Job Functions:

Approximate Salary:

Job Satisfaction:

Job Dissatisfaction:

Opportunities for Advancement:

Options Available to Broaden Employment Opportunities:

LESSON 1-3
Laboratory Safety

LESSON OBJECTIVES

After studying this lesson, you should be able to:

- Explain why safety rules must be observed.
- List three classifications of laboratory hazards.
- Give two examples of each type of hazard.
- List a way to prevent or correct each type of hazard.
- Explain what should be done if an accident occurs in the laboratory.
- Explain what is meant by universal precautions and give the reasons for using them.
- State eleven safety precautions for the handling of biological specimens.
- Describe proper laboratory clothing.
- State eighteen basic rules of laboratory safety.
- Define the glossary terms.

GLOSSARY

acquired immunodeficiency syndrome / a form of immune deficiency induced by infection with human immunodeficiency virus; AIDS

autoclave / a device which uses pressurized steam for sterilization

biological safety hood / a special cabinet which draws air away from the worker, providing a safe work area for the handling of infectious agents

carcinogen / a substance which has the ability to produce or cause cancer

fume hood / a device which draws contaminated air out of an area and either cleanses and recirculates it or discharges it to the outside

human immunodeficiency virus / a retrovirus which has been identified as the cause of AIDS; HIV

universal precautions / precautions to be used in the handling of all patients and biological specimens in order to prevent exposure of health care workers to infectious or harmful agents

14

INTRODUCTION

Safety is a topic that should be foremost in the minds of health care providers, both employers and employees. The goal of health care workers should be to provide quality patient care in an environment which is safe to both workers and patients.

Changes in health care workers' awareness of the importance of safety precautions in health care settings have come largely as a result of the discovery of **acquired immunodeficiency syndrome** (AIDS), a viral disease which has been found worldwide. However, there have always been certain hazards associated with providing health care, for example, potential exposure of workers to infectious agents such as the hepatitis virus or tuberculosis organism.

This lesson identifies physical, chemical, and biological hazards which workers may encounter in the clinical laboratory. The lesson also outlines safety precautions that are mandatory for proper operation of a clinical laboratory. Most of these precautions are also applicable to other health care settings such as surgery units, doctors' or dentists' offices, dialysis centers, or nursing care facilities.

PHYSICAL HAZARDS

Physical hazards may be present in what is thought of as ordinary equipment or surroundings. Electrical equipment is one major source of physical hazards. All electrical equipment must be properly grounded following the manufacturer's instructions. When even minor repair is undertaken, such as replacing a bulb in a microscope, the instrument must be disconnected from the electrical supply before work is begun. All electrical cords and plugs must be kept in good repair. There must be no frayed cords or exposed wires.

Fire is another potential danger in the laboratory. If Bunsen burners or other open flames are used, care must be taken to insure that loose clothing and long hair cannot catch on fire (Figure 1–2). Smoking must not be permitted in laboratories. Flammable chemicals should be stored in a flameproof cabinet, away from heat sources. All laboratory workers should know the location and

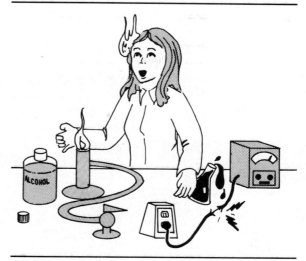

Figure 1–2. Physical hazards. Keep electrical equipment in good repair and observe safety precautions when using Bunsen burners.

proper use of the fire extinguishers. They must also know the fire escape route and the procedure to follow if the exit is blocked by fire. A fire blanket should be readily available. It is important to have periodic inspections of fire extinguishing equipment and frequent fire drills.

All instruments must be used only as the instructions dictate. Any instrument with moving parts must be used with care. A centrifuge lid should not be opened until the centrifuge has completely stopped. **Autoclaves,** which use pressurized steam to sterilize materials, present special hazards. Manufacturer's instructions should be followed carefully (see Lesson 1–4). Thermal gloves should be worn to prevent burns when removing items from the autoclave.

Only glassware which is free of cracks and chips should be used. Any broken or chipped items should be immediately discarded into rigid cardboard or plastic containers, *never* in plastic bags alone. Puncture-proof containers may be made from carefully sealed cardboard boxes or purchased commercially.

CHEMICAL HAZARDS

Chemicals present a variety of hazards. Chemicals may be flammable, may be caustic and cause

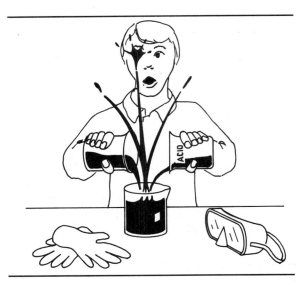

Figure 1–3. Chemical hazards. Wear safety goggles and gloves when handling harsh chemicals to prevent splashing the chemical on skin or in eyes.

burns, or may be poisonous or carcinogenic. Occasionally, laboratory procedures require reagents which contain radioisotopes.

Some of the chemicals used in laboratory work are strong acids or bases which are capable of causing severe skin burns. They must be used with caution to avoid splashes which would damage the eyes or burn the skin (Figure 1–3). Goggles and gloves should be worn when handling such strong chemicals to prevent skin or eye contact in the event of an accidental splash. Any chemicals which do contact the skin should be washed off immediately with water for approximately five minutes unless the label says otherwise. An eyewash station should be located in the lab.

Flammable liquids and concentrated acids and bases should be stored in a safe place in proper containers. Most suppliers now label chemical containers with information listing the hazards that the chemical presents, the procedure to follow if an accident occurs, and the proper storage and disposal of the chemical.

Toxic fumes are produced by some laboratory chemicals. These should be used only in a **fume hood,** an enclosed cabinet which will draw the fumes away from the worker.

Few **carcinogens,** or cancer-causing agents, are used in the clinical laboratory. However, it's wise to avoid direct skin contact or breathing of dust of any chemicals. Although radioisotopes are usually present only in trace amounts when in a clinical reagent, gloves should be used when handling, and disposal should be made according to manufacturer's recommendations as well as state and federal guidelines. Personnel using radioisotopes should have special training in radiation safety.

All chemicals and solutions should be disposed of properly. Some laboratory chemicals can be safely poured directly into the drain (to avoid splashes), followed by lots of water. However, it is very important that explicit directions be provided by the laboratory supervisor for the disposal of each chemical. Some chemicals may require special disposal (such as in a toxic waste landfill) by toxic waste personnel. The laboratory must have a written policy for the handling, use, and disposal of all hazardous chemicals used in the laboratory. Because employees have a right to know of the hazards to which they may be exposed, a listing of the hazards specific chemicals pose as well as the procedures to be followed in case of accidental exposure or emergency must also be available to workers.

BIOLOGICAL HAZARDS

Biological specimens and reagents derived from blood components present a special problem because they may contain infectious agents which are potentially harmful but are not readily evident. The two most important diseases which are of concern are hepatitis and AIDS. Viral hepatitis can be transmitted by exposure to infected blood, body fluids, or blood components. AIDS is caused by **human immunodeficiency virus** (HIV) and may be transmitted in the following ways: by sexual contact with an infected person; by parenteral, mucous membrane, and nonintact skin exposure to infected blood or blood components; and from an infected mother to her newborn.

Universal Precautions

The Centers for Disease Control (CDC), a branch of the Public Health Service, U.S. Department of

Health and Human Services, has researched and compiled data from other researchers regarding the transmission of infectious diseases such as AIDS and hepatitis. The CDC has issued recommendations for preventing human immunodeficiency virus (HIV) and hepatitis virus transmission in health care settings. Because it is not possible to know whether or not each patient or patient specimen is infected with HIV or other pathogens, the CDC has recommended "universal blood and body fluid precautions" to be used in the care and handling of *all* patients or patient specimens.* These **universal precautions** are recommended for use with all patients regardless of whether or not they have been tested for HIV or hepatitis. (This differs from earlier CDC recommendations which called for precautions only when a patient was suspected of being infected with a blood-borne pathogen or had tested positive.)

Use of Protective Barriers

It should be emphasized that, for optimum safety, health care workers must use appropriate barrier precautions when handling all patients and patient specimens. These precautions, which are listed below, apply to handling blood and any body fluid. Although blood is the most important source of blood-borne pathogens, other body fluids such as cerebrospinal fluid, pleural fluid, synovial fluid, peritoneal fluid, pericardial fluid, and amniotic fluid should be considered potentially infectious.

The risk of transmission of blood-borne pathogens can be minimized if health care workers adhere to the following general precautions:

1. Use protective barriers to prevent exposure of skin or mucous membranes to blood and all body fluids. Barriers may include gloves, mask, face shield, goggles or safety glasses, or gown, depending on the situation. These barriers

should be changed after each patient contact and disposed of properly. (Techniques for donning mask, gown and gloves are described in Lesson 1–9.)
2. Wash hands immediately after removing gloves. Any contaminated skin surface should be washed immediately and thoroughly. (Handwashing technique is described in Lesson 1–9.)
3. Use precautions to avoid injuries from sharp, contaminated objects such as needles or scalpels. Needles should not be recapped by hand. These should be disposed of only in rigid, puncture-resistant biohazard containers.

Rules for Handling Biological Specimens

Special rules to follow when handling biological specimens include:

1. Do not contaminate the outside of specimen containers, labels, or request forms.
2. Phlebotomists should wear gloves when obtaining blood. Gloves should also be worn when handling and processing specimens.
3. Use a **biological safety hood** or cabinet when handling specimens in a manner where aerosols may be generated. These cabinets have a face shield and draw air away from the worker.
4. Mouth pipetting should not be allowed in the laboratory. Only automatic (mechanical or electrical) pipets or pipets with safety bulbs should be used when transferring reagents and specimens. If mouth pipetting is necessary, special filters are available which can be attached to the mouthpiece of the pipet.
5. Many laboratory reagents are made from blood components. These reagents must be considered potentially harmful and should be handled using the same precautions as for biological specimens. (Although most reagents are now tested for hepatitis and HIV antibodies by the manufacturers, the reagents should be handled with care since no test can give 100% assurance of safety.)
6. Biological specimens and any contaminated articles must be placed in special biohazard

---

*Detailed information regarding universal precautions is available from the state health department or by consulting the following publications of the U.S. Department of Health and Human Services (prepared by the CDC, Atlanta, GA): *Morbidity and Mortality Weekly Report* (MMWR) 36, no. 2S, August 21, 1987; and *MMWR* 37, no. 24, June 24, 1988.

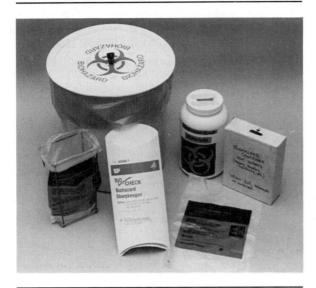

Figure 1–4. Examples of biohazard containers. Clockwise from top left: large container for non-sharp objects, two homemade rigid containers for sharp objects, autoclave bag for non-sharp objects, commercial container for sharp objects, and commercial holder for autoclave bag.

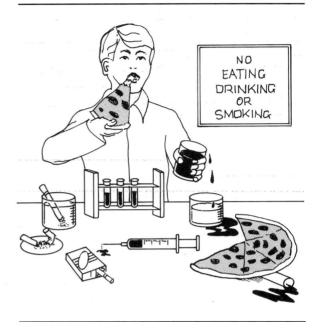

Figure 1–5. Biological hazards. Dispose of sharp contaminated objects properly; wipe up spills promptly with disinfectant; and do not eat, drink or smoke in the laboratory work area.

bags or containers (Figure 1–4). Sharp objects such as lancets, needles, microscope slides, and glass capillaries must be placed in rigid, non-glass, puncture-proof containers suitable for autoclaving or incineration. Contaminated articles such as cotton balls, gloves, gauze, and paper towels may be placed in plastic biohazard bags. These biohazard bags and containers must be disposed of by incineration, or sterilized by autoclaving before disposal, usually in a landfill. (Regulations for disposal of biohazardous materials vary from state to state; therefore, it is necessary to follow each state's guidelines.)

7. The bacteriology laboratory presents additional hazards and special precautions are necessary. All organisms must be handled as if they can cause disease. All waste must be autoclaved before disposal, or incinerated.

8. Hands must be washed before and after each procedure using biological materials. Easily obtainable disinfectants for the hands are Hibiclens® by Stuart Pharmaceuticals, or a dilute solution of tincture of green soap. Both can be purchased at medical supply and drug stores.

9. Protective clothing should be replaced if it becomes contaminated, and removed before leaving the workplace.

10. Eating, drinking and smoking must be prohibited in the laboratory work area (Figure 1–5).

11. The laboratory work area should be disinfected before and after each use and anytime a spill occurs. An appropriate solution is a 5–10% solution of sodium hypochlorite (chlorine bleach) or a good commercial disinfectant such as Amphyll®.

LABORATORY CLOTHING

It is important that proper clothing be worn when working in the laboratory. This may include a uniform along with a laboratory coat, jacket, or apron to protect clothing and skin from spills of chemicals, stains and biological specimens. Gloves should be worn during phlebotomy, when handling specimens or strong chemicals, and any time contamination may occur. If splashes are likely to happen, laboratory safety goggles should be worn. Long hair should be pinned back to prevent contact with open flames or equipment with moving parts. Loose jewelry, such as long chains and bracelets, may get caught in equipment and should not be worn. Shoes should be comfortable and should have a closed toe to protect feet from spills or sharp objects.

TEACHER/SUPERVISOR RESPONSIBILITY

In 1971, the Occupational Safety and Health Act was passed by the federal government; many states have also passed safety legislation. These laws are designed to insure that employers provide safe workplaces. Adherence to the laws is monitored by the Occupational Safety and Health Administration (OSHA).

As of August 1, 1988, all laboratories are required by OSHA to have a written Hazardous Communication Program. Employees or students have a "right to know" whether the possibility of exposure to hazardous substances exists in the workplace. It is the responsibility of the teacher, supervisor, or employer to insure that a student or worker has been given proper orientation and training in safety procedures and handling of hazardous materials before any work is performed in the laboratory. The official OSHA guidelines must be consulted to insure that the laboratory's policies are in compliance with the OSHA regulations. Students or workers must be provided with safety equipment and should be monitored for adherence to safety rules and precautions. Students or workers must also report all accidents to the supervisor immediately. It is helpful to require the student or worker to sign a safety agreement form (Appendix A) when the training session has been completed. Periodic continuing education sessions on safety will reinforce the importance of safety.

GENERAL LABORATORY RULES

Although there are certain hazards present in the clinical laboratory, it is possible for the laboratory to be a safe work environment. Each worker must be responsible, use safe work habits, and observe all safety rules, whether or not they are posted (Figure 1–6).

No set of rules can cover all the precautions that should be observed in a laboratory setting. Also,

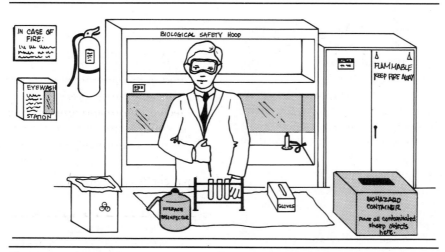

Figure 1–6. A safe laboratory. The laboratory can be a safe workplace when safety rules are followed.

nothing can replace the use of good common sense. However, there are several good, general principles which should always be observed:

1. Refrain from horseplay.
2. Avoid eating, drinking, smoking, gum chewing, or applying makeup in the work area.
3. Wear a laboratory jacket or coat and closed-toe shoes.
4. Pin long hair away from the face and neck to avoid contact with chemicals, equipment, or flames.
5. Avoid wearing chains, bracelets, rings, or other loose hanging jewelry.
6. Use gloves when handling blood, biological specimens, and hazardous chemicals or reagents.
7. Use universal precautions in handling of patients and biological specimens, including human blood and diagnostic products made from human blood.
8. Disinfect work area before and after laboratory procedures and at any other time necessary.
9. Wash hands before and after laboratory procedures, after removing gloves, and any other time necessary.
10. Wear safety glasses when working with strong chemicals and when splashes are likely to occur.
11. Wipe up spills promptly and appropriately for the type of spill.
12. Avoid tasting, smelling, or breathing the dust of any chemicals.
13. Follow the manufacturer's instructions for operating equipment.
14. Handle equipment with care and store it properly.
15. Report any broken or frayed electrical cords, exposed electrical wires, or damaged equipment.
16. Discard any broken glassware into a safe container.
17. Allow visitors only in the nonworking area of the laboratory.
18. Report any accident to the supervisor immediately.

LESSON REVIEW

1. Why must safety rules be strictly observed?
2. Name the three classifications of laboratory hazards. Give two examples of each type of hazard and tell how each might be avoided or corrected.
3. What should be done if an accident occurs in the laboratory?
4. What is the major hazard present when handling blood, body fluids, or blood-derived reagents?
5. Describe what is meant by observing universal precautions and state the purpose of using protective barriers.
6. Give eleven safety rules to follow when working with biological specimens.
7. What type of clothing should be worn by laboratory workers?
8. State eighteen general rules of laboratory safety and explain the importance of each.
9. Define acquired immunodeficiency syndrome, autoclave, biological safety hood, carcinogen, fume hood, human immunodeficiency virus, universal precautions.

STUDENT ACTIVITIES

1. Re-read the information on laboratory safety.
2. Review the glossary terms.
3. Make a poster warning of a laboratory hazard or listing basic safety rules.
4. Use the worksheet to make a safety check of the laboratory. Check for frayed cords, exposed wires, fire extinguishers, safety posters, posting of fire exit routes, etc. Inspect the chemicals present in the laboratory. Are they labeled with appropriate instructions? Note the procedure to follow in case of skin contact or chemical spill.
5. Practice the procedure for fire and the use of fire extinguishers; learn the fire escape route.
6. Design a set of rules for the proper handling of a patient blood sample. Include the procedures for handling from the time of collection, through transporting and testing of the sample, to disposal.
7. Write to the local health department, state health department, or U.S. Department of Health and Human Services for information regarding the handling of biohazardous materials.

Worksheet

NAME_____ DATE _____

LESSON 1–3 LABORATORY SAFETY

Use this worksheet to make a safety check of the laboratory. For each item listed below, determine if conditions are satisfactory, S, or unsatisfactory, U, (safe or unsafe). If unsatisfactory, make recommendation(s) for correction in the spaces indicated.

    I.   Safety Check for Physical Hazards.

        A. Examine all electrical instruments (microscopes, spectrophotometers, etc.) for frayed wires and proper storage conditions (storage away from water and harsh chemicals, use of dust covers, etc.). Evaluate conditions and record recommendations for each instrument examined.

Instrument	S U (check one)	Observation/Recommendation
_____	__ __	_____
_____	__ __	_____
_____	__ __	_____
_____	__ __	_____

        B. Make a fire safety check of the lab.

          1. Are fire extinguishers present? _____
            When was the last date of inspection? _____
            Do extinguishers have instructions for use posted with them? _____
               Fire extinguishers: S___   U___
          2. Is a fire exit route posted? _____
            Is it up-to-date? _____
            Walk the fire exit route. Was it easy to follow? _____
            Could all exit doors be opened? _____
               Fire exit route: S___   U___
          Recommendation(s) for improving fire safety: _____
          _____
          _____

   II. Safety Check for Chemical Hazards.

        A. Examine the chemicals in the laboratory.

          1. Are all clearly labeled? _____
          2. Do the labels contain information on storage, disposal, and procedure in case of spills or accidental exposure? _____
          3. Are chemicals labeled "flammable" stored away from fire (Bunsen burners)? _____

    4. Where are concentrated acids and bases stored? _____
      Chemical storage: S___   U___
  B. Is a fume hood present? _____
      When was it last checked for proper air flow? _____
      Fume hood: S___   U___
  C. Is an eyewash station present? _____
      Are instructions for use posted? _____
      Eyewash station: S___   U___
  Recommendation(s) for improving chemical safety: _____
  _____
  _____

III.   Safety Check for Biological Hazards.
     Examine the laboratory for biological hazards.
     A. Are safety rules posted? _____
     B. Where are blood specimens discarded? _____
       Where are contaminated gloves, gowns, cotton, etc., discarded? _____
     C. Where are used needles and lancets discarded? _____
       Is the container puncture-proof? _____
     D. How are containers of contaminated material disposed of when full? _____
     E. Are gloves available for use by workers? _____
       What other safety barriers are provided? _____
     F. How are work surfaces disinfected? _____
       How are hands disinfected? _____
       How are reusable items such as hemacytometers cleaned? _____
        Disposal of biological specimens: S___   U___
        Disposal of sharp, contaminated objects: S___   U___
        Availability of safety barriers: S___   U___
        Disinfection procedures: S___   U___
     Recommendation(s) for improving safety regarding biological hazards: _____
     _____
     _____

IV.   Laboratory Safety Policy.
     Inquire about the laboratory's policy regarding employee orientation and training in the safe handling of hazardous substances.
     A. Is a written Hazard Communication Program available in the laboratory? _____
     B. Does the laboratory administration follow appropriate "employee right to know" policies in the safety orientation and training programs? _____
     C. Are written records kept of employee safety training sessions? _____
       Are all employees asked to sign safety agreement forms after safety training? _____
       Laboratory safety policy   S___   U___
     Recommendation(s) for improving laboratory safety policy: _____
     _____
     _____

LESSON 1-4
Laboratory Glassware and Equipment

LESSON OBJECTIVES

After studying this lesson, you should be able to:
- Identify five basic types of glassware used in the laboratory and explain the use of each.
- Identify two types of glass pipets and explain the proper use of each.
- Describe proper care and cleaning procedures for laboratory glassware.
- Explain the operation of automatic pipets.
- List precautions to be observed in the use of laboratory glassware.
- Explain the proper use of a centrifuge.
- Explain the function of a pH meter.
- Discuss the operation of an autoclave.
- List three rules for using a laboratory balance.
- Explain how deionized water and distilled water are made.
- Define the glossary terms.

GLOSSARY

centrifuge / an instrument which may be used to spin biological samples at high speeds to separate particulate matter from the liquid portion of the sample

critical measurements / measurements made when the accuracy of the concentration of a solution is important; measurements made using glassware manufactured to strict standards

deionized water / water which has had most of the ions removed

distilled water / the condensate collected after water has been boiled to remove impurities

meniscus / the curved surface of a liquid in a container

noncritical measurements / measurements which are estimates; measurements made in containers which estimate volume (such as the Erlenmeyer flask)

pH / an expression of the degree of acidity or alkalinity of a solution

reagents / substances or solutions which are used in laboratory analyses

rotor / the part of the centrifuge which holds the samples and rotates during the operation of the centrifuge

solute / a liquid, gas, or solid which is dissolved in a liquid to make a solution

solvent / that liquid into which the solute is dissolved

TC / to contain

TD / to deliver

INTRODUCTION

Most laboratory procedures require the use of some type of laboratory glassware and general laboratory equipment. The glassware and equipment may be used in a specific procedure or in the preparation of **reagents,** solutions used in laboratory analyses. This lesson explains the uses of basic laboratory glassware, deionized and distilled water, and basic laboratory equipment such as centrifuges, automatic pipets, pH meters, autoclaves, and laboratory balances.

GLASSWARE

Basic laboratory glassware includes beakers, flasks, test tubes, graduated cylinders and pipets.

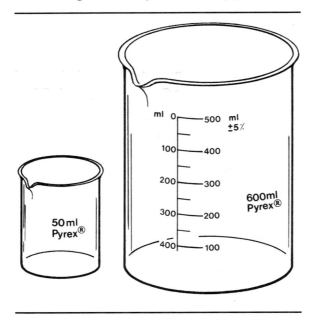

Figure 1–7. Beakers with markings

Beakers

Beakers are wide-mouthed, straight-sided jars which have a pouring spout formed out of the rim (Figure 1–7). They are useful for estimating the amount of liquids or mixing solutions, or for simply holding liquids. On the side of each beaker are markings. These indicate the approximate capacity in milliliters (ml). Many beakers have additional markings to indicate volume increments of 50 ml to 100 ml. Beakers have many functions in a laboratory, but they must be used only for **noncritical measurements,** or estimated measurements.

Flasks

Three commonly used flasks are the Erlenmeyer, Florence, and volumetric flasks (Figure 1–8). The Erlenmeyer flask has a flat bottom and sloping sides which gradually narrow in diameter so that the top opening is bottle-like. The opening may be plain, to be stoppered with a cork, or it may have threads for a cap. Erlenmeyer flasks range from 50 ml capacity to 2000 ml capacity. They may be used to hold liquids, to mix solutions, or to measure noncritical volumes. Markings on the side indicate the capacity in mls. In addition, some also have 50 ml to 100 ml increment marks. These are called *graduated flasks* and are convenient for estimating volumes or making noncritical measurements.

The Florence flask has a flat bottom and rounded sides which give rise to a long cylindrical neck. The only markings are the total capacity in milliliters. These flasks usually range in size from the 50 ml to the 2000 ml capacity. The uses of the Florence flask are similar to those of beakers and

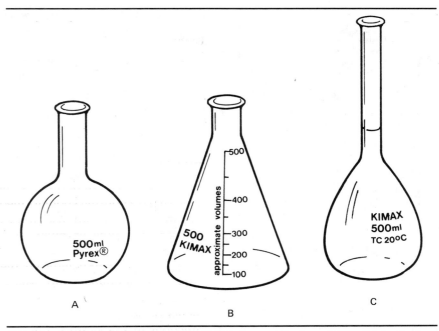

Figure 1–8. Flasks A) Florence flask, B) Erlenmeyer flask, and C) Volumetric flask

Erlenmeyer flasks. Only noncritical measurements are made in a Florence flask.

The volumetric flask is the one to be used for making **critical measurements,** measurements which require accuracy. Volumetric flasks are manufactured to strict standards and guaranteed to contain a certain volume at a particular temperature. They are most often used to prepare solutions when the accuracy of the concentration is important. When used, a portion of water or other **solvent** is placed into the flask. An exact amount of **solute** is measured into the flask. The remaining solvent is then added until it approaches the line. The last portion is added slowly until the bottom of the **meniscus,** or curved liquid surface, is level with the marking on the neck of the flask when viewed at eye level (Figure 1–9).

Test Tubes

Test tubes are available in a variety of sizes and shapes and are used in many laboratory procedures (Figure 1–10). They may function as containers for liquid samples such as blood, urine, or

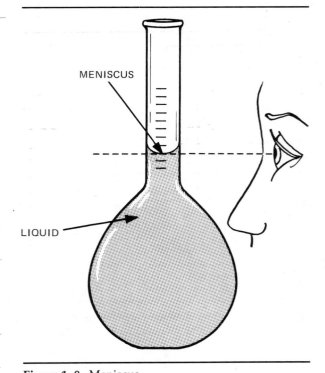

Figure 1–9. Meniscus

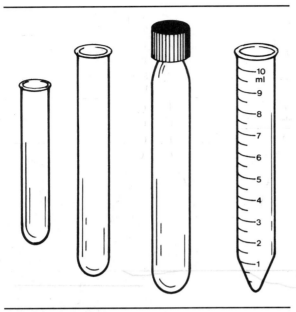

Figure 1–10. Test tubes

of glass pipets: volumetric or transfer (Figure 1–11) and graduated or measuring (Figure 1–12). Volumetric pipets are tubes with a mouthpiece on one end, a round or oval bulb in the center, and a tapered tip on the other end. These are usually labeled **TD** which indicates that they are manufactured to deliver a specified volume of liquid in a certain time period. They are used whenever the accuracy of a transferred volume is critical. To use a volumetric pipet, a pipet bulb is attached to the mouthpiece. The liquid is suctioned up into the pipet to the marking on the stem above the center bulb. The outside of the pipet stem is wiped dry with tissue. The pipet is held nearly vertical, and the tip is placed on the surface of the container into which the liquid is to be transferred. The suction is released and the liquid is allowed to flow into the container. The tip is left in contact with the container surface a few seconds to completely drain the pipet. (A small drop will remain in the pipet tip.)

Graduated pipets are long tubes with a total capacity marking near the mouthpiece. Graduated pipets are usually labeled TD. They may have a frosted band around the top indicating that the last drop of liquid is blown out after the contents are drained. Pipets without a frosted band (non blowout) are used as described in volumetric pipets. Graduated pipets are graduated to the tip with markings indicating uniform increments. Graduated pipets may be used to

serum. In some procedures, the reaction may take place in the test tube itself. Sometimes a test method requires that the contents be heated in the test tube. This should be done with caution after checking to insure that the test tube is made of heat-resistant glass.

Pipets

Pipets are used often in laboratory work to measure and transfer liquids. There are two basic types

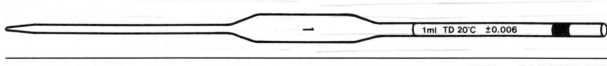

Figure 1–11. Volumetric pipet

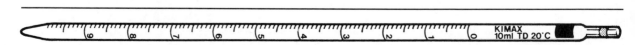

Figure 1–12. Serological pipet, a type of graduated pipet

transfer total capacity or a partial volume. One commonly used graduated pipet is the serological pipet, which is usually a blowout type (marked TD and having a frosted band). To use a serological pipet, a pipet bulb is attached. The liquid is suctioned up to the line as for the volumetric pipet. The outside stem of the pipet is wiped dry with tissue. To deliver the total volume from the pipet, the liquid is allowed to drain out while the pipet is held almost vertically. The last remaining drops are forced out by using the bulb.

In laboratory work, it is often necessary to accurately measure or transfer very small volumes. Micropipets, which can be calibrated for 0.5 ml or less, are available for this purpose (Figure 1–13). Micropipets may be of a semi-automated type. These can be pre-set to draw up and dispense a specific volume. They may also be of the manual type in which the sample is drawn up to a certain mark. An example is the Sahli pipet (0.02 ml) which is used for hemoglobin determinations. Micropipets are often labeled **TC** (to contain). This means that they must be rinsed in order to dispense the stated volume of the pipet.

Graduated Cylinders

Graduated cylinders are upright, straight-sided tubes with a flared base to provide stability. They

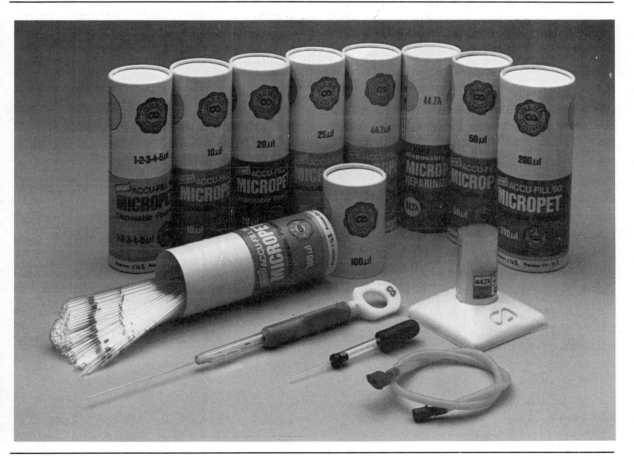

Figure 1–13. Micropipets *(Photo courtesy of Becton Dickinson & Co.)*

are used in the laboratory to make noncritical volume measurements (Figure 1–14). In size they range from 10 ml to 2000 ml capacity. Markings on the side indicate the total capacity and various increments in ml. Liquids are measured in a graduated cylinder by pouring the liquid into the cylinder until the meniscus meets the desired volume mark. Graduated cylinders are commonly used to measure the volume of 24-hour urines.

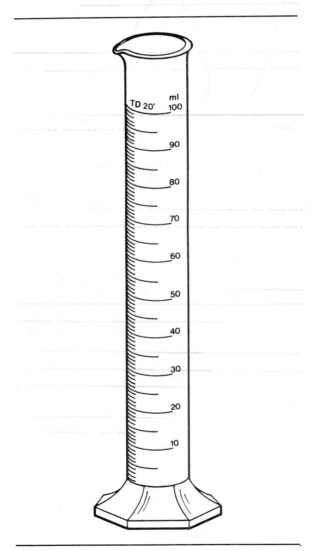

Figure 1–14. Graduated cylinder with markings

CARE AND CLEANING OF GLASSWARE

Good quality laboratory glassware is expensive and must be handled with care. Glassware should be stored in a place which offers protection from dust and accidental breakage. Pipets with tips which have been chipped or broken are no longer accurate. Glassware which is chipped or cracked should be discarded to avoid injuries to laboratory workers. Before glassware is heated, it must be checked to insure it is heat-resistant. Pyrex® and Kimax® are two types of heat-resistant glassware.

Glassware should be washed in a good laboratory detergent and rinsed thoroughly. Residues of detergent left in glassware are detrimental to laboratory results. A tap-water rinse followed by a distilled-water rinse is sufficient in most instances. However, rinsing up to twelve times with distilled water is required for some glassware used in sensitive procedures.

Stubborn deposits can usually be removed by soaking the glassware in laboratory detergent overnight. More persistent problems may require the use of an acid cleaning solution. This can be a dangerous procedure and must not be attempted by a student. The majority of cleaning problems can be avoided if glassware is rinsed with water immediately after it is used. If liquids are allowed to dry in the glassware, cleaning is difficult. Larger pieces of glassware may be inverted and allowed to air dry. Smaller pieces, such as pipets and test tubes, are dried by placing them inverted into a drying oven.

Precautions
■ Insure that the correct glassware is being used for the task.
■ Check pipettes for broken or chipped tips.
■ Check beakers, flasks, and cylinders for chips and cracks to avoid cuts and other injuries.
■ Rinse glassware with water after use.
■ Always use a clean pipet for each measurement.
■ Use clean glassware for measurements.

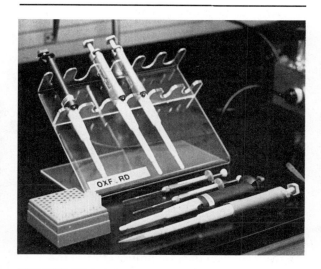

Figure 1–15. Examples of mechanical automatic pipetters *(Photo courtesy of John Estridge)*

LABORATORY EQUIPMENT

Automatic Pipets

Automatic pipets are used in most laboratories. With these pipets, pre-set volumes can be transferred by depressing and releasing a plunger on the pipet (see Figure 1–15). Pipetting with an automatic pipet is preferred over manual pipetting because it eliminates the need for mouth pipetting or using safety bulbs. When used according to manufacturer's instructions, automatic pipets deliver volumes with excellent accuracy and precision.

Several types of automatic pipets are available. Some use disposable plastic tips which are changed with every sample (Figure 1–15). Others have a reusable glass capillary tip with a teflon plunger. Since the tips on both styles of automatic pipets have no markings to indicate the volume contained, automatic pipets must be cleaned and calibrated regularly to confirm accuracy. Some automatic pipets deliver only one volume while others are adjustable within a narrow range, such as 20–200 µl or 1–20 µl. All mechanical pipets should be stored vertically, tip end down.

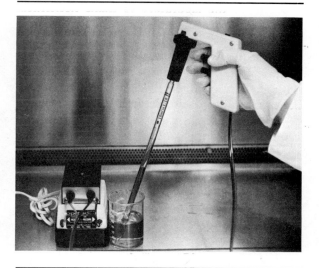

Figure 1–16. Example of electrical automatic pipetter *(Photo courtesy of John Estridge)*

Another type of automatic pipet is an electrical or battery-operated device which is used with regular graduated and volumetric glass pipets of various sizes (Figure 1–16). The mouthpiece of the glass pipet fits into the holder. Suction

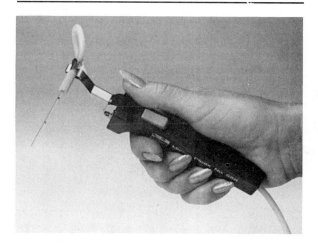

Figure 1–17. The Micro-Pipex pipet filler can be used with micropipets such as Sahli and blood cell diluting pipets, as well as with capillary tubes. *(Photo courtesy of ISOLAB, Inc. and TIP Industries, Inc.)*

is produced by a pump, and aspirating and dispensing are controlled by buttons. These pipets are easy to use and allow the use of glass pipets to dispense many different volumes.

Semiautomated devices are available for use with micropipets (Figure 1–17). One such device, the Micro-Pipex, is available from ISOLAB, Inc. This can be used for dispensing volumes with capillary micropipets as well as with larger pipets such as blood cell diluting pipets and the Sahli pipet. By using devices such as this, the need for mouth pipetting is eliminated.

Centrifuges

Centrifuges are instruments used to spin samples at high speeds, forcing the heavier particles to the bottom of the container. The most frequent laboratory use of the centrifuge is to separate the cellular components of blood from the liquid so that the liquid may be used for testing.

Centrifuges vary in size, capacity, and speed capability. *Clinical centrifuge* is the name given to tabletop models which can be used for urinalysis or serum separation. These usually have a speed capacity of from 0–3000 rpm (revolutions per minute), and will hold tubes ranging from 5 to 50 ml sizes, depending on the adapters. A serofuge is a small centrifuge used in blood banking and serology to spin serological tubes (usually 13 × 75 mm).

Microcentrifuges, or microfuges, are also becoming widely used. These will spin special microtubes (0.5–1.5 ml capacity) at high speeds, usually about 12,000 rpm. The microhematocrit centrifuge is a variation of the microfuge; it spins capillary tubes at high speeds so that hematocrits can be measured.

Other types of centrifuges include high speed centrifuges which rotate at speeds from 0–20,000 rpm and ultracentrifuges which rotate at speeds over 50,000 rpm. These centrifuges are specially equipped so that samples may be kept cool while being centrifuged. Centrifuges such as these are typically used only in research laboratories and are not required for routine clinical testing.

As with other instruments, the manufacturer's instructions must always be followed when using a centrifuge. Some general rules to follow in the operation of all centrifuges are:

1. Do not operate centrifuges with the lids open.
2. Balance the contents of the centrifuge before operating. For example, if there is only one sample to be centrifuged, a tube identical in size and volume of solution contained must be placed in the **rotor** opposite the sample tube. (The rotor is the part of the centrifuge which holds the tubes and rotates during the operation of the centrifuge.) For every sample placed in the rotor, there must be a balancing sample placed directly opposite.
3. Do not open the centrifuge lid until the rotor has stopped spinning.
4. Spin samples with lids on to avoid creating aerosols.
5. Use only tubes that are specified as appropriate for that particular centrifuge.

Autoclaves

Autoclaves are devices used to sterilize items by heating them under pressurized steam; they are like large pressure cookers. In an autoclave, the items are heated under a pressure of 15 lb/sq. in. to a temperature of 121°C for 15 to 20 minutes. This has proven sufficient to kill contaminants and infectious agents such as fungal and bacterial spores and viruses.

Most autoclaves are programmed to operate automatically, using a timed cycle. Items to be sterilized are placed in the autoclave chamber, which is surrounded by a metal jacket containing steam. The door, which has a seal to prevent the escape of steam, must be securely locked before the sterilizing process is initiated. When the autoclave is turned on, the chamber fills with steam which drives air out. A valve closes and the pressure builds to the set value, usually 15 lb. After the temperature reaches 121°C, the items are heated for 15 to 20 minutes. The steam is then released slowly so that pressure will gradually decrease to atmospheric pressure. When atmospheric pressure is reached, the chamber is vented and the door may be opened carefully, avoiding any escaping steam. The sterile items may then be removed using tongs or heat-proof gloves.

Because of the presence of steam under pressure, great care must be used when operating an autoclave. When sterilizing liquids, they must be in loosely capped, heat-resistant containers which are no more than half full. These containers should be placed in a heat-proof tray or pan to catch overflow. The pressure must be reduced slowly to prevent boiling over. Condensation may form on dry items which are sterilized; many autoclaves have a drying cycle to eliminate this moisture. As with any other laboratory instrument, instructions must be followed carefully.

Autoclaves are used for sterilizing items such as glassware, pipets, media, surgical instruments, and water. They may also be used to decontaminate biohazardous materials before disposal, such as blood specimens, cultures of bacteria, or filled biohazard containers.

Laboratory Balances

There are several types of balances or scales used in laboratories. They differ in the amounts that can be weighed and the sensitivity of measurements. Measurements which only need to be made to 0.01 g may be weighed on smaller, less expensive balances such as a triple beam or double beam balance. Measurements of as little as 0.0001 or 0.00001 g may be made using single pen balances of great sensitivity. The manufacturer's instructions must be followed when using laboratory balances to weigh substances. Some general rules to keep in mind are:

1. Keep balances clean; wipe up any spills promptly.
2. Avoid jarring the instrument. Position it on a sturdy, draft-free, vibration-free counter. Do not move it from place to place.
3. Use the balance gently and appropriately. Do not try to weigh 0.005 g on a balance that is only accurate to 0.01 g.

pH Meters

In most laboratory tests it is critical that the reagents used be of the proper pH. The **pH** is an expression of the degree of acidity or alkalinity of a solution. This is determined by measuring the hydrogen ion concentration using a pH meter. The pH scale goes from 0–14. Seven represents a neutral point; values above 7 indicate alkaline solutions, values below indicate acid solutions. A pH change of a whole increment, such as a change from pH 5 to pH 6, actually represents a ten-fold change in hydrogen ion concentration since the numbers of the pH scale represent logarithms.

pH meters use a glass electrode to measure pH. The meter must be calibrated using a solution of known pH before each pH measurement. The pH values may be displayed digitally or on a galvanometer type scale. Special care must be taken in the handling, maintenance, and storage of the electrode so that it will not dry out or be broken. Manuals which come with the meters give detailed instructions for use.

DISTILLED AND DEIONIZED WATER

In many laboratory procedures, reagents must be made or reconstituted from a powder. Tap water is not suitable for use in making most reagents because it contains impurities. **Distilled water** is therefore usually required for reagent preparation. Distilled water is the condensate collected after water has been boiled to remove impurities. Water that has been double distilled has most of the contaminants removed.

Deionized water is prepared by passing water through a resin bed to remove ions. If charcoal is included in the bed, other contaminants will be removed. Good quality distilled or deionized water for laboratory use has a low electrical conductivity.

A small distillation apparatus can be installed easily in most laboratories. Often, distilled water will be passed through a deionizing cartridge and the resulting water will be deionized distilled water. Alternatively, distilled water for making reagents can be purchased.

Distilled and deionized water should be stored in a clean, dust-free container of borosilicate glass or plastic. Stored water should be replaced frequently. Unless a procedure specifically calls for tap water, all aqueous reagents should be made using distilled or deionized water.

LESSON REVIEW

1. Name three types of laboratory flasks.
2. Name three pieces of glassware which may be used to hold liquids.
3. Which pieces of glassware are used to make critical measurements?
4. Name two types of glass pipets and explain the difference between them.
5. Do broken pipet tips affect the accuracy of the pipet?
6. The last drop is forced out of which type of pipet?
7. Why is immediate rinsing of glassware important after use?
8. Why must glassware be handled with care?
9. Why is it important that glassware be rinsed free of detergent?
10. What is the major use for volumetric flasks?
11. Explain the difference in distilled and deionized water. Why are these used in the laboratory?
12. Describe two types of automatic pipets.
13. What rules should be followed when using a laboratory balance?
14. Explain the function of a pH meter.
15. Give five general rules to follow when operating a centrifuge.
16. Why must one be careful when using an autoclave?
17. Define centrifuge, critical measurements, deionized water, distilled water, meniscus, noncritical measurements, pH, reagents, solute, solvent, TC, and TD.

STUDENT ACTIVITIES

1. Re-read the information on laboratory glassware and equipment.
2. Review the glossary terms.
3. Measure out 100 ml of water in one beaker and transfer it to another beaker or flask. Does it also measure 100 ml?
4. Measure 100 ml of water in an Erlenmeyer flask and transfer it to a volumetric flask. Is the volume exactly 100 ml?
5. Practice dispensing volumes from volumetric and serological pipets.
6. Practice filling a graduated cylinder to various levels and reading the meniscus.

Depending on which instruments are available, complete the activities in numbers 7–10. Read the instruction manual carefully before attempting to use an instrument. Then be sure to follow the instructions carefully when using that instrument.

7. If a pH meter is available, practice measuring the pH of a solution such as saline. Note how the pH changes when a few drops of 0.1% HCl are added to the solution, or a few drops of 0.1% NaOH. Dilute the solution in half by adding one part water to one part solution. Now measure the pH. Did it change? How can the result be explained?
8. If a balance is available, practice weighing a chemical, or a substance such as salt or sugar. Note the capacity of the balance; what is the largest weight that can be measured? What is the smallest increment that can be read (1 g, 0.1 g, 0.01 g, etc.)?
9. If a centrifuge is available, practice centrifuging a sample. Be sure to use appropriate balance tubes. Note the speed scale; what is the maximum rpm the centrifuge can achieve? What size tubes can the centrifuge handle safely?
10. If automatic pipets are available, practice dispensing liquids using the procedure recommended by the manufacturer.

LESSON 1–5
The Microscope

LESSON OBJECTIVES

After studying this lesson, you should be able to:
- Locate and name the parts of a microscope and explain the function of each.
- Explain the use of the coarse and fine adjustments.
- Use the low power objective to view an object.
- Use the high power objective to view an object.
- Use the oil immersion objective to view an object.
- Adjust the condenser and diaphragm.
- Clean the oculars and objectives.
- Explain the proper care and storage of the microscope.
- Define the glossary terms.

GLOSSARY

binocular / having two oculars or eyepieces

coarse adjustment / adjusts position of microscope objectives; used to initially bring objects into focus

condenser / apparatus located below the microscope stage which directs light into the objective

eyepiece / ocular

fine adjustment / adjusts position of microscope objectives; used to sharpen focus

iris diaphragm / regulates the amount of light which strikes the object being viewed through the microscope

lens / a transparent material curved on one or both sides which spreads or focuses light

lens paper / a special nonabrasive material used to clean optical lenses

microscope arm / the portion of the microscope which connects the lenses to the base

microscope base / the portion of the microscope which rests on the table and supports the instrument

monocular / having one ocular

nosepiece / revolving unit to which microscope objectives are attached

objective / magnifying lens which is closest to the object being viewed with a microscope

ocular / eyepiece of the microscope, contains a magnifying lens

stage / platform on which object to be viewed microscopically is placed

working distance / distance between the microscope objective and the slide when the object is in sharp focus

INTRODUCTION

The microscope is used in many laboratory departments. By using the microscope, it is possible to view structures or cells which are too small to be seen with the naked eyes. The microscope is used to evaluate stained blood smears and tissue sections, perform cell counts, examine urine sediment, observe cellular reactions, and observe and interpret smears containing microorganisms.

The microscopist must be skilled in using the microscope if maximum information is to be gained from studying prepared slides. Because the microscope is a delicate, expensive instrument, special care must be taken in its use, cleaning, and storage.

COMPOUND MICROSCOPES

The microscope used most in clinical laboratories is the compound bright-field microscope, which has two lens systems. The **lens** system nearest the eye is in the ocular (eyepiece). The other system is in the objectives, which are close to the object being viewed.

A microscope may be monocular or binocular. A **monocular** microscope has only one eyepiece for viewing objects. It is used frequently in schools because of its low cost. A **binocular** microscope has two eyepieces. It is used in most laboratories because both eyes are used to view an object, which reduces eyestrain.

PARTS OF THE MICROSCOPE

Microscopes may differ slightly from one model to another. However, there are some parts which are common to all microscopes. Figure 1–18 shows a monocular microscope and Figure 1–19 shows a binocular microscope with the parts labeled.

Oculars and Objectives

Located at the top of the microscope are the **oculars** or **eyepieces.** They are attached to a barrel or tube that is connected to the **microscope arm.** The oculars, through which the object is viewed, contain magnifying lenses which magnify objects. The usual magnification is ten times ($10\times$), but oculars are also available in $15\times$ and $20\times$. The underside of the arm contains a revolving **nosepiece** to which the objectives are attached. Most microscopes have three **objectives** or magnifying lenses: the low power objective which magnifies $\times 10$; the high power objective which magnifies $\times 40$, 43, or 45; and the oil immersion objective which magnifies $\times 95$, 97, or 100. Each objective is marked with color-coded bands and the degree of magnification. To determine the degree of magnification in use, multiply the magnification listed on the ocular (usually $10\times$) by the magnification listed on the objective being used. For example, an object viewed with a $10\times$ ocular and high power ($43\times$) objective would be magnified 430 times ($430\times$).

Condenser and Diaphragm

The arm of the microscope connects the objectives and eyepiece(s) to the **microscope base** which supports the microscope. The base also contains the light or mirror which supplies light to the object viewed. The light or mirror has a movable

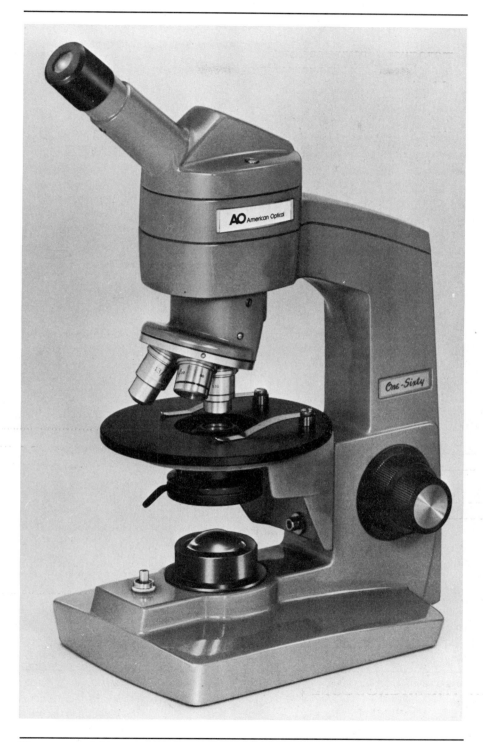

Figure 1–18. Monocular microscope *(Photo courtesy of Reichert Scientific Instruments)*

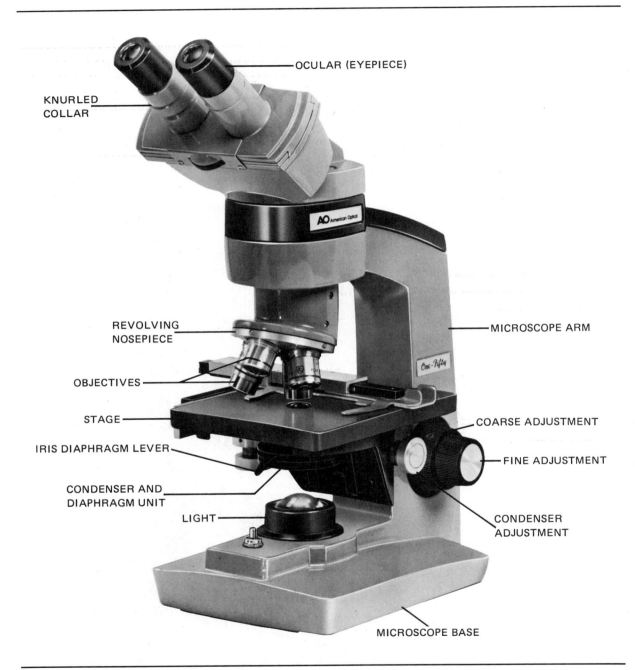

Figure 1–19. Parts of a microscope *(Photo courtesy of Reichert Scientific Instruments)*

condenser and iris diaphragm located above it. The condenser may be lowered or raised. It focuses or directs the available light into the objective. The iris diaphragm, located in the condenser unit, regulates the amount of light which strikes the object being viewed (much like the shutter of a camera). The iris diaphragm may be adjusted by a movable lever.

Coarse and Fine Adjustments

The two focusing knobs may also be located just above the base. The coarse adjustment is used to focus with the low power objective only. The fine adjustment is used to give a sharper image after the object is brought into view with the coarse adjustment. The working distance is the distance between the objective and the slide when the object is in sharp focus. The higher the magnification of the objective, the shorter the working distance will be. The coarse adjustment should not be used when using the higher magnifications. This is to prevent the objective from accidentally striking the slide and becoming damaged.

Stage

The stage of the microscope is supported by the arm and is located between the nosepiece and the light source. The stage serves as the support for the object being viewed, usually a prepared microscope slide, and has a clip to keep the slide stationary. Some stages are movable by using knobs located just below the stage. This moves the stage left and right or backward and forward. Other stages are fixed (immovable) and the slide must be moved manually to view different areas.

USING THE BRIGHT-FIELD MICROSCOPE
Adjustment of Oculars for Binocular Microscopes

The oculars of binocular microscopes must be adjusted for each individual's eyes. The distance between the oculars should be adjusted (as when using binoculars) so that one image is seen. The object is then brought into sharp focus with the coarse and fine adjustments, while looking through the right ocular with the right eye. The right eye is then closed and the knurled collar on the left ocular is used to bring the object into sharp focus while viewing the object through the left ocular with the left eye.

Use of Low Power Objective

The low power objective is used for initially locating objects and for viewing large objects. A slide is secured, specimen side up, on the stage with the clips. The low power objective is rotated into position, and the microscope light is turned on. The coarse adjustment is used to decrease the distance between the objective and the slide while watching to see when the objective stops moving. Then, while looking through the ocular, the coarse adjustment is used to move the objective and slide apart until the objects on the slide may be seen. (In some microscopes, the coarse adjustment raises and lowers the objectives. In other microscopes, the stage is raised and lowered when the coarse adjustment is turned.) A clearer image is then achieved by focusing with the fine adjustment.

Use of High Power Objective

The high power (43×) objective is used when greater magnification is needed. After initial focusing with the low power objective, the high power objective is used by carefully rotating it into position. The fine adjustment is used to bring the object into sharp focus. Most microscopes are parfocal and therefore require only slight changes in the fine adjustment. The coarse adjustment should not be used when the high power objective is in position. The high power objective is used in procedures such as cell counts and viewing urine sediments.

Use of Oil Immersion Objective

The oil immersion objective is used to view stained blood cells, tissue sections, and stained slides containing microorganisms. After initial focusing with low power, the objective is slightly rotated to the side. A drop of immersion oil is placed on the slide directly over the condenser. The oil immersion objective is then carefully rotated into the drop of oil, taking care not to allow any other objective to contact the oil. The fine adjustment is used to focus the object. The coarse adjustment should not be used when the oil immersion objective is in position. Immersion oil should never be used on any objective other than the one marked oil immersion.

When examination of the slide is completed, the low power objective is rotated into position and the slide is removed from the stage. All oil should be cleaned from the objective with **lens paper.**

Light Adjustment

The condenser and diaphragm must be adjusted according to the objective being used and the type of specimen being observed. When viewing objects with the oil immersion lens, the condenser should be raised until it is almost touching the slide. The diaphragm should be completely open to give maximum light. When looking at objects with low power, the condenser may need to be lowered somewhat to reduce the brightness of the light and increase contrast. The condenser should be raised and diaphragm opened when viewing most stained preparations with high power. However, the condenser may need to be lowered somewhat when viewing unstained fluids, such as urine sediments or cell dilutions for counting. This gives more contrast between the constituents being viewed and the background.

OTHER TYPES OF MICROSCOPES

The compound microscope described in this lesson uses bright-field microscopy to view objects. With this type of microscopy, the background against which objects are viewed is bright or lighted. This is well-suited for viewing stained specimens, such as stained blood smears. However, some other types of specimens may be better viewed using other types of microscopy.

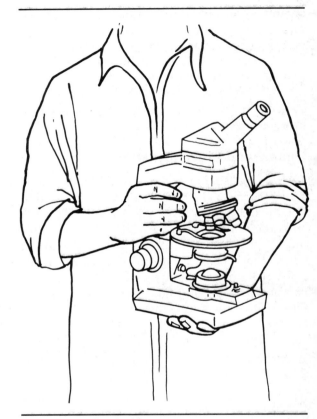

Figure 1–20. Transporting the microscope

Phase-Contrast Microscopes

The phase-contrast microscope provides a way of viewing unstained cells, which are transparent. By using special objectives and a special condenser, ordinary light microscopes can be equipped for phase-contrast microscopy. These are useful for viewing unstained specimens such as urine sediments and for performing platelet counts using the hemacytometer.

Fluorescent Microscope

The fluorescent microscope enables objects which have been stained with fluorescent dyes to be observed. When these dyes are combined with antibodies, it is possible to identify specific areas of reaction within a cell or on a cell surface. The fluorescent microscope may be used to identify organisms such as mycobacteria and to detect the presence of antibodies in certain diseases such as syphilis.

Electron Microscope

The electron microscope enables objects too small to be seen with bright-field microscopes to be viewed. Objects as small as .001 µm can be viewed by passing an electron beam through them. This microscope is very expensive and requires lengthy specimen preparation and special expertise to operate. It is rarely used in clinical medicine other than in centers performing medical research.

CARE OF THE MICROSCOPE

Care of Lenses

The microscope lenses should be cleaned with lens paper before and after each use. Other material such as laboratory tissue may scratch the lenses. It is especially important that lenses never be left with oil on them. Oil will soften the cement (glue) which holds the lens in the objective.

Transporting the Microscope

A microscope should be left in a permanent position on a sturdy lab table in an area where it will not get bumped. However, if the microscope must be moved, it should be held securely with one hand supporting the base and the other hand holding the arm (Figure 1–20). The microscope should be placed gently on tabletops, to avoid jarring.

Storage of Microscope

When the microscope is not being used, it should be left with the low power objective in position and the nosepiece in the lowest position. The stage should be centered so that it does not project from either side of the microscope. The microscope should be stored in a plastic dust cover.

Precautions

- Avoid jarring or bumping the microscope.
- Use the coarse adjustment only with low power objective.
- Use oil each time the oil immersion lens is used.
- Use immersion oil on the oil immersion objective only.
- Move or transport the microscope with one hand under the base and the other hand gripping the arm.
- Clean all oculars and objectives with lens paper after each use.
- Store microscope covered in a protected area.

LESSON REVIEW

1. Explain the functions of the iris diaphragm and condenser.
2. Name the three objectives on a microscope.
3. Explain the uses of the coarse and fine adjustments.
4. What is the proper method of cleaning a microscope after use?
5. How should a microscope be stored when not in use?
6. When is the oil immersion lens used?
7. When is immersion oil used on a slide?
8. Define binocular, coarse adjustment, condenser, eyepiece, fine adjustment, iris diaphragm, lens, lens paper, microscope arm, microscope base, monocular, nosepiece, objective, ocular, stage, and working distance.

STUDENT ACTIVITIES

1. Re-read the information on the microscope.
2. Review the glossary terms.
3. Locate and identify the parts of a microscope.
4. Practice using a microscope using the procedure as outlined in the Student Performance Guide.

Student Performance Guide

NAME _____

DATE _____

LESSON 1–5
THE MICROSCOPE

Instructions

1. Practice using the microscope.
2. Demonstrate the proper use of the microscope satisfactorily for the instructor. All steps must be completed as listed on the instructor's Performance Check Sheet.
3. Complete a written examination satisfactorily.

Materials and Equipment

- hand disinfectant
- microscope (monocular or binocular)
- lens paper
- prepared slides
- immersion oil
- surface disinfectant

Note: Procedure will vary slightly according to microscope design. Consult operating procedure in microscope manual for specific instructions.

Procedure			S = Satisfactory U = Unsatisfactory
You must:	**S**	**U**	**Comments**
1. Wash hands			
2. Assemble equipment and materials			
3. Clean the ocular(s) and objectives with lens paper			
4. Use the coarse adjustment to raise the nosepiece unit			

You must:	S	U	Comments
5. Raise the condenser as far as possible by turning the condenser knob			
6. Rotate the 10×, or low power, objective into position, so that it is directly over the opening in the stage			
7. Turn on the microscope light. If using a mirror, position the light about ten inches in front of the microscope so that it shines directly on the mirror. Adjust the mirror position so that a bright light is reflected upward into the center of the condenser			
8. Open the diaphragm until maximum light comes up through the condenser			
9. Place slide on stage and secure with clips. The condenser should be positioned so that it is almost touching the bottom of the slide			
10. Locate the coarse adjustment			
11. Look directly at the stage and 10× objective and turn the coarse adjustment until the objective is as close to the slide as it will go. Stop turning when the objective no longer moves. *Note:* Do not lower any objective toward a slide while looking through the ocular(s)			
12. Look into the ocular(s) and slowly turn the coarse adjustment in the opposite direction (as step 11) to raise the objective until the object on the slide comes into view			
13. Locate the fine adjustment			
14. Turn the fine adjustment to sharpen the image			

Note: If a binocular microscope is used, the oculars must be adjusted for each individual's eyes.
  a. Adjust distance between oculars so that one image is seen (as when using binoculars)
  b. Use coarse and fine adjustments to bring object in to focus while looking through the right ocular with right eye
  c. Close the right eye, look into the left ocular with left eye, and use the knurled collar on the left ocular to bring the object into sharp focus. (Do not turn coarse or fine adjustment at this time.)
  d. Look into oculars with both eyes to observe that object is in clear focus. If not, repeat the procedure			

You must:	S	U	Comments

15. Scan the slide by either method:
   a. Use the stage knobs to move the slide left and right and backward and forward while looking through the ocular(s), or
   b. Move the slide with the fingers while looking through the ocular(s) (for microscope without movable stage)			

16. Rotate the high power (40×) objective into position while observing the objective and the slide to see that the objective does not strike the slide			
17. Look through the ocular(s) to view the object on the slide; it should be almost in focus			
18. Locate the fine adjustment			
19. Look through the ocular(s) and turn the fine adjutment until the object is in focus. Do not use the coarse adjustment.			
20. Scan the slide as in step 15, using the fine adjustment if necessary to keep the object in focus			
21. Rotate the oil immersion (100×) objective into position while looking directly at the objective to see that it does not strike the slide			
22. Locate the fine adjustment			
23. Look through the ocular(s) and turn the fine adjustment until the object is in view			
24. Rotate the oil immersion objective to the side slightly (so that no objective is in position)			
25. Place one drop of immersion oil on the portion of the slide which is directly over the condenser			
26. Rotate the oil immersion objective back into position being careful not to rotate the 40× objective through the oil			
27. Look to see that the oil immersion objective is touching the drop of oil.			
28. Look through the ocular(s) and slowly turn the fine adjustment until the image is clear. Use only the fine adjustment to focus the oil immersion objective			
29. Scan the slide using the procedure in step 15			

You must:	S	U	Comments
30. Rotate the 10× objective into position (do not allow 40× objective to touch oil)			
31. Remove the slide from the microscope stage and gently clean the oil from the slide with lens paper			
32. Clean the oculars, 10× objective, and 40× objective with clean lens paper			
33. Clean the 100× objective to remove all oil			
34. Clean any oil from the microscope stage and condenser			
35. Turn off the microscope light and disconnect			
36. Position the nosepiece in the lowest position using the coarse adjustment			
37. Center the stage so that it does not project from either side of the microscope			
38. Cover the microscope and return it to storage			
39. Clean work area			
40. Wash hands			

Comments:

Student/Instructor:

Date:_____ Instructor:_____

LESSON 1–6
Introduction to Medical Terminology

LESSON OBJECTIVES

After studying this lesson, you should be able to:
- Define stem words from a selected list.
- Define prefixes from a selected list.
- Define suffixes from a selected list.
- Identify some common abbreviations of medical laboratory terms from a selected list.
- Pronounce some commonly used medical terms.
- Define the glossary terms.

GLOSSARY

prefix / modifying word or syllable(s) placed at the beginning of a word
stem / main part of a word; root word
suffix / modifying word or syllable(s) placed at the end of a word
terminology / special terms used in any specialized field

INTRODUCTION

Most specialized fields have a unique vocabulary or **terminology.** Medical terminology is the study of terms or words used in medicine. It is necessary for health care workers to know, understand, and be able to use medical terms in order to carry out instructions and to communicate effectively.

This lesson is only an introduction to the structure of medical terms and to abbreviations that are frequently used in the medical laboratory. Learning medical vocabulary is a long process. Knowledge of medical terms will evolve and expand as the terms are used while working in health care delivery systems. The proper use of medical terminology is as much a part of the job of laboratory and health care workers as other job functions. Each individual will gain confidence in using medical terminology by using the terms in daily activities.

STRUCTURE OF MEDICAL TERMS

Most medical terms are a combination of word parts—prefixes, suffixes, and stems—which are clues to the meaning of the word. A **prefix** is a word or syllable(s) which modifies the stem and is placed at the beginning of the word. A **suffix** is a word or syllable(s) placed at the end of the word and usually describes what happens to the stem. The **stem** or root is the main part of the word. These word parts are usually connected by a vowel such as "o" or "a."

Most of the stems, prefixes, and suffixes are derived from Latin or Greek words and have a specific meaning. By combining various prefixes, stems, and suffixes, many medical terms with precise meanings may be formed. Not all terms will have all three word parts. Some words may have only a prefix and a stem or a stem and suffix. All terms, though, will have a stem or root word. If the meanings of commonly used word parts are known, then a new term can often be analyzed to determine the general idea of its meaning. For example, hyperproteinuria can be broken into three word parts: hyper, protein, uria. "Hyper" means an increased amount. "Uria" refers to "in the urine." Therefore, the term means a condition with an increased amount of protein in the urine. By combining these parts to make a word, a medical shortcut has been created. One word can describe what would normally take a sentence or sometimes a paragraph. These medical terms, although shorter than sentences, have precise meanings. Sometimes a slight modification, such as alteration of one or two letters, can change the meaning of a word. For example, a macrocyte is a cell larger than normal while a microcyte is a cell smaller than normal. It is very important to spell, pronounce, and use medical terms correctly so that the intended meaning is conveyed.

Prefixes

Prefixes, placed before stem words, give more information about the stem, such as location, time, size, or number. For example, *intra*vascular means inside the vessel, and *pre*natal refers to something that happens before birth. Table 1–1 contains a list

Table 1–1. Selected prefixes commonly used in medical terminology

Prefix	Definition	Example of Term	Prefix	Definition	Example of Term
a, an	absent, deficient	anemia	end(o)	inside, within	endoparasite
ab	away from	absent	enter(o)	intestine	enterotoxin
ad	toward	adrenal	epi	upon, after	epidermis
ambi	both	ambidextrous	equi	equal	equilibrium
aniso	unequal	anisocytosis	hemi	half	hemisphere
ante	before	antenatal	hyper	above, excessive	hyperglycemia
ant(i)	against	antibiotic	hypo	under, deficient	hypoventilation
auto	self	autograft	infra	beneath	infracostal
baso	blue	basophil	inter	among	intercostal
bi	two	binuclear	intra	within	intracranial
bio	life	biology	iso	equal	isotonic
brady	slow	bradycardia	macr	large	macrocyte
circum	around	circumnuclear	mal	bad, abnormal	malformation
co, com, con	with, together	concentrate	medi	middle	median
contra	against	contraception	mega	huge, great	megaloblast
de	down, from	decay	melan	black	melanoma
di	two	dimorphic	meta	after, next	metamorphosis
dia	through	dialysis	micro	small	microscope
dipl	double	diplococcus	mon(o)	one, single	monoxide
dis	apart, away from	disease	morph	shape	morphology
dys	bad, difficult, improper	dysphagia	neo	new	neoplasm
e, ecto, ex	out from	ectoparasite	necro	dead	necropsy

Table 1–1 *(cont.)*

Prefix	Definition	Example of Term	Prefix	Definition	Example of Term
neutro	neutral	neutrophil	quad(r)	four	quadrant
olig	few	oliguria	retro	backward	retroactive
orth	straight, normal	orthopedic	semi	half	semiconscious
pan	all	pandemic	steno	narrow	stenosis
para	beside	paraplegic	sub	under	subcutaneous
per	through	percolate	super, supra	above	superinfection
peri	around	pericardium	syn	together	synergistic
phago	to eat	phagocyte	tachy	swift	tachycardia
poly	many	polyuria	tetra	four	tetramer
post	after	post-op	therm	heat	thermometer
pre, pro	before	prenatal	trans	through	transport
pseudo	false	pseudoappendicitis	tri	three	trimester
psych(o)	mind	psychology	uni	one	unicellular
py(o)	pus	pyuria			

of commonly used prefixes and the definition of each. A sample term using the prefix is also given.

Stems

The stem gives the major subject of the term. For example, in the term *appendi* citis, the stem is appendix. Therefore, appendicitis means an inflammation of the appendix. In the term endo*card* itis, the root or stem is "card," referring to heart; the term literally means an inflammation within the heart. A list of commonly used stem words and the meaning of each is given in Table 1–2.

Suffixes

Suffixes are attached to the end of a stem. Suffixes usually tell what is happening to the subject of the stem. They often indicate a condition, operation, or symptom. For example, in the term append*ectomy*, "ectomy" is a suffix which means to cut out

or remove by excision. Therefore, an appendectomy is the surgical removal of the appendix. A list of commonly used suffixes and their definitions is given in Table 1–3.

PRONUNCIATION

It is not enough to just understand written medical terms. You also need to pronounce them correctly to communicate effectively with others. Correct pronunciation may be easy for some frequently used terms or short terms, but more difficult for some of the longer terms. Although most terms are derived from Greek and Latin, the Latin and Greek pronouncing rules cannot always be relied on for the proper pronunciation. Your medical dictionary can give you a guide to common usage but even authors disagree on some standard pronunciations. By listening to others who work with you, you can learn how words are commonly pronounced in your area. Pronuncia-

Table 1–2. Selected stems commonly used in medical terminology

Stem	Definition	Example of Term	Stem	Definition	Example of Term
adeno	gland	lymphadenitis	lip	fat	lipoma
alg	pain	analgesic	lith	stone	cholelithiasis
arter	artery	arteriogram	mening	membrane covering brain	meningitis
arthr	joint	arthritis			
audio	hearing	auditory	myel	marrow	myelogram
brachi	arm	brachial	myo	muscle	myositis
bronch(i)	air tube in lungs	bronchitis	nephro	kidney	nephron
cardi	heart	myocardium	neur	nerve	neurectomy
calc	stone	calcify	noct	night	nocturia
carcin	cancer	carcinogen	onc	tumor	oncology
caud	tail	caudate	oo	egg	oogenesis
ceph(al)	head	encephalitis	ophthal	eye	ophthalmologist
chol	bile, gall bladder	cholesterol	os, osteo	bone	osteosarcoma
chondr	cartilage	chondroplasia	oto	ear	otitis
chrom	color	chromogen	path	disease	pathogen
cran	skull	craniotomy	ped	child	pediatrician
cut	skin	subcutaneous	phleb	vein	phlebitis
cyan	blue	cyanosis	phob	fear	phobia
cyst	bladder, bag	cystocele	phot	light	photosensitive
cyt(o)	cell	monocyte	pneum	air	pneumonitis
dactyl	finger	arachnodactyly	pod	foot	pseudopod
dent, dont	teeth	orthodontist	pulm	lung	pulmonary
derm	skin	dermatitis	ren	kidney	adrenal
edema	swelling	edematous	rhin	nose	rhinoplasty
erythro	red	erythrocyte	scler	hard	sclerosis
febr	fever	afebrile	sep	poison	septic
gastr(o)	stomach	gastritis	soma(t)	body	somatic
genito	reproductive	genital	sperm	seed	spermatogenesis
gloss	tongue	glossitis	stoma	mouth, opening	stomatitis
glyco	sweet	glycosuria	therm	temperature	thermometer
gran	grain	granulocyte	thorac	chest	thoracotomy
hem(a), haem	blood	hematology	thromb	clot	thrombocyte
hepat(o)	liver	hepatitis	tome	knife	microtome
histo	tissue	histology	tox	poison	toxin
hydro	water	hydrocephalic	ur(o), uria	urine	hematuria
hystero	uterus	hysterectomy	vas	vessel	intravascular
iatro	physician	podiatrist	ven	vein	intravenous
leuk	white	leukocyte			

tion will be improved and confidence will be gained by practicing the pronunciation of terms.

ABBREVIATIONS

Abbreviations are used commonly in medicine to avoid having to repeatedly write or say several syllables. A short list of common abbreviations used in the medical laboratory is shown in Table 1–4. This table does not include abbreviations used in prescriptions, nursing care, and other areas of health care. A worker should be familiar with abbreviations so that physician's orders or instructions can be carried out correctly.

Table 1–3. Selected suffixes commonly used in medical terminology

Suffix	Definition	Example of Term	Suffix	Definition	Example of Term
algia	pain	neuralgia	osis	state, condition, increase	leukocytosis
blast	primitive, germ	erythroblast	ostomy	create an opening	ileostomy
centesis	puncture, aspiration	amniocentesis	otomy	cut into	phlebotomy
cide	death, killer	bacteriocide	opathy, pathia	disease	adenopathy
ectomy	excision, cut out	gastrectomy	penia	lack of	leukopenia
emesis	vomiting	hematemesis	phil	affinity for, liking	eosinophil
emia	in the or of the blood	bilirubinemia	phyte	plant	dermatophyte
ferent	carry	afferent	plastic, plasia	to form or mold	hyperplasia
genic	origin, producing	pyogenic	pnea	breathing	apnea
ia, iasis	state, condition	iatrogenic	poiesis	to make	hemopoiesis
iole	small	bronchiole	rrhage	excessive flow	hemorrhage
itis	inflammation	pharyngitis	rrhea	flow	diarrhea
lysis	free, breaking down	hemolysis	scope, scopy	view	arthroscope
oid	resembling, similar to	blastoid	stasis	same, standing still	hemostasis
(o)logy	study of	pathology	troph(y)	nourishment	hypertrophy
oma	tumor	hepatoma			

Table 1–4. Abbreviations commonly used in a medical laboratory

A	absorbance	GTT	glucose tolerance test
AIDS	acquired immunodeficiency syndrome	GU	genitourinary
ALP, AP	alkaline phosphatase	Hb, Hgb	hemoglobin
ALT	alanine aminotransferase	HCl	hydrochloric acid
AST	aspartate aminotransferase	HCO_3	bicarbonate
BP	blood pressure	Hct	hematocrit
BUN	blood urea nitrogen	HDL Chol	high density lipoprotein cholesterol
C	Centigrade, Celsius	HIV	human immunodeficiency virus
CBC	complete blood count	H_2O	water
cc, ccm	cubic centimeter	HPF	high power field
CK	creatine kinase	IM	infectious mononucleosis
Cl	chloride	IU	international unit
cm	centimeter	IV	intravenous
CNS	central nervous system	K	potassium
CO	carbon monoxide	L	liter
CO_2	carbon dioxide	LD, LDH	lactate dehydrogenase
crit	hematocrit	LDL Chol	low density lipoprotein cholesterol
CSF	cerebral spinal fluid	LPF	low power field
cu mm	cubic millimeter, mm^3	MCH	mean corpuscular hemoglobin
E.U.	Ehrlich units	MCHC	mean corpuscular hemoglobin concentration
F	Fahrenheit	MCV	mean corpuscular volume
FUO	fever of unknown origin	meq	milliequivalent
g, gm	gram	mg	milligram
GGT	gamma glutamyl transferase	MI	myocardial infarction
GI	gastrointestinal	mL, ml	milliliter

Table 1–4. *(cont.)*

MLT	medical laboratory technician	RBC	red blood cell
mm	millimeter	RF	rheumatoid factors
mmol	millimole	S.I.	Le Système International d'Unités (International System of Units)
MT	medical technologist		
Na	sodium	sp. gr.	specific gravity
NaCl	sodium chloride, saline	Staph	*Staphylococcus*
nm	nanometer	stat	immediately
O.D.	optical density	Strep	*Streptococcus*
pH	a number indicating the relative acidity of a solution	UA	urinalysis
		µl	microliter
PP	post-prandial	µmol	micromole
RA	rheumatoid arthritis	WBC	white blood cell

LESSON REVIEW

1. What is a prefix?
2. What is a suffix?
3. What is a stem?
4. Name the stems used for cell, heart, head, skin, chest, kidney, muscle, liver, stomach.
5. Name ten common suffixes and give a meaning for each.
6. Name ten common prefixes and give a meaning for each.
7. List ten abbreviations frequently used in the medical laboratory.
8. Define prefix, stem, suffix, and terminology.

STUDENT ACTIVITIES

1. Re-read the lesson on medical terminology.
2. Review the glossary terms.
3. Practice pronouncing the word parts and medical terms in Tables 1–1 through 1–3. Look up pronunciations of ten terms and practice saying them out loud.
4. Study the definitions for prefixes, suffixes, and stems listed in the tables.
5. Study the abbreviations listed in Table 1–4.
6. Use each of the prefixes, suffixes, or stems in a word not on the list.
7. Look up the meanings of the examples of medical terms listed in Tables 1–1 through 1–3.

LESSON 1–7
The Metric System

LESSON OBJECTIVES

After studying this lesson, you should be able to:
- Discuss the importance of the proper use of metric units.
- Name prefixes commonly used to denote smaller or larger metric units.
- Convert English units to metric units.
- Convert metric units to English units.
- Convert units within the metric system.
- Perform measurements of distance, volume, and weight using metric units.
- Define the glossary terms.

GLOSSARY

gram / basic metric unit of weight or mass
liter / basic metric unit of volume
meter / basic metric unit of distance or length
SI units / standardized units of measure; international units

INTRODUCTION

The metric system is the system of measurements used internationally for scientific work. In European countries, the metric system is also used in everyday life. Milk is purchased by the liter. Body weight is measured in kilograms. If the weather report predicts a high of 34°C for the day, the European knows not to wear a coat because it will be a hot day. This is because the temperature is measured on the centigrade or Celsius scale.

In the United States, use of the metric system is encouraged. However, the English system is still used for most measurements and observations made in everyday life. We drive our cars at fifty-five miles per hour. We report our weight in pounds and our height in feet and inches. We cook using measures such as teaspoon, cup, and pint. However, the English system is not accurate enough for most scientific measurements. Therefore, a student of science must know and be able to use the metric system in laboratory observations and measurements.

IMPORTANCE OF MEASUREMENTS

Units of measurement are used frequently in medicine. They are used to measure vital statistics such as height, weight, and temperature; the amount of fluid intake and output; and dosages of medication. In the laboratory, measurements are used to indicate numbers of cells or quantities of substances in a patient's blood, serum, or other body fluids. Very small quantities can be measured accurately and easily using the metric system. These measurements are then compared to normal values and the patient's condition is assessed. The results may be used to establish a diagnosis and to prescibe therapy. Therefore, it is important that all measurements are made correctly and accurately.

COMMON MEASUREMENTS

Measurements that are commonly determined include the:

- concentration of a substance
- weight of a substance or object
- volume of a solution or object
- size or length of an object
- temperature
- time

The weights, volumes, and sizes or lengths of objects can be most accurately measured using the metric system. In the United States, body temperatures are commonly measured on the Fahrenheit scale. Laboratory temperatures are measured on the centigrade or Celsius scale. Fortunately, laboratory time is measured in seconds, minutes, and hours as is the time of day.

THE METRIC SYSTEM

The metric system is named because it is based on a fundamental unit of distance, the **meter.** In the metric system, the **meter (m)** is the basic unit used to measure distance. The **gram (g)** is the basic unit used to compare mass or weight. And, the **liter (l)** is the basic unit used to measure volume.

The metric system uses decimal notations and the units are divided into increments of ten. This means that units larger or smaller than the basic units (meter, liter, and gram) can be obtained by multiplying or dividing by increments of ten (or by a power of ten).

Prefixes may be added to the basic units to indicate larger or smaller units (Table 1–5). For example, "kilo" means 1,000. Therefore, a kilometer (km) is 1,000 meters or 10^3 meters; a kilogram (kg) is 1,000 grams, and a kiloliter (kl) is 1,000 liters. Although "kilo" is the prefix most commonly used for large units, "deca" may be used to indicate the unit times ten, as in decaliter. Or, "hecto" may indicate the unit times one hundred. The prefixes and their definitions are the same for the three basic units.

In laboratory analyses, it is more common to measure units smaller than the basic units. Table 1–5 lists the prefixes and the multiple of the basic unit which each represents. Two common prefixes used are "milli," which means one-thousandth (.001 or 10^{-3}), and "centi," which means one-hundredth (.01 or 10^{-2}). A milliliter is .001 liter or 10^{-3} liter. In chemistry, solutions may be made by adding milligrams (mg) of substances to milliliters (ml) of solvent. Substances such as glucose may be measured in mg per 100 ml (or mg per deciliter) of serum. In hematology, blood cells are counted per cubic millimeter or per liter of blood.

Other prefixes commonly used to denote size are "micro," which denotes one millionth or 10^{-6}, and "nano" which is 10^{-9}. (See Table 1–5 for abbreviations and prefixes.) Small samples are measured in microliters (μl) or 10^{-6} liter. Wavelengths of light are measured in nanometers (nm) or 10^{-9} meter.

Converting Units

It may be necessary to convert units within the metric system or to convert English units to metric or metric units to English units. For this reason, it is helpful to have a general idea of the metric equivalents of commonly used English measures.

Table 1–5. Commonly used prefixes in the metric system

Abbreviation	Prefix	Meaning	Multiple of Basic Unit	Weight Gram (g)	Length Meter (m)	Volume Liter (L)
k	kilo	1000	10^3	kg	km	kl
h	hecto	100	10^2	hg*	hm*	hl*
da	deca	10	10^1	dag*	dam*	dal*
d	deci	.1	10^{-1}	dg*	dm*	dl
c	centi	.01	10^{-2}	cg*	cm	cl*
m	milli	.001	10^{-3}	mg	mm	ml
μ	micro	.000001	10^{-6}	μg	μm	μl
n	nano		10^{-9}	ng	nm	nl*
p	pico		10^{-12}	pg	pm*	pl*

*Units not commonly used in the laboratory

Equivalents are listed in Tables 1–6 and 1–7. To convert units from one system to another, simply multiply by the factor listed. For example, since one inch is equal to 2.54 centimeters (cm), twelve inches would equal 12 × 2.54, or 30.48 cm. To convert metric units to English units, use Table 1–7 in the same manner. Since one kg equals 2.2 pounds, the weight in pounds of a patient weighing 70 kg may be determined by multiplying 70 × 2.2 to equal 154 pounds.

In laboratory work, it is more common to need to convert units within the metric system. To make these conversions, the worker needs to know equivalents, such as how many milliliters or microliters are in a liter, or how many milligrams are in a gram. These conversions can be made by using the information in Table 1–8.

Metric units may be converted to larger units such as grams to kilograms or milliliters to liters; the decimal in the original unit is moved to the left for the appropriate number of spaces. Example: To convert 50 g to kg, multiply by .001 or move the decimal to the left three places: 50 g = .050 kg. To convert centimeters to meters, multiply by .01

Table 1–6. Conversion of English units to metric units

	English Unit	English Abbreviation	Multiply By	To Get Metric Unit	Metric Abbreviation
Distance	1 mile	mi	= 1.6	kilometers	km
	1 yard	yd	= 0.9	meters	m
	1 inch	in	= 2.54	centimeters	cm
Mass	1 pound	lb	= 0.454	kilograms	kg
	1 pound	lb	= 454	grams	g
	1 ounce	oz	= 28	grams	g
Volume	1 quart	qt	= 0.95	liters	l
	1 fluid ounce	fl. oz.	= 30	milliliters	ml
	1 teaspoon	tsp	= 5	milliliters	ml

Table 1–7. Conversion of metric units to English units

	Metric Unit	Metric Abbreviation	Multiply By	To Find English Unit	English Abbreviation
Distance	1 kilometer	km	= 0.6	miles	mi
	1 meter	m	= 3.3	feet	ft
	1 meter	m	= 39.37	inches	in
	1 centimeter	cm	= 0.4	inches	in
	1 millimeter	mm	= .04	inches	in
Mass	1 gram	g	= .0022	pounds	lb
	1 kilogram	kg	= 2.2	pounds	lb
Volume	1 liter	l	= 1.06	quarts	qt
	1 milliliter	ml	= .03	fluid ounces	fl. oz.

Table 1–8. Common metric equivalents

Mass	10^{-3} kg	= 1 gram	= 10^3 mg	= 10^6 µg
	10^{-3} g	= 1 mg	= 10^3 µg	= 10^6 ng
	10^{-9} g	= 1 ng	= 10^3 pg	
Volume	10^{-3} kl	= 1 liter	= 10^3 ml	= 10^6 µl
	10^{-3} l	= 1 ml	= 10^3 µl	= 10^6 nl
	10^{-1} l	= 1 dl	= 10^2 ml	
Length	10^{-3} km	= 1 meter	= 10^3 mm	= 10^6 µm
	10^{-3} m	= 1 mm	= 10^3 µm	= 10^6 nm
	10^{-2} m	= 1 cm	= 10 mm	= 10^4 µm
	10^{-3} mm	= 1 nm	= 10 Å	

or move the decimal two places to the left: 160 cm = 1.6 meters.

Metric units may be converted to smaller units, such as g to mg or liters to microliters; the decimal in the number is moved to the right the appropriate number of spaces. To convert 5 g to mg, multiply by 1000 or move the decimal to the right three places: 5 g = 5000 mg. Scientific notation is often used to make the numbers less bulky and easier to compute. For example, five grams equals 5,000,000 µg or 5.0×10^6 µg.

SI UNITS

Even though the metric system is used internationally to obtain laboratory measurements, the method of reporting results differs from country to country or even within countries. This can be confusing when one is trying to compare laboratory data. For example, the concentration of protein may be expressed as g/L in some laboratories or g/dl in others.

An effort is being made to standardize the reporting of laboratory values by using an international system of units called **SI units** (Table 1–9). Blood cell counts have traditionally been expressed as the number of cells per cubic millimeter (cu mm) of blood. In the SI system, however, they are expressed as number of cells per liter of blood. Chemical substances such as bilirubin or glucose which were expressed as mg per deciliter (dl) or per 100 ml, are now expressed as mg or g per liter or as micromoles (µmol) or millimoles (mmol) per liter. It is imperative that the proper units of measurement be included with all laboratory results. For example, a glucose reported simply as 5.6 would cause great concern in a lab that measures blood glucose in mg/dl. The normal value should be around 80–100 mg/dl and 5.6 would be extremely low. However, in labs where blood glucose is measured in mmol/liter, 5.6 would be a normal finding.

Common Equivalents

There are a few units which have been commonly used in the laboratory but are being phased out in favor of more appropriate terms. Since these units

Table 1–9. International system of units (SI units)

Common Usage	SI Equivalent
micron (μ)	micrometer (μm; 10^{-6} meter)
cubic micron (μ³)	femtoliter (fl; 10^{-15} liter)
micromicrogram (μμg)	picogram (pg; 10^{-12} gram)
microgram (mcg)	microgram (μg; 10^{-6} gram)
Angstrom (Å)	$nm \times 10^{-1}$
millimicron (mμ)	nanometer (nm; 10^{-9} meter)
lambda (λ)	microliter (μl; 10^{-6} liter)

Test	Old Unit	SI Unit
Cell counts	cells/mm³ or cells/cumm	cells/μl or cells/liter
Hematocrit	% (Ex: 41%)	Percent expressed as decimal (Ex: 0.41)
Hemoglobin	g/dl	g/liter
MCV	μ³	fl
MCH	μμg	pg
MCHC	%	g/dl (or g/l)

are still used by some laboratories and appear in older books or manuals, one needs to understand the equivalents of these units. A milliliter (ml) may also be called a cc (cubic centimeter), especially when referring to dosages. A cubic centimeter may be written as cc, cu cm, or cm³. A microliter (μl), which is one-thousandth of a ml, may also be called a cubic millimeter (cu mm or mm³). Micron is the old term referring to micrometer. Lambda (λ) is the term previously used for microliter and wavelength of light; nanometer is now used for wavelength.

TEMPERATURE CONVERSIONS

The two temperature scales used in medicine are the Fahrenheit scale and the Celsius or centigrade scale. The Fahrenheit scale is used for measuring body temperature. The Celsius scale is used in the laboratory for measuring temperatures of reaction and incubation and boiling points. The method of converting from one temperature scale to another is discussed in Lesson 1–8, Laboratory Math.

LESSON REVIEW

1. What is the basic metric unit of distance or length?
2. What is the basic metric unit of volume?
3. What is the basic metric unit of weight?
4. What are the meanings of kilo, micro, milli, nano, centi?
5. Why is the metric system preferred over the English for scientific measurements?
6. Convert the following English measurements to metric units:
   3 inches = _____ cm or _____ mm
   5 qt. = _____ liters or _____ ml
   64 oz. = _____ g or _____ kg or _____ mg
7. Convert the following units:
   12 mg = _____ μg or _____ g
   50 ml = _____ μl or _____ cc or _____ dl
8. Define gram, liter, meter, and SI units.

STUDENT ACTIVITIES

1. Re-read the information on the metric system.
2. Review the glossary terms.
3. Practice measuring metric volumes, lengths, and weights and converting metric units using the worksheets.

Metric
Worksheet—Distance

NAME _____   DATE _____

LESSON 1–7 THE METRIC SYSTEM

Obtain a meter stick or metric ruler and an English ruler from the instructor. Use the information in Tables 1–5 through 1–9 to answer the questions below.

1. Look at the meter stick. Locate the cm and mm divisions. How many centimeters are in a meter? _90_
   How many mm in a cm? _10_ How many mm in a meter? _900_

2. Draw the indicated length of line beside each number beginning at the dot.
   - 35 mm
   - 6 cm
   - 83 mm
   - (1.2 dm)

3. Measure the lines above using a ruler marked in English units (inches):
   - 35 mm   = _1 3/8_ inches
   - 6 cm   = _2 3/8_ inches
   - 83 mm   = _3 5/16_ inches
   - 1.2 dm = _____ inches

   Which of the measurements (English or metric) do you feel is the most accurate? _metric_

4. How many mm in one inch? _25.4_   One mm = _.04_ inch
   How many cm in one inch? _2.54_   One cm = _.4_ inch

   Convert the following units:
   - 4 inches = _10.16_ cm
   - 0.5 inches = _1.27_ cm   What number did you multiply by to obtain the answers? _2.54_
   - 38 cm   = _15.2_ in.
   - 7 cm   = _2.8_ in.   What number did you multiply by to obtain the answers? _.4_
   - 3.5 inches = _88.9_ mm $(3.5 \times 2.54 \div .10 = 88.9)$
   - 35 mm   = _1.4_ in. $(3.5 cm \times .4 = 1.4 in)$

5. How many inches are in a meter? _32.4_ What English unit of measure is the closest in size to the meter? _yard_

6. Measure your height or the height of another student using the meter stick. What is the height in cm? _157.48_ in meters? _55.8_ Convert the height in cm to inches: _62.992_ Now measure the height in inches and compare the results.

55

Metric Worksheet—Weight

LESSON 1–7 THE METRIC SYSTEM

Use Tables 1–5 through 1–9 to answer the questions below.

1. What is the basic metric unit of weight? _____gram_____

2. How many mg in a g? _____ How many µg in a g? _____ How many g in a kg? _____

3. Convert the following units:

   300 mg = _____ g = _____ kg
    50 mg = _____ g = _____ kg
   4000 mg = _____ g = _____ kg
   200 µg = _____ g
   750 µg = _____ mg
    80 g   = _____ kg

   What decimal rule did you follow to make the conversions?_____

   _____

4. Convert the following units:

   0.4 kg = _____ mg = _____ µg
   9.2 g   = _____ mg = _____ µg
   0.6 g   = _____ µg
   10 mg = _____ µg = _____ pg
   280 mg = _____ µg = _____ pg

   What decimal rule did you follow in making the conversions? _____

   _____

5. Weigh yourself or another student. What is the weight in g? _____ in kg? _____

6. A man who weighs 165 pounds would weigh _____ kg.

7. A child who weighs 32 pounds would weigh _____ kg or _____ g.

8. Is a man who is 178 cm tall and weighs 135 kg overweight, underweight, or of normal weight?

   _____

9. If scales are available, weigh 10 ml of water in a container. How much does the water weigh? _____
   Does one milliliter of water weigh approximately 1 gram?
   Yes _____ No _____

Metric Worksheet—Volume

NAME_____ DATE _____

LESSON 1–7 THE METRIC SYSTEM

Obtain a medicine cup, a 50 ml graduated cylinder, and a 50 ml beaker from the instructor. Use Tables 1–5 through 1–9 to answer the questions below.

1. What is the basic unit of volume in the metric system? _____
2. How many ml in a liter? _____ dl in a liter? _____ µl in a liter? _____
3. Convert the following units:

    45 cc = _____ liter = _____ ml
   550 ml = _____ liter
     4 dl = _____ liter
    60 µl = _____ liter = _____ ml
   0.1 dl = _____ liter
 6,700 ml = _____ liter

   What decimal rule did you follow to make the conversions? _____
_____

4. Convert the following units:

   0.3 liter = _____ dl = _____ ml
   5 liters = _____ ml
   7 ml   = _____ µl
   3 dl   = _____ ml = _____ µl
   0.1 dl   = _____ ml

   What decimal rule did you follow to make the conversions? _____
_____

5. What English unit is closest in volume to the liter? _____
6. Convert the following English units:

   3.5 pints = _____ ml = _____ l
    3 quarts = _____ ml = _____ l
    5 fl. oz. = _____ ml = _____ l

7. If gasoline is $1.20 per gallon at station A and 30 cents a liter at station B, which has the cheapest gasoline?
_____

8. Fill the medicine cup to the one ounce mark with water. Transfer the water to a 50 ml graduated cylinder. How many milliliters of water was in the one fluid ounce?_____
Fill the medicine cup again with water and transfer the one fl. oz. to a 50 ml beaker. Which gives the most accurate measurement, the beaker or the graduated cylinder?_____

LESSON 1-8
Laboratory Math

LESSON OBJECTIVES

After studying this lesson, you should be able to:
- Convert Celsius temperatures to Fahrenheit.
- Convert Fahrenheit temperatures to Celsius.
- Prepare percent solutions.
- Prepare laboratory dilutions.
- Use proportions to prepare laboratory solutions.

GLOSSARY

Celsius / temperature scale having the freezing point of water at zero (0°) and the boiling point at one hundred (100°); indicated by "C"; also called centigrade

Fahrenheit / a temperature scale having the freezing point of water at 32° and the boiling point at 212°; indicated by "F"

ratio / relationship in degree or number between two things

saline / an isotonic solution of sodium chloride in distilled water; usually made in either a 0.85 or 0.90% concentration for use in medical laboratory procedures; may be referred to as normal or physiological saline.

INTRODUCTION

Some form of math is used in most laboratory exercises no matter how simple the procedure. The math principles may be used directly in the procedure. Or, math may be used indirectly, as in the preparation of test reagents and in the research and development of the procedures themselves. It is not sufficient just to understand the fundamentals of laboratory math. One must also be able to use math principles correctly if laboratory results are to be accurate.

The Direct Use of Math

The direct use of math in a procedure could involve making a dilution of the blood or serum being analyzed. For example, to do a white blood cell count, the blood must first be diluted to a 1/20 concentration.

Indirect Uses of Math

In some instances, math is not used in an obvious way in a laboratory procedure. One example is in

58

Problem: Convert 98.6° F (normal body temperature) to Celsius (C) degrees.

Formula: $C = \dfrac{5}{9}(F-32)$

Solution: $C = \dfrac{5}{9}(98.6-32)$

$C = \dfrac{5}{9}(66.6)$

$C = 36.99$ or 37

Answer: 98.6° F is equal to 37° C

Figure 1–21. Example of Fahrenheit temperature converted to Celsius

Problem: Convert 37° C to Fahrenheit (F) degrees.

Formula: $F = \dfrac{9}{5}(C) + 32$

Solution: $F = \dfrac{9}{5}(37) + 32$

$F = 66.6 + 32$

$F = 98.6$

Answer: 37° C is equal to 98.6° F

Figure 1–22. Example of Celsius temperature converted to Fahrenheit

the preparation of the reagents. The concentration of laboratory reagents is often expressed as a percentage (%). A good example is the 70% solution of ethyl alcohol used to cleanse the skin at the site of puncture before blood collection. **Saline,** a solution of .85% NaCl, is widely utilized in medical laboratory procedures. In serology and blood banking, a reagent commonly used is a 2% concentration of red blood cells. The directions for some reagents may also express the concentration as a proportion, such as two parts of Solution "A" to three parts of Solution "B."

TEMPERATURE CONVERSION

Converting temperatures from **Celsius** (C) to **Fahrenheit** (F), or vice versa, also employs math. The temperature scale most widely used in laboratory work is Celsius (a temperature scale in which the freezing point of water is 0° and the boiling point is 100°). In scientific work, the required temperature for a specific reaction is almost always expressd in Celsius degrees. There are, however, instances in which one might need to convert Celsius to Fahrenheit (a temperature scale in which the freezing point of water is 32° and the boiling point is 212°) or vice versa. Normal human body temperature is usually stated as 98.6° Fahrenheit. A laboratory procedure may require that a test be run at normal body temperature, but the equipment in the laboratory is calibrated in Celsius

degrees. This makes it necessary that the 98.6°F be converted to Celsius degrees (Figure 1–21). This can be accomplished by the use of the formula:

Celsius degrees = 5/9(F–32)

The normal body temperature may then be expressed as 37°C. Conversely, the normal body temperature, 37°C, can be converted to Fahrenheit degrees (Figure 1–22) by using the formula:

Fahrenheit degrees = 9/5(C) + 32

A temperature conversion chart is shown in Appendix D.

PROPORTION

Proportion is used when reagents are prepared by adding together a specific amount of one solution with a specific amount of another solution. An example would be instructions which direct that two parts (measures) of solution "A" be added to three parts (measures) of solution "B" to prepare the final solution, "C." The formula to determine the actual volumes required of solutions "A" and "B" is:

$$\frac{(C)}{(A) + (B)} = V$$

where: C = Total volume of final solution
A = Total parts of solution A
B = Total parts of solution B
V = Total volume of one part

Problem: A buffer is made by adding 2 parts of "solution A" to 5 parts of "solution B." How much of solution A and solution B would be required to make 70 ml of the buffer?

Formula: $\dfrac{\text{Total volume required (C)}}{\text{parts of "A" + parts of "B"}}$ = volume of one part (V)

Solution: $\dfrac{70 \text{ ml required}}{2 \text{ parts "A" + 5 parts "B"}}$ = volume of one part

$\dfrac{70}{7}$ = 10 ml = volume of one part (V)

2 parts of solution "A" = 2 × 10 = 20 ml
5 parts of solution "B" = 5 × 10 = 50 ml

Answer: The buffer would be made by mixing 20 ml of solution A with 50 ml of solution B to give a total volume of 70 ml.

Figure 1–23. Preparing a solution using proportions

When measuring the bilirubin level in serum, a Diazo reagent is used. This reagent is prepared by adding 0.3 parts of Diazo reagent B to ten (10) parts of Diazo reagent A. Buffer solutions are also often prepared using proportions. An example is illustrated in Figure 1–23.

Proportion can also be used to determine how much of a solution of a specific concentration is required to prepare a second solution of a lower concentration. The 2% solution of acetic acid used in white blood cell counts can be prepared using proportions. If a 10% solution of acetic acid is available, the 2% solution can be prepared from that concentration (Figure 1–24). The general formula is:

$$C_1 \times V_1 = C_2 \times V_2$$

In this formula C_1 refers to the concentration of solution one and V_1 to its volume. The C_2 and V_2 refer to the concentration and volume of solution two.

PERCENTAGE SOLUTIONS

The concentrations of many laboratory reagents are expressed in percentage. Percentage solutions may be made by weighing out a specific amount of a solute for each 100 ml of solvent, usually distilled water. This is called a weight to volume percentage (w/v). One example of this type is the 0.85% saline (sodium chloride) solution which is used in many serological and bacteriological procedures. One hundred ml of 0.85% saline can be prepared by placing about 50 ml of distilled

Problem: Prepare 100 ml of a 2% solution of acetic acid using a 10% acetic acid solution.

Formula: $C_1 V_1 = C_2 V_2$ C_1 = concentration of first solution

Solution: $(2)(100 \text{ ml}) = (10)(V_2)$ C_2 = concentration of second solution

$200 \text{ ml} = 10(V_2)$ V_1 = required volume of first solution

$\dfrac{200}{10}\text{ml} = V_2$ V_2 = required volume of second solution

$20 \text{ ml} = V_2$

Answer: Twenty ml of 10% acetic acid are added to 80 ml of distilled water to make 100 ml of a 2% solution of acetic acid.

Figure 1–24. Using the formula: $C_1 \times V_1 = C_2 \times V_2$ to prepare a solution

Problem: Prepare 500 ml of 0.85% saline.

Solution: 1. A 0.85% solution contains 0.85 g of the solute in every 100 ml of solution.
2. Therefore, to prepare 500 ml, 5×0.85 g or 4.25 g of sodium chloride (NaCl) must be used.
3. To prepare the solution:
    a. Weigh out 4.25 g of NaCl
    b. Fill a 500 ml volumetric flask approximately half full with distilled water
    c. Add 4.25 g of NaCl and swirl gently to dissolve
    d. Fill the flask to the line with distilled water

Figure 1–25. Preparation of a weight to volume (w/v) percentage solution

Problem: Prepare one liter of 2% acetic acid from concentrated (glacial) acetic acid.

Solution: 1. A 2% solution of acetic acid contains 2 ml of acetic acid in each 100 ml of solution.
2. Therefore, one liter of 2% acetic acid contains $2 \text{ ml} \times 10$, or 20 ml of acetic acid.
3. To prepare the solution:
    a. Fill a one-liter volumetric flask approximately half full of distilled water
    b. Add 20 ml of concentrated acetic acid and swirl to mix
    c. Fill the flask to the line with distilled water

Figure 1–26. Preparation of a volume to volume (v/v) percentage solution

water into a 100 ml volumetric flask, adding 0.85 grams of sodium chloride and then adding the water up to 100 ml; thus 100 ml of 0.85% saline contains 0.85 g sodium chloride. In a similar manner 500 ml of 0.85% saline could be prepared (Figure 1–25).

Another type of percentage is called volume to volume (v/v), in which a certain volume of one liquid is added to a specific volume of another. A 1% solution of hydrochloric acid can be prepared by adding one ml of the concentrated acid to 99 ml of water. Another example is the preparation of one liter of 2% acetic acid (Figure 1–26).

RATIOS

A **ratio** is the relationship in number or degree between two things. Dilutions, which are ratios, express the relationship between a part of a solution and the total solution. Dilutions are used frequently in the laboratory, especially in hematology and serology (Figure 1–27). One procedure for performing the white blood cell count requires that a 1 to 20 (1:20) dilution of the blood be made in order to count the cells. This is accomplished by adding 0.5 units of blood to 9.5 units of the diluting fluid. The

Problem: Prepare 10 ml of a 1:10 dilution of serum using saline as the diluent.

Solution: 1. A 1:10 dilution contains one part of a substance combined with 9 parts of a diluent to give a total of 10 parts.
2. Add 1 ml of serum to 9 ml of saline to form 10 ml of a 1:10 dilution of the serum.
3. If 50 ml were required, 5 ml of serum would be added to 45 ml saline.

Figure 1–27. Preparation of a 1:10 dilution

total volume is equal to 0.5 plus 9.5 (0.5 + 9.5) or 10 parts. The relationship between the 0.5 and the total volume is expressed as the ratio of $\frac{10}{.5}$, a dilution factor of 20, or a dilution of 1:20.

LESSON REVIEW

1. Give an example of a percentage solution used in the laboratory.
2. Why are temperature conversions sometimes necessary?
3. Give the formulas for conversion of degrees F to degrees C.
4. What is the dilution when 1 part is added to 9 parts?
5. What are the two formulas used to solve proportion problems?
6. How is a 1% (v/v) solution prepared?
7. How is a 5% (w/v) solution prepared?
8. Define Celsius, Fahrenheit, ratio, and saline.

STUDENT ACTIVITIES

1. Re-read the information on laboratory math.
2. Review the glossary terms.
3. Find examples of temperature in Celsius degrees, percent solutions, and dilutions or ratios in a chemistry or similar textbook.
4. Practice preparing solutions in the laboratory as instructed by the teacher.
5. Practice the calculations for percentage solutions, proportions, and ratios using the worksheets.

Laboratory Math Worksheet—Proportions

NAME_____ DATE _____

LESSON 1–8 LABORATORY MATH

1. In the lab a procedure calls for 200 ml of a 2% solution of red cells. A 50% solution is available. How much of the 50% solution is needed? How would the solution be prepared?

2. A 1% solution of hydrochloric acid is required for a procedure. A 5% solution is available. How much of the 5% will be required to make 500 ml of a 1% solution?

3. A procedure calls for acetic acid and water with the proportions being two parts of acetic acid to three parts of water. One hundred ml are needed. How much acetic acid and how much water are required?

4. One liter of 70% alcohol is needed. How much 95% alcohol is required to make the 70% solution?

$$1000 \, ml$$
$$(95)(X) = (70)(1000)$$
$$95x = 70,000$$
$$x = 736.8 \, ml$$

736.8 ml = Alchohol
263.2 = dist. water
_____
1000 ml of 70% alcohol

5. Two hundred ml of 2% acetic acid are needed. How many ml of 5% acetic acid are requied to make the 2% solution?

Laboratory Math Worksheet—Percentage Solutions

NAME_____ DATE _____

LESSON 1–8 LABORATORY MATH

1. How would 100 ml of a 10% solution of sodium chloride be prepared?

2. For a lab procedure, 50 ml of a 2% solution of red cells are needed. How is the solution prepared?

    50 ml = total volume

    2% × 50m   2% = .02
    *   C × V*

3. Give the instructions for the preparation of 300 ml of a 5% solution of acetic acid using concentrated (glacial) acetic acid.

    5% × 300
    *   15 acetic acid*
    *   285 saline*

4. If 250 ml of a 4% solution of hydrochloric acid (HCl) are needed for a procedure, how could it be prepared from a 10% solution of HCl?

5. Give the instructions for preparing one liter of a 3% solution of sodium chloride.

Laboratory Math Worksheet—Ratios

NAME_____ DATE _____

LESSON 1–8 LABORATORY MATH

1. A 1 to 25 dilution of blood is required for a procedure. How is it prepared?

2. The red blood cell count requires that blood be diluted so that 0.5 parts are diluted to a total of 100 parts. What is the dilution?

3. How could a 1:10 dilution of serum be prepared?

4. If 0.5 ml of serum is added to 4.5 ml of saline, what is the dilution?

5. If 0.5 ml of blood is added to 9.5 ml of saline, what is the dilution?

LESSON 1–9
Isolation Techniques for the Laboratory Worker

LESSON OBJECTIVES

After studying this lesson, you should be able to:
- Discuss the role of the infection control department in the hospital.
- Explain why isolation techniques are used.
- List five types of isolation and explain the basis for each classification.
- Demonstrate proper handwashing technique.
- Demonstrate proper gowning technique.
- Demonstrate the proper method of putting on a mask.
- Demonstrate proper gloving technique.
- Demonstrate proper removal and disposal of mask, gown and gloves.
- Demonstrate double-bagging technique for the transport of contaminated items.
- Define the glossary terms.

GLOSSARY

carrier / a person who harbors an organism and has no symptoms or signs of disease, but is capable of spreading the organism to others

enteric isolation / type of isolation used for patients with intestinal infections

infection / the condition in which the body or tissue is invaded by a pathogenic organism

isolation / the practice of limiting the movement and social contact of a patient who is potentially infectious or who must be protected from exposure to infectious agents

microbe / a microscopic single-celled organism

nonpathogenic / unable to cause disease in a normal individual

nosocomial infection / infection acquired in a hospital or health-care facility

pathogen / a microorganism or substance which is capable of causing disease

protective isolation / reverse isolation

respiratory isolation / type of isolation for patients infected with organisms that are easily transmitted through the air

reverse isolation / a type of isolation designed to protect highly susceptible patients from exposure to infectious agents; protective isolation

strict isolation / type of isolation for patients with highly contagious diseases

wound or skin isolation / type of isolation for patients with skin infections or open wounds

INTRODUCTION

Microbes are single-celled microscopic organisms that are present in the environment and in and on the human body. Microbes include bacteria, viruses, protozoa, and fungi. Most microbes are **nonpathogenic,** meaning that they do not normally cause disease. Some microbes are capable of causing diseases. These are called **pathogens.**

Infection is the condition occurring when the body is invaded by a pathogenic agent which may, under favorable conditions, multiply and cause disease. Three components must be present in order for infection to occur: 1) a source of microorganisms; 2) a susceptible person or host; and 3) a method of transmission of the microbe from the source to the susceptible host. The source may be an infected person or animal, the environment, or contaminated articles or equipment. The method of transmission may be: direct contact; inhaling dust or droplets containing microbes, or air droplets produced by coughing or sneezing; exposure to infectious body fluids; ingestion of contaminated water or food; or vectors such as insects.

Infections usually cause disease symptoms such as fever, redness, fluid accumulation, or pain. However, infections may also be present in a person who feels well and has no symptoms of illness. This person, in some instances, may be a **carrier,** a source of infection for others. A small percentage (approximately 5%) of hospitalized patients in the United States develop **nosocomial infections.** These are infections acquired in the hospital. The infections may be acquired through contact with infected personnel, visitors or equipment.

Within the hospital, it is the task of the infection control department to monitor contagious diseases and prevent their spread. This department is also responsible for setting standards to insure that patients do not acquire infections while in the hospital. This can be accomplished by setting guidelines for the handling of patients who are contagious or who are highly susceptible to infection, that is, those who have little resistance or immunity. One method used is **isolation,** which includes separation of the patient from other persons, and limiting contact with that patient. Every health care institution has an infection control program based on regulations of agencies such as CDC, Joint Commission for Accreditation of Health Care Organizations (JCAHO), and state regulatory agencies. This lesson provides general guidelines for isolation techniques that apply to laboratory workers such as phlebotomists or other personnel who must obtain a blood sample from the patient in isolation, and who normally have only limited exposure to the patient. Other texts should be consulted for guidelines for nursing personnel, since more extensive patient contact is required. The student or worker must be sure to follow the rules and guidelines of the particular institution.

TYPES OF ISOLATION

Each institution has regulations regarding the isolation classifications and the procedures to be followed for each type. A typical classification

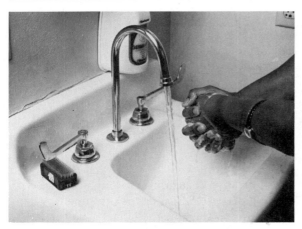

A. Interlace the fingers to clean between them.

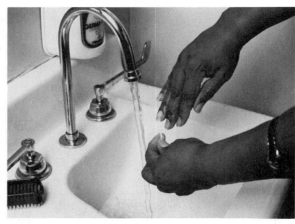

B. Use the blunt edge of an orange stick to clean under the fingernails.

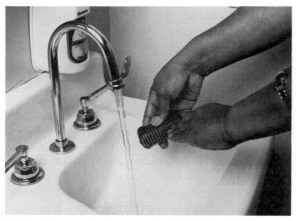

C. Another way to clean under the fingernails is to use a hand brush.

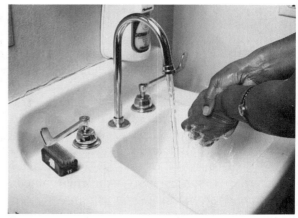

D. Rinse hands thoroughly with the fingertips down.

Figure 1–28. Handwashing technique

scheme would include: 1) wound or skin isolation; 2) enteric isolation; 3) respiratory isolation; and 4) strict or complete isolation. Institutions may also have an isolation procedure for protecting susceptible patients from infection. This is called **reverse** or **protective isolation.**

Wound or Skin Isolation

Wound or **skin isolation** is required if the patient has a skin infection or open wound. Workers (or

visitors) are usually required to wear gloves and gown when entering the patient's room.

Enteric Isolation

Enteric isolation is used for patients who have intestinal infections. These are usually caused by ingestion of pathogens such as *Salmonella, Shigella,* or hepatitis virus, and are usually accompanied by symptoms such as diarrhea or dysentery. Usually all persons entering the patient's room are re-

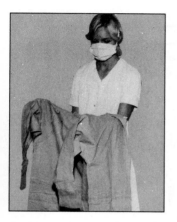
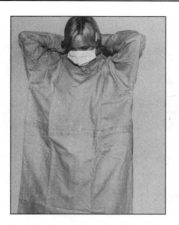
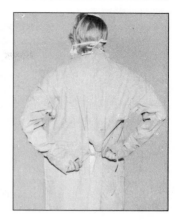

A. After tying on the mask, put on the gown outside the patient's room/unit.

B. Slip fingers inside the neck-band and tie gown.

C. Reach behind, overlap the ends of the gown so the uniform is covered, and secure the waist ties.

Figure 1–29. Putting on a clean mask and cover gown before entering the patient's room

quired to wear gown and gloves. All waste is left in the patient's room for later disposal, and bathroom facilities are used only by the patient.

Respiratory Isolation

Respiratory isolation is used when patients are infected with organisms easily transmitted through the air, such as tuberculosis, meningococcal meningitis, and measles. Patients should be in rooms with closed doors. Persons entering the room must wear a mask. Any contaminated supplies must be disposed of inside the patient's room.

Complete or Strict Isolation

Complete isolation is necessary for patients with certain contagious diseases such as smallpox, chicken pox, and bacterial pneumonias. The patient should be kept in a closed room. Persons entering the room must wear mask, gown and gloves. Items taken into the room must be disposed of inside the room.

Reverse or Protective Isolation

Reverse or protective isolation is used for patients who are very susceptible to disease. Examples include: patients with extensive burns; patients with immunodeficiencies; patients who have had chemotherapy or tissue transplants; and certain dialysis patients, intensive care patients, and newborns. These patients require a private room. Persons entering must wear a mask and sterile gown and gloves. Articles brought into the room must be clean or sterile. Used articles may be removed from the room since the patient is not infectious.

PROCEDURES FOR SPECIFIC TECHNIQUES

This lesson gives general procedures for handwashing and donning and removing protective barriers such as gloves, masks, and gowns. Health care facilities will have specific instructions and necessary supplies located outside the room of each patient requiring isolation techniques.

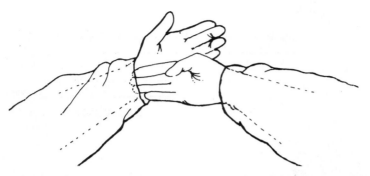

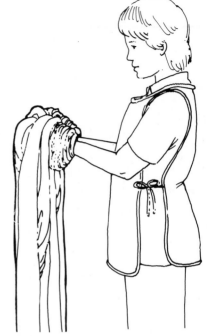

A. Slip fingers of the right hand inside the left cuff of the gown and pull the gown as shown, over the left hand. Do not touch the outside of the gown with the right hand.

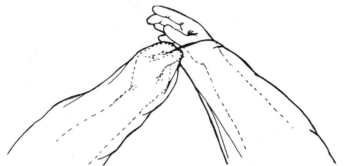

C. As the gown is removed, fold with the contaminated side inward and then roll.

B. Using the gown-covered left hand, pull the gown down over the right hand.

Figure 1–30. Removing the contaminated gown

Handwashing

Handwashing is the most important procedure in isolation techniques, just as it is in maintaining safety in the laboratory (Lesson 1–3). Proper handwashing should be the first and last step of all procedures. Handwashing does not sterilize the hands, but removes surface contaminants, dead skin and surface organisms. Hands and wrists should be lathered in warm water and scrubbed front and back and between fingers, rubbing thoroughly. The scrubbing process should last at least 1–2 minutes. Fingernails may be cleaned using a fingernail brush or an orange stick. The hands are then rinsed from the arm or wrist toward the tips of the fingers while holding hands in a downward position (Figure 1–28, page 68). The faucet should be turned on and off using a clean towel or tissue to avoid contaminating hands with organisms or substances which may be present on the faucet handles.

Masks

Masks should be put on after hands are washed, avoiding touching the skin with hands. Most masks have two ties, one for the upper neck and one for the head. Masks should only be worn for 15–20 minutes before changing into another mask. They should not be allowed to dangle around the neck (Figure 1–29, page 69).

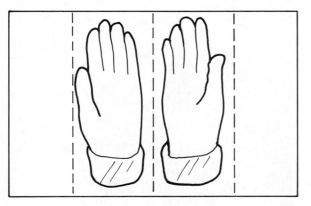

A. Illustration of gloves in a newly-opened sterile pack.

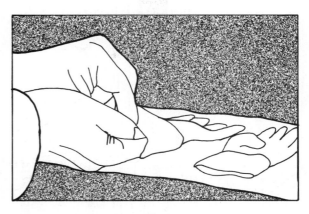

B. Picking up first glove by the cuff to insert first hand.

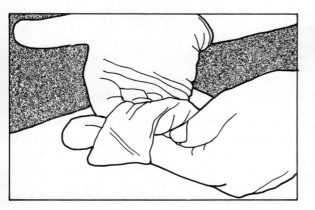

C. Using the sterile gloved hand to don second glove.

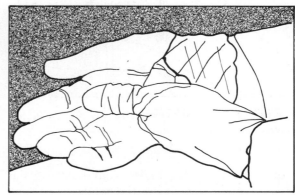

D. Adjusting gloves.

Figure 1–31. Donning sterile gloves

Gown

Laboratory coats should be removed before donning gowns. The gown should be touched only on the inside surface and should cover all clothing when tied (Figure 1–29). Gowns are removed by turning the inside of the gown to the outside and folding the contaminated outer side inward (Figure 1–30).

Gloves

Gloves required for isolation cases must be clean. Some types of isolation, such as reverse isolation, may require sterile gloves. The cuff or wrist area of gloves should be pulled over sleeve ends of the gown so that all skin or clothing is covered. It is best to avoid wearing sharp rings or jewelry which may puncture gloves. If sterile gloves are

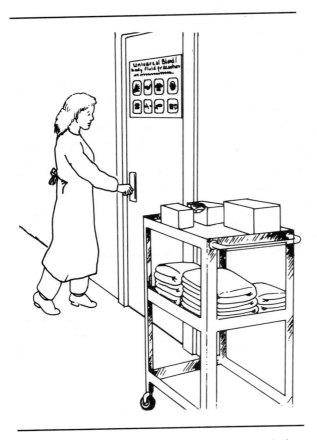

Figure 1–32. A clean cover gown is put on before entering the patient's room

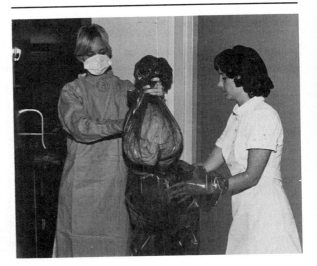

Figure 1–33. Double-bagging technique. The cuff made at the top of the bag protects the hands of the health care worker who is holding the bag open to receive the bag of contaminated articles from the patient's room.

required, the worker must avoid touching the outside of the gloves with the hands when donning them. This is accomplished by carefully opening the sterile package, picking up a glove by the cuff, and carefully inserting hand into glove (Figure 1–31, page 71). The second glove is then picked up by placing the gloved fingers under the cuff and holding the glove while the hand is inserted. The cuffs are then unfolded by sliding the gloved fingers under the cuff. Sterile gloves should always be used to handle sterile equipment or instruments.

Entering and Exiting the Room

The procedure used for entering and exiting the patient's room differs according to the type of isolation. In general, most supplies are located on a cart outside the patient's room and are put on before entering (Figure 1–32). Only items which will be used for the patient should be taken into the room. Phlebotomists should leave trays and requisition slips outside the room to avoid contamination of these items. Equipment such as tourniquets and writing pens are left in the room for future use. When exiting the room, the used supplies are left in a special disposal container usually located inside the room. Exceptions to this procedure include reverse isolation, where disposables are usually left in a container outside the room for disposal.

Double-Bagging

Contaminated articles must be appropriately bagged, labeled and disposed of following the hospital's infectious waste disposal guidelines. In some instances it may be necessary to double-bag the contaminated items. To accomplish double-bagging, a person in the patient's room places the contaminated materials into a bag and seals it. A second worker is outside the room with a clean, open bag, held so that the top edges of the bag are folded down over the hands to prevent possible contamination (Figure 1–33). The sealed bag is placed into the open bag which is then sealed securely and labeled by the worker outside the room. Some laboratory specimens may have to be double-bagged in this manner for transport.

UNIVERSAL BARRIER PRECAUTIONS

Laboratory workers should observe universal barrier precautions in the laboratory, in patient's rooms, and in all other health care situations. These precautions are discussed in depth in Lesson 1–3, Laboratory Safety. It is mandatory that personnel use precautions to prevent exposure to all blood and body fluids, whether known to be infectious or not. These precautions include using proper handwashing techniques; wearing gloves when handling all biological specimens, containers, or possibly contaminated articles; wearing goggles if aerosols or splashes are likely to occur; careful handling of sharp objects and disposal in a puncture-proof container; and cleaning spills immediately with an appropriate disinfectant such as a 1:10 dilution of chlorine bleach.

LESSON REVIEW

1. What is the function of the infection control department in the hospital?
2. State two reasons for using isolation techniques.
3. Name five types of isolation. Give an example of a condition requiring each type of isolation. Explain how isolation procedures vary for each type.
4. Explain the proper method of handwashing. When is handwashing performed?
5. Explain the proper technique of putting on and removing a gown.
6. Explain how to put on gloves.
7. Why is it necessary to double-bag some items? How is this done?
8. Define carrier, enteric isolation, infection, isolation, microbe, nonpathogenic, nosocomial infection, pathogen, protective isolation, respiratory isolation, reverse isolation, strict isolation, and wound or skin isolation.

STUDENT ACTIVITIES

1. Re-read the information on isolation techniques for the laboratory worker.
2. Review the glossary terms.
3. Practice the procedures for proper handwashing and donning and removal of mask, gown, and gloves, as outlined on the Student Performance Guide.
4. Demonstrate the technique of double-bagging as outlined in the Student Performance Guide.

Student Performance Guide

NAME _____

DATE _____

LESSON 1–9
ISOLATION TECHNIQUES
FOR THE
LABORATORY WORKER

Instructions

1. Practice the procedures for handwashing; donning mask, gown, and gloves; and for double-bagging.
2. Demonstrate the procedures for handwashing; donning mask, gown, and gloves; and for double-bagging satisfactorily for the instructor. All steps must be completed as listed on the instructor's Performance Check Sheet.
3. Complete a written examination satisfactorily.

Materials and Equipment

- sink for handwashing
- hand disinfectant or soap
- clean paper towels
- disposable masks
- disposable gowns
- disposable gloves (sterile gloves optional)
- disposal receptacle for used items
- biohazard bags or other plastic bags with materials for labeling

Note: The following procedures are intended as general guidelines for laboratory workers who must have contact with patients in isolation. The appropriate institutional policy manual must be consulted for specific instructions.

Procedure	S	U	S = Satisfactory U = Unsatisfactory
You must:	**S**	**U**	**Comments**
1. Assemble equipment and materials			
2. Turn on warm water using a paper towel to turn the faucet handle, and discard the towel			
3. Dispense soap onto hands and rub fronts and backs of hands and between fingers vigorously for 1–2 minutes. (If using bar soap, keep the bar in the hands during the entire lathering process)			
4. Rinse hands holding them fingertips-downward under warm running water			
5. Use clean towel to dry hands and turn off faucet. Dispose of towel, touching only the clean side			
6. Pick up a mask and place it over mouth and nose, being careful not to touch the face with the fingers			
7. Tie the ends of the mask around the head and neck			
8. Slip arms into the sleeves of a gown, being careful to touch only the inside of gown			
9. Secure gown at neck and back of waist with ties, being careful that clothing is completely covered			
10. Put on gloves, avoiding touching the outside of the gloves with the hands			
11. Pull the cuffs of the gloves over the sleeves of the gown. *Note:* If using sterile gloves, open the package being careful not to touch the outside of the gloves. Pick up the right glove by the cuff and insert the right hand. Pick up and hold the left glove by inserting fingertips of gloved right hand into the cuff of the left glove. Insert the left hand into glove. Position glove cuffs over wrists by using fingertips to push cuff toward elbow.			
12. With the help of an assistant, double-bag an isolation bag following steps a–c. a. Place the "contaminated" item into a bag and seal or tie it closed			

You must:	S	U	Comments
b. Place the sealed bag into another bag held by the assistant outside the door of the room. The second bag should be held with the top folded down over the assistant's hands to prevent possible contamination of hands			
c. The assistant should then seal, label, and dispose of the double-bagged item appropriately			
13. Remove the gloves by folding them down and turning inside out			
14. Discard gloves into receptacle for contaminated materials			
15. Untie neck and waist ties of gown			
16. Wash hands following steps 2–5			
17. Untie mask, touching only the ties			
18. Hold the mask by the ties only and discard into proper receptacle			
19. Remove gown by slipping hands back into gown sleeve, touching only inside of gown			
20. Fold the gown down over arms inside-out and discard into appropriate receptacle			
21. Wash hands following steps 2–5			
22. Leave room using clean paper towel to turn door knob			

Comments:

Student/Instructor:

Date:_____ Instructor:_____

UNIT 2
Basic Hematology

UNIT OBJECTIVES

After studying this unit, you should be able to:
- Perform a capillary puncture.
- Perform a microhematocrit.
- Perform blood dilutions using blood diluting pipets.
- Use a hemacytometer.
- Perform a manual red cell count and calculate the results.
- Perform a manual white cell count and calculate the results.
- Perform a hemoglobin determination.
- Make a blood smear.
- Stain a blood smear.
- Identify blood cells from a stained smear.
- Perform a differential leukocyte count.

OVERVIEW

Blood is composed of formed elements suspended in a fluid called plasma. These formed elements include erythrocytes (red blood cells), leukocytes (white blood cells), and thrombocytes (platelets). These cellular elements are produced and mature in the bone marrow. They are then released into the bloodstream where they play important roles in oxygen transport, blood clotting and providing immunity.

Hematology is the study of the formed elements of blood and the blood-forming tissues. The cellular elements of blood may be studied by counting the cells, as in red cell and white cell counts. Cellular elements may also be studied from stained blood smears. From these smears, the percentages of cell types and the morphology (the structure and form) of cells can be determined.

A blood sample adequate for most hematological tests may be obtained from capillaries by finger puncture. If a larger sample is required, blood is obtained from a vein by venipuncture. Venous blood samples are usually collected in a tube containing an anticoagulant which prevents clotting. When a blood sample has had anticoagulant added, the liquid portion is called plasma. When blood is collected without an anticoagulant, it forms a clot and the liquid portion remaining is called serum. Anticoagulated blood is used for most hematological tests.

One of the most frequently requested tests in the hematology laboratory is the CBC, or complete blood count. The CBC is a combination of tests that usually includes a red cell count, white cell count, hemoglobin, hematocrit, differential count, estimation of platelet numbers, and observation of blood cell morphology. In this unit, you will be introduced to basic procedures. These will include performing the tests comprising a CBC, collecting a capillary blood specimen, and using medical laboratory instruments and equipment.

The examination of blood can provide important information. It can help in the diagnosis and treatment of many blood diseases such as the leukemias and anemias. It also aids in the diagnosis and management of diseases that originate in other body systems.

Test results are relied upon for the diagnosis and treatment of disease. Therefore, it is vital that the tests are performed with accuracy, precision, and utmost attention to proper procedure. It takes practice and skill to perform most of the basic hematology procedures in a reliable manner.

LESSON 2–1
Capillary Puncture

LESSON OBJECTIVES

After studying this lesson, you should be able to:

- Identify sites for capillary punctures.
- Choose and prepare a site for capillary puncture.
- Perform a capillary puncture.
- Collect a blood specimen from a capillary puncture.
- List the precautions to be observed when performing a capillary puncture.
- Define the glossary terms.

GLOSSARY

anticoagulant / agent which prevents blood coagulation

capillary / a minute blood vessel which connects the smallest arteries to the smallest veins

capillary tube / a glass tube of very small diameter used for laboratory procedures

heparin / an anticoagulant used in certain laboratory procedures

lancet / a sterile, sharp-pointed blade used to perform a capillary puncture

lateral / toward the side

INTRODUCTION

A **capillary** is a small blood vessel connecting the small arteries (arterioles) to the small veins (venules). Because of the capillary's small diameter, capillary puncture is an efficient means of collecting a blood specimen when only a small amount of blood is required. It may also be used when the patient has a condition which would make venipuncture difficult. Capillary blood is a good specimen because the cell distribution resembles that normally found in the circulating blood. Blood cell counts, the microhematocrit, and the blood smear are some of the procedures which can be performed using a capillary blood sample.

79

PUNCTURE SITES

The puncture sites used to obtain capillary blood are the finger, heel, and ear lobe. In adults and children, the normal puncture site is the ring finger because it usually is not calloused. The puncture is made at the tip of the fleshy pad and slightly to the side (Figure 2–1) using a sterile, sharp-pointed blade called a **lancet.** If the tips of the fingers are heavily calloused or thickened, a special lancet may be used. Although the ear lobe may be used as a puncture site, the blood from there may not have normal cell distribution. In infants, the **lateral** or side portion of the heel pad is usually used. If possible, previous puncture sites should always be avoided.

Preparation of Puncture Site

The area selected for a capillary puncture must be carefully prepared. The puncture site will be warm if circulation is adequate. Coolness of the skin indicates decreased circulation. If this is so, the patient's hands may be gently massaged or placed in warm water for a few minutes. Alcohol-soaked gauze or cotton should be used to cleanse and disinfect the puncture site. The site should then be allowed to air dry or should be wiped dry with sterile gauze. This allows the blood to form a well-rounded drop following puncture—something it will not do on moist skin.

PERFORMING THE PUNCTURE

Gloves must be worn by the person performing the puncture. The patient's hand and finger should be held so that the puncture site is readily accessible (Figure 2–1). The skin near the chosen site should be pulled taut. A sterile lancet is then used to pierce the site to a depth of 2–3 mm. Capillary punctures may also be performed using semi-automated devices such as the Autolet® or Monojector™. The puncture should be performed in one quick, steady motion. The first drop of blood that appears is wiped away because it contains tissue fluid.

The second and following drops of blood are used for samples. Depending on the tests to be performed, the blood may be collected in blood-diluting pipets or in capillary tubes. **Capillary tubes** are glass tubes of small diameter used to collect blood from a capillary puncture. It may be

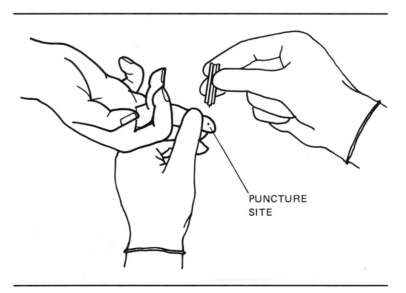

PUNCTURE
SITE

Figure 2–1. Capillary puncture

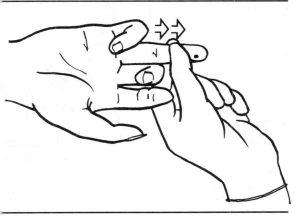

Figure 2-2. Massaging the finger gently to increase blood flow

necessary to massage the finger to increase blood flow. However, pressure should not be applied near the puncture site (Figure 2-2). Squeezing the finger will force tissue fluid into the blood sample and dilute it. The capillary tube should be held in an almost horizontal position and should be filled 2/3 to 3/4 full. (Figure 2-3).

TYPES OF CAPILLARY TUBES

Two types of capillary tubes are available: tubes coated with **heparin,** an anticoagulant, and uncoated tubes. The **anticoagulant** is necessary to prevent clotting of capillary blood. Tubes which are heparinized have a red ring on one end. Precalibrated tubes are usually heparinized. Heparinized capillary tubes should always be used when collecting capillary blood samples. Uncoated or plain capillary tubes have a blue ring on one end. These are used to test venous blood collected with an anticoagulant.

Precautions

■ Gloves must be worn when performing a capillary puncture.
■ Circulation around the puncture site must be adequate.
■ The puncture site should be cleansed thoroughly.
■ The puncture site must be dry because blood will spread and will not form a drop on moist skin.
■ The puncture should be performed quickly and to a depth of 2–3 mm to assure good blood flow.
■ The finger should not be squeezed; tissue fluid will dilute the blood sample.
■ Capillary samples must be collected quickly to prevent blood clotting.

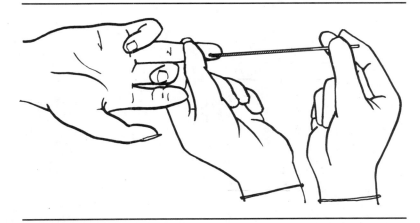

Figure 2-3. Collecting capillary blood into a capillary tube

LESSON REVIEW

1. What are the usual puncture sites for adults; for infants?
2. How is a capillary puncture site prepared?
3. What is a capillary vessel?
4. Why would a capillary puncture be performed?
5. Why is the first drop of blood wiped away?
6. What is the procedure if the patient has cold hands?
7. List the precautions that must be observed when performing a capillary puncture.
8. Define anticoagulant, capillary, capillary tube, heparin, lancet, and lateral.

STUDENT ACTIVITIES

1. Re-read the information on capillary puncture.
2. Review the glossary terms.
3. Practice using the capillary tubes by filling them from a tube of well-mixed anticoagulated blood.
4. Practice performing a capillary puncture as outlined on the Student Performance Guide.

Student Performance Guide

NAME _____

DATE _____

LESSON 2–1
CAPILLARY PUNCTURE

Instructions

1. Practice the procedure for performing a capillary puncture.
2. Demonstrate the procedure for a capillary puncture satisfactorily for the instructor. All steps must be completed as listed on the instructor's Performance Check Sheet.
3. Complete a written examination successfully.

Materials and Equipment

- gloves
- hand disinfectant
- lancets (sterile, disposable)
- sterile cotton balls or gauze squares
- 70% alcohol or alcohol swabs
- capillary tubes (heparinized)
- sealing clay or disposable plastic caps
- pre-calibrated capillary tubes (optional)
- surface disinfectant
- biohazard container
- puncture-proof container for sharp objects

Procedure	S = Satisfactory U = Unsatisfactory		
You must:	**S**	**U**	**Comments**
1. Wash hands with disinfectant and put on gloves			
2. Assemble equipment and materials			
3. Explain the procedure to the patient			
4. Select and warm the puncture site			

83

You must:	S	U	Comments
5. Cleanse the puncture site with alcohol-soaked gauze or cotton			
6. Allow the site to air dry or wipe with dry sterile gauze or cotton			
7. Position the puncture site, holding the skin taut with one hand and holding the lancet in the other hand.			
8. Perform the capillary puncture, using a quick, firm stab			
9. Wipe the first drop of blood away with sterile gauze or cotton			
10. Massage the finger gently to produce the second drop of blood			
11. Fill a capillary tube two-thirds to three-quarters full using the second drop of blood (fill to the line if using precalibrated capillary tubes)			
12. Fill a second tube in the same manner			
13. Place the clean end of the capillary tubes into the sealing clay or seal with plastic sealing cap			
14. Apply pressure to the puncture site by pressing with dry sterile gauze or cotton			
15. Place used lancet and used capillary tubes into a puncture-proof container for sharp objects			
16. Discard used gauze or cotton into biohazard container			
17. Clean and return equipment to proper storage			
18. Clean work area with surface disinfectant			
19. Remove gloves and discard into biohazard container. Wash hands with hand disinfectant			

Comments:

Student/Instructor:

Date:_____ Instructor:_____

LESSON 2–2
Microhematocrit

LESSON OBJECTIVES

After studying this lesson, you should be able to:
- Prepare a microhematocrit sample.
- Centrifuge a microhematocrit sample.
- Determine the microhematocrit value.
- Explain what the microhematocrit measures.
- List the normal values for a microhematocrit.
- List conditions that affect the microhematocrit value.
- List precautions that should be observed in performing the microhematocrit.
- Define the glossary terms.

GLOSSARY

buffy coat / a light-colored layer of leukocytes and platelets which forms on the top of the red cell layer when a sample of blood is centrifuged or allowed to stand

EDTA / ethylene diamine tetraacetic acid; commonly used anticoagulant for hematological studies

hematocrit / the volume of erythrocytes packed by centrifugation in a given volume of blood and expressed as a percentage; abbreviated "crit" or Hct

microhematocrit / a hematocrit performed on a small sample of blood

microhematocrit centrifuge / a machine which spins capillary tubes at a high speed to cause rapid separation of liquid from solid components

plasma / the liquid part of the blood in which the cellular elements are suspended

INTRODUCTION

The **microhematocrit** is a commonly performed test. It may be performed separately or as part of a complete blood count (CBC). It is a simple procedure requiring only two to three drops of blood, which makes it an ideal test to follow the progress of anemic or bleeding patients.

The microhematocrit is a variation of a test called the **hematocrit.** The hematocrit is a test that is performed using one milliliter of blood in a Wintrobe tube (named for the person who developed the test). The test is based on the principle of separating the cellular elements of the blood from the liquid part, the **plasma.** In both hematocrit and microhematocrit procedures, the separation process is speeded up by centrifugation. After centrifugation, the red cells will be at the bottom of the tube, the white cells and platelets in the center, and the plasma at the top. The layer containing the white cells and platelets has a whitish-tan appearance and is commonly referred to as the **buffy coat** (Figure 2–4). From this separation the hematocrit or microhematocrit is determined by comparing the concentration of red cells to the volume of the whole blood sample. Laboratory personnel often refer to a hematocrit as a "crit" or abbreviate it with the letters Hct.

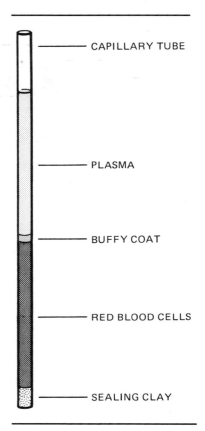

CAPILLARY TUBE

PLASMA

BUFFY COAT

RED BLOOD CELLS

SEALING CLAY

Figure 2–4. Diagram of packed cell column

PERFORMING THE MICROHEMATOCRIT

The blood sample may be obtained from a capillary puncture or from a tube of venous blood which has had the anticoagulant **EDTA** added. The blood is drawn by capillary action into capillary tubes of very small diameter (Figure 2–5) which are sealed (Figure 2–6). To do this, the clean end of the tube is placed in sealing clay. This makes a tight seal and prevents contamination of the clay with blood. Tubes may also be sealed using disposable plastic sealing caps.

The tube is then placed in a special **microhematocrit centrifuge** (Figures 2–7, 2–8). The sealed ends of the tubes are placed against the rubber gasket and the open ends toward the center. After being centrifuged for the prescribed time (usually 3–5 minutes), the hematocrit percentage is read by placing the tube on a special microhematocrit reader (Figure 2–9). Some centrifuges, such as the Clay Adams Readacrit, have a built-in reading scale (Figure 2–7). Special precalibrated capillary tubes must be used with this type of centrifuge. Microhematocrits should be performed in duplicate. The average of the two results is reported.

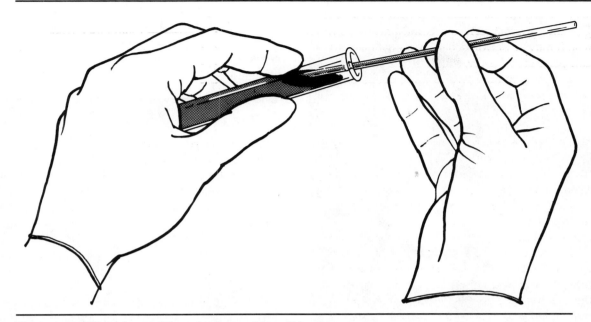

Figure 2–5. Filling the capillary tube from a tube of blood

The two values should not vary by more than ±2 percent.

NORMAL VALUES

The normal microhematocrit value varies with the sex and age of the patient (Table 2–1). The values range from a low of 32% for a one-year-old to a high of 60% for a newborn.

Factors that Influence Microhematocrit Values

The values obtained for microhematocrits can be influenced by physiological or pathological factors and by the handling of the specimen during

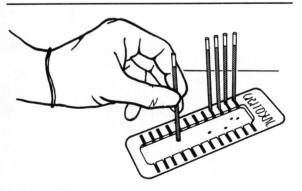

Figure 2–6. Sealing the capillary tube with sealing clay

Table 2–1. Normal microhematocrit values

Age	Microhematocrit Values (%)	
	Average	Range
Adult males	47	42–52
Adult females	42	36–48
Children (both sexes):		
Newborn	56	51–60
One year	35	32–38
Six years	38	34–42

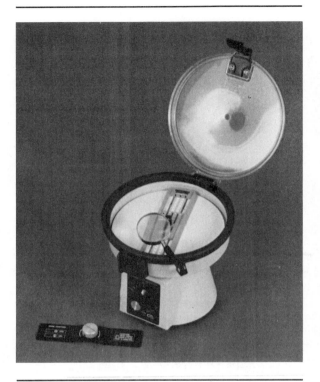

Figure 2–7. Microhematocrit centrifuge with built-in reader *(Photo courtesy of Clay Adams Division of Becton Dickinson & Co.)*

the test procedure. Improper blood collection or the use of inadequately mixed blood can cause unreliable results.

A low microhematocrit value can indicate an anemia or the presence of bleeding in a patient. An increased value may be caused by dehydration in the patient or by a condition such as polycythemia.

AUTOMATION

The hematocrit is now frequently determined by electronic means. Some instruments calculate the hematocrit using the values from the red cell count and the red cell volume. Other instruments use the principle of electrical current conductance. Red

cells conduct less current than the plasma in which they are suspended. Therefore, a blood sample with a high hematocrit (increased red cells) will have a lower conductance than one with a low hematocrit.

Precautions

■ The recommended speed and time of centrifugation must be strictly followed.
■ The clay seal must be tight or the contents of the tube may leak out.
■ The sealed end of the capillary tube must be placed against the rubber gasket in the centrifuge.
■ The inner centrifuge lid must be closed securely before closing the outer lid, to prevent breaking glass tubes.
■ The microhematocrit should be read at the top of the red cell layer—not at the top of the buffy coat.

LESSON REVIEW

1. Explain the microhematocrit procedure.
2. What does the microhematocrit measure?
3. Why must the capillary tube be sealed securely?
4. By what action does blood enter the capillary tube?
5. What is the usual length of time for centrifugation?
6. Name a condition which could cause a decreased microhematocrit value.
7. Give the normal values of microhematocrit for males, females, and newborns.
8. What precautions should be observed when performing a microhematocrit?
9. Define buffy coat, EDTA, hematocrit, microhematocrit, microhematocrit centrifuge, and plasma.

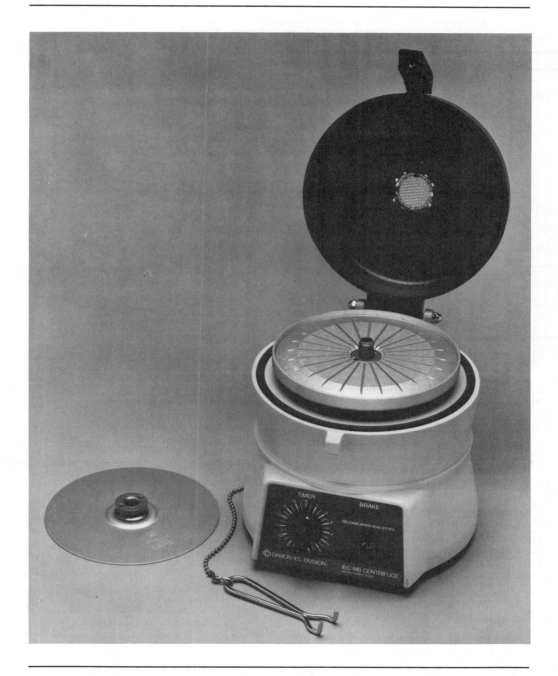

Figure 2–8. Microhematocrit centrifuge without reader *(Photo courtesy of International Equipment, Division of Damon)*

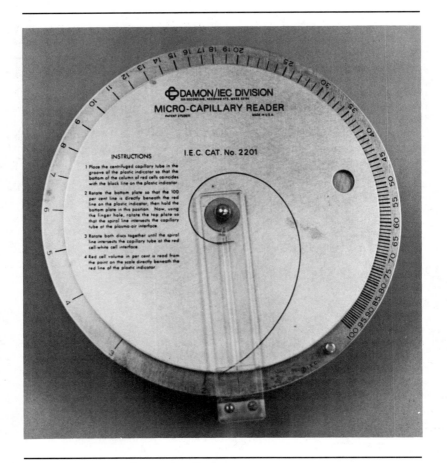

Figure 2–9. Microhematocrit reader *(Photo courtesy of International Equipment Company, Division of Damon)*

STUDENT ACTIVITIES

1. Re-read the information on microhematocrit.
2. Review the glossary terms.
3. Practice performing a microhematocrit test on several blood samples as outlined on the Student Performance Guide.
4. Repeat the microhematocrit procedure on a blood sample, lengthening or shortening the centrifugation time. Record the results and give the reason for the different values obtained in the previous microhematocrit.
5. Demonstrate the importance of using well-mixed blood: perform a microhematocrit on a well-mixed sample; allow the sample tube to stand upright two minutes and perform another microhematocrit without re-mixing the blood. Compare the results and explain the difference.

Student Performance Guide

NAME _____

DATE _____

LESSON 2–2
MICROHEMATOCRIT

Instructions

1. Practice the microhematocrit procedure.
2. Demonstrate the microhematocrit procedure satisfactorily for the instructor. All steps must be completed as listed on the instructor's Performance Check Sheet.
3. Complete a written examination successfully.

Materials and Equipment

- gloves
- hand disinfectant
- capillary tubes, plain and with heparin
- pre-calibrated capillary tubes (optional)
- sealing clay or disposable plastic sealing caps
- microhematocrit centrifuge and reader
- tube of anticoagulated venous blood
- paper towels or soft laboratory tissue
- 70% alcohol or alcohol swabs
- gauze or cotton balls, sterile
- blood lancets, sterile, disposable
- surface disinfectant
- biohazard container
- puncture-proof container for sharp objects

Note: Consult the instruction manual for the centrifuge being used. Refer to the specific procedure being performed.

Procedure			S = Satisfactory U = Unsatisfactory
You must:	**S**	**U**	**Comments**
1. Wash hands with disinfectant and put on gloves			
2. Assemble equipment and materials			
3. Fill two capillary tubes using a tube of EDTA anticoagulated blood: a. Mix the tube of blood thoroughly by rocking tube from end to end gently 20 to 30 times			
b. Remove cap from tube, avoiding contamination of hands with blood			
c. Tilt the tube so that blood is very near the top edge of the tube			
d. Insert a plain capillary tube beneath the surface of the blood and fill to two thirds by capillary action (if using pre-calibrated tubes, fill to the line) *Note:* Wipe the outside of the filled capillary tube with tissue, if necessary, to remove excess blood			
e. Seal the tube by placing the clean end into the tray of sealing clay or using plastic sealing cap			
f. Fill a second tube in the same manner			
4. Fill two capillary tubes from a capillary puncture: a. Wash hands with disinfectant and put on gloves			
b. Assemble equipment and materials			
c. Perform a capillary puncture			
d. Wipe away the first drop of blood			
e. Place one end of a heparinized capillary tube into the second drop of blood			
f. Allow the tube to fill two thirds by capillary action. A slight downward angle of the tube may be necessary (if using pre-calibrated tubes, fill to the line)			
g. Fill a second tube in the same manner			
h. Wipe the outside of the filled capillary tube with soft tissue, if necessary, to remove excess blood			
i. Seal the capillary tube by placing the clean end into the tray of sealing clay (the sealing clay will stay cleaner if dry/clean end of the capillary tube is sealed)			
5. Check to see if the interior sealing clay edge appears level in tubes			

You must:	S	U	Comments
6. Place tubes into the microhematocrit centrifuge with sealed ends securely against the gasket (balance the centrifuge by placing the tubes opposite each other)			
7. Fasten both lids securely			
8. Set the timer and adjust the speed if necessary			
9. Centrifuge for the prescribed time			
10. Allow centrifuge to come to a complete stop and unlock lid			

11. Determine the microhematocrit values using one of the following methods:
A. A centrifuge which requires calibrated tubes and has a built-in scale:
  (1) Position the tubes as directed by the manufacturer's instructions to obtain the microhematocrit value
B. A centrifuge which can accept any microhematocrit tubes:
  (1) Remove capillary tubes from centrifuge carefully
  (2) Place tube on the microhematocrit reader provided
  (3) Follow instructions on the reader to obtain the hematocrit value			

12. Average the values from the two tubes and record the hematocrit			
13. Discard capillary tubes and used lancets into a puncture-proof container for sharp objects			
14. Clean and return equipment to proper storage			
15. Clean the work area with surface disinfectant			
16. Remove and discard gloves and wash hands with hand disinfectant			

Comments:

Student/Instructor:

Date:_____ Instructor:_____

LESSON 2-3
Blood Diluting Pipets

After studying this lesson, you should be able to:
- Identify the parts of a blood diluting pipet.
- Explain the function of a blood diluting pipet.
- Dilute a blood sample using the white blood cell diluting pipet.
- Dilute a blood sample using the red blood cell diluting pipet.
- Dispense drops one at a time from a filled blood diluting pipet.
- Clean a blood diluting pipet.
- Calculate the dilutions made with red and white blood cell diluting pipets.
- Explain the proper care of a blood diluting pipet.
- List the precautions to be observed when using blood diluting pipets.
- Define the glossary terms.

GLOSSARY

aspiration / act of drawing in by suction

capillary action / the action by which a fluid will enter a tube or pipet because of the attraction between the glass and liquid

cell diluting fluid / diluting solution which will not damage the cells being counted

erythrocyte / red blood cell; RBC; transports oxygen to the tissue and carbon dioxide (CO_2) to the lungs

leukocyte / white blood cell; WBC; protects from disease

micropipet / pipet which holds a very small volume

red cell diluting pipet / pipet used to dilute blood for a red cell count; RBC pipet

white cell diluting pipet / pipet used to dilute blood for white cell count; WBC pipet

INTRODUCTION

Before blood cells may be counted microscopically, blood must be diluted. This is because cellular elements in the blood are so concentrated. Blood diluting pipets are valuable pieces of equipment which are used to dilute blood and other body fluids. To use the reusable Thoma-style pipets, blood (or other sample) and a **cell diluting fluid** are mixed within the pipet. A count is then performed using the diluted sample, a counting chamber, and a microscope. The Thoma-style pipets are used mostly for **erythrocyte, leukocyte,** and platelet counts. However, they may also be used for sperm counts, counting cells in spinal fluid, synovial fluids, or other body fluids. Red and white cell pipets are shown in Figure 2–10.

PARTS OF A BLOOD DILUTING PIPET

Blood diluting pipets have three basic parts: (1) a long calibrated stem into which the sample and diluting fluid are aspirated, (2) the bulb in which the contents are mixed, and (3) the short stem to which a suction device or pipet filler is attached (Figure 2–10). Various mechanical pipetting aids are available which may be used to aspirate liquids into blood diluting pipets. Some examples of these are the Pipet Pump (Bel-Art) and the Micro-Pipex (ISOLAB, Inc.). The Micro-Pipex is pictured in Figure 1–17, Lesson 1–4. Blood diluting pipets may differ in the markings on the stems and the size of the mixing bulb. Only pipets manufactured according to specifications of the National Institute of Standards and Technology (NIST) and certified by NIST to have a ±1% accuracy should be used for clinical work. (NIST was formerly the National Bureau of Standards.)

The Red Cell Diluting Pipet

The **red cell diluting pipet** is used to dilute blood for a red cell or erythrocyte count (Figure 2–11). The 0.5 mark on the long stem is the mark to which blood is drawn. The 101 mark on the short stem is the mark to which diluting fluid (mixed with sample) is drawn. The red bead identifies the pipet as an RBC pipet and also mixes the contents.

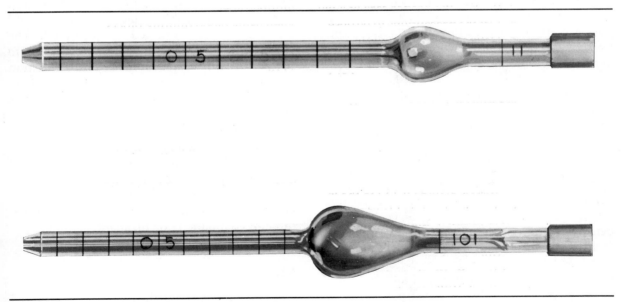

Figure 2–10. Red (bottom) and white (top) cell diluting pipets *(Photo courtesy of Reichert Scientific Instruments)*

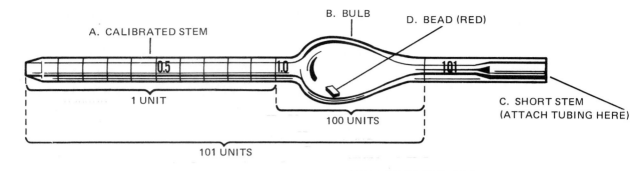

Figure 2–11. Parts of a red cell diluting pipet

The bulb is the area where sample and diluting fluid are combined in exact proportions and mixed.

The White Cell Diluting Pipet

The **white cell diluting pipet,** shown in Figure 2–10, is used to dilute blood for a white cell or leukocyte count. The pipet is designed like the RBC pipet except that it holds a smaller volume and makes a lower dilution. The 0.5 mark on the long stem is the mark to which blood is drawn. The 11 mark is the mark to which diluting fluid (mixed with blood) is drawn. In the bulb the blood and diluting fluid are combined in exact proportions and mixed. The white or clear bead aids in mixing the contents and in identifying the WBC pipet.

USING A BLOOD DILUTING PIPET

Blood diluting pipets are all used in a similar manner. The important steps in using a pipet are: filling the pipet, mixing the contents, and dispensing the diluted sample. Pipets must be clean and dry when used in order to make accurate dilutions. When a pipet is completely dry, the mixing bead will roll freely in the bulb.

Cell counts provide valuable information to the physician. It is important that the cell counts be as accurate as possible. Therefore, it is important that blood dilutions be performed carefully and precisely. If anticoagulated venous blood is used, it must be mixed by gentle inversion 20–30 times before sampled. (Do not shake!)

Filling the Pipet

Both sample and diluting fluid are aspirated into the pipet using a pipetting aid attached to the short stem. The pipetting aid is attached to the pipet and the tip of the pipet is placed into the sample. The sample is then carefully and slowly drawn up to the 0.5 mark by **aspiration** or **capillary action** (Figure 2–12). The excess sample is then wiped from the outside of the pipet tip with soft tissue, taking care not to touch the tip of the pipet, thereby withdrawing some of the sample. Diluting fluid is then carefully aspirated to the 11 or 101 mark (Figure 2–13). The pipet should be slowly rotated while fluid is aspirated. It is important that the dilutions are accurate. Therefore, the sample must be drawn exactly to the 0.5 mark and the diluting fluid exactly to the 11 or 101 mark.

Mixing Fluids

Once the pipet is filled, the index finger is placed over the pipet tip and the pipet filler is carefully

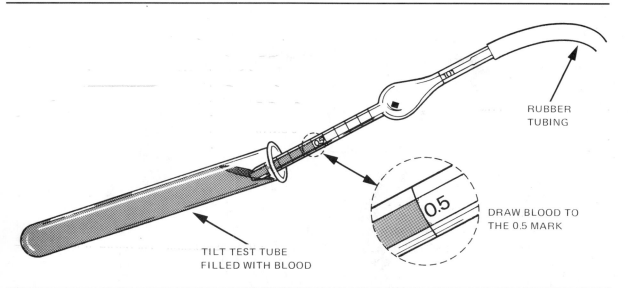

RUBBER
TUBING

DRAW BLOOD TO
THE 0.5 MARK

0.5

TILT TEST TUBE
FILLED WITH BLOOD

Figure 2–12. Aspirating a sample using the RBC pipet

removed while the pipet is held in a horizontal position. The contents of the pipet are then mixed by using hand rotation or a pipet shaker. For hand mixing, the pipet is held carefully so that the thumb covers one end of the pipet and the middle or index finger covers the other end (Figure 2–14). The pipet is then rotated in a figure-eight motion for two or three minutes. If an automatic shaker is used, the pipet should be carefully inserted into the shaker (Figure 2–15). The timer should be set for the proper shaking time (at least two minutes).

Dispensing Fluids

Fluid should be dispensed from the pipet as soon as shaking is completed to avoid settling of the contents. The pipet should be held as shown in Figure 2–16 with the index finger over the short stem of the pipet to control the flow of the fluid. Four to five drops of fluid should be expelled from the pipet onto gauze, cotton, or paper towel which should then be discarded. These first drops consist mostly of diluting fluid and do not contain the

proper cell concentration. The next drop in the pipet may then be introduced into a counting chamber for the cell count.

CALCULATING DILUTIONS FOR THE RBC PIPET

The long stem of most RBC pipets has ten divisions. Some types have a mark for each ten divisions; others have only a 0.5 and 1.0 mark. The 0.5 mark represents 0.5 unit and the 1.0 mark represents 1.0 unit. The bulb of the RBC pipet contains 100 units of volume; therefore, 101 units of volume are contained from the tip of the pipet to the 101 mark. When a sample is drawn into the pipet bulb and mixed, the dilution occurs only in the bulb. (The stem contains only diluting fluid and is not considered.) Therefore, the sample is diluted to a total volume of 100 units (Figure 2–11). Example: Draw 0.5 unit of blood into the pipet stem and dilute by drawing diluting fluid to the 101 mark. The mixing bulb now has 0.5 unit of blood

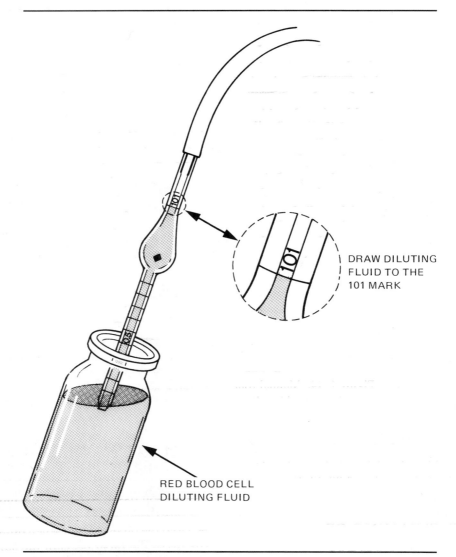

DRAW DILUTING
FLUID TO THE
101 MARK

RED BLOOD CELL
DILUTING FLUID

Figure 2–13. Diluting a sample using the RBC pipet

in 100 units of the total diluted sample. The dilution factor may be determined by dividing 100 by 0.5. The dilution factor is 200, or a 1:200 dilution of the sample has been made. Many dilutions are possible if the pipet being used is marked in 0.1 unit divisions. The formula below is used to calculate the dilution factor for the blood diluting pipets:

$$\frac{bulb\ units}{blood\ units} = dilution\ factor$$

CALCULATING DILUTIONS FOR THE WBC PIPET

The WBC pipet is similar to the RBC pipet except that the bulb contains 10 units of volume. There-

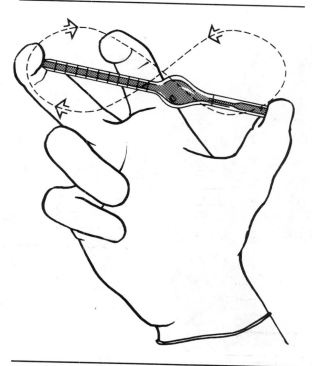

Figure 2–14. Manual rotation of blood diluting pipet using figure-eight motion

fore, a sample drawn to the 0.5 mark and diluted to the 11 mark would contain 0.5 unit of sample in ten units of total diluted sample, a 1:20 dilution.

CARE AND CLEANING OF BLOOD DILUTING PIPETS

Blood diluting pipets should be cleaned thoroughly after each use. The pipet may be cleaned using a suction apparatus (Figure 2–17). The pipet should be cleaned with laboratory detergent (do not use soap), rinsed with distilled water, and dried with acetone. Pipets should be handled gently; they break easily, particularly at the point where the bulb joins the stem. They should be transported carefully and stored so that the tips are protected and will not become chipped.

Precautions

■ Wipe blood from outside surface of pipet using a soft tissue, avoiding touching the tip of the pipet.

■ Hold the pipet upright when filling and keep the tip of the pipet beneath the surface of the fluid to avoid entry of air bubbles into the pipet. Air bubbles will alter the dilution. If air bubbles occur, the filling procedure must be repeated using a clean, dry pipet.

■ Do not draw blood sample past the 0.5 mark (or diluting fluid past the 11 or 101 mark) since this will affect the accuracy of the dilution. If this occurs, repeat the filling procedure using a clean, dry pipet.

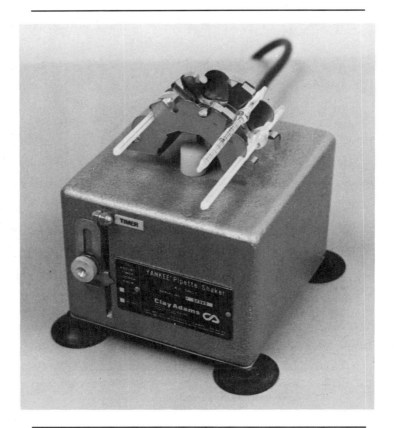

Figure 2–15. Automatic pipet shaker *(Photo courtesy of Clay Adams Division of Becton Dickinson & Co.)*

■ Always use a clean, dry pipet to perform a dilution.
■ Store used pipets in dilute chlorine bleach until they can be cleaned. Do not allow sample to dry in the pipet.
■ Do not use a pipet with a chipped tip.

SELF-FILLING BLOOD DILUTING MICROPIPETS

Self-filling, self-measuring disposable systems such as Unopette® are available for counting erythrocytes, leukocytes, and platelets. These disposable systems consist of the **micropipet,** pipet shield, and a sealed plastic reservoir containing a premeasured volume of diluting fluid (Figure 2–18). The sample is collected in the micropipet, introduced into the reservoir, and the contents are mixed and dispensed from the reservoir. Correct use of these self-filling, self-measuring systems usually provides a more accurate dilution than the blood diluting pipets. Use of these systems eliminates mouth-pipetting.

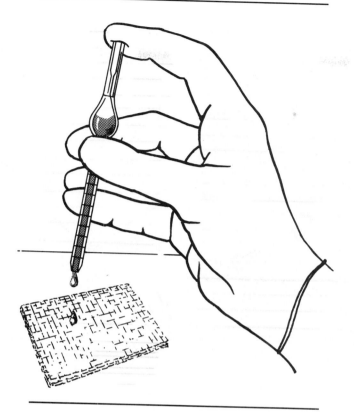

Figure 2–16. Dispensing four to five drops from blood diluting pipet onto a gauze pad

LESSON REVIEW

1. Draw and label the parts of the RBC pipet.
2. Draw and label the parts of the WBC pipet.
3. How should a blood diluting pipet be cleaned?
4. What dilution is made when the blood sample is drawn to the 0.5 mark and diluting fluid to the 101 mark in the RBC pipet?

5. Explain the proper care of blood diluting pipets.
6. List precautions to be observed when using blood diluting pipets.
7. Define aspiration, capillary action, diluting fluid, erythrocyte, leukocyte, micropipet, red cell diluting pipet, and white cell diluting pipet.

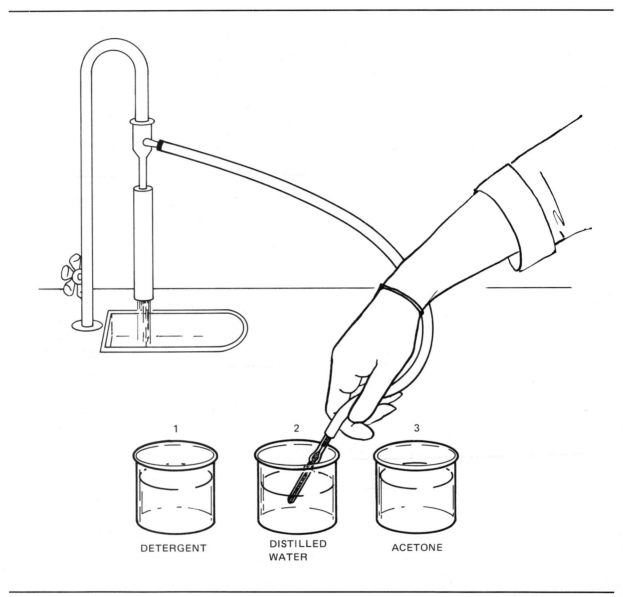

1

2

3

DETERGENT

DISTILLED
WATER

ACETONE

Figure 2–17. Cleaning a blood diluting pipet using suction apparatus

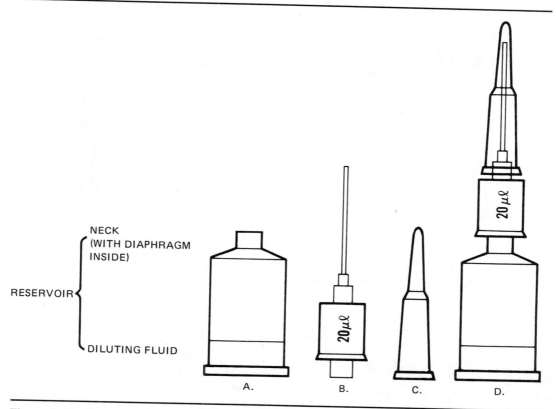

Figure 2–18. Parts of a disposable blood diluting unit such as Unopette®. A) Pre-filled reservoir containing pre-measured diluting fluid and sealed with diaphragm, B) capillary pipet with overflow chamber and capacity marking, C) pipet shield, and D) assembled unit

STUDENT ACTIVITIES

1. Re-read the information on blood diluting pipets.
2. Review the glossary terms.

3. Practice the procedure for using the WBC and RBC blood diluting pipets as outlined on the Student Performance Guide.

Student Performance Guide

NAME _____

DATE _____

LESSON 2–3
BLOOD DILUTING PIPETS

Instructions

1. Practice the procedure for using the red cell and white cell blood diluting pipets.
2. Demonstrate the red and white blood diluting pipet procedures satisfactorily for the instructor. All steps must be completed as listed on the instructor's Performance Check Sheet.
3. Complete a written examination successfully.

Materials and Equipment

- gloves
- hand disinfectant
- WBC pipet
- RBC pipet
- blood or diluted red food coloring
- diluting fluid or water
- pipet filler
- paper towels or gauze
- pipet shaker (optional)
- suction apparatus for cleaning (optional)
- laboratory detergent
- distilled water
- acetone
- soft laboratory tissue
- surface disinfectant
- biohazard container
- chlorine bleach

Procedure			S = Satisfactory U = Unsatisfactory
You must:	**S**	**U**	**Comments**
1. Wash hands with disinfectant and put on gloves			
2. Assemble equipment and materials			
3. Connect the pipet filler to the end of the WBC pipet having the 11 mark			
4. Hold a tube of well-mixed blood or diluted red food coloring in the opposite hand and tilt the tube so that the sample is near the lip of the tube (Figure 2–12)			
5. Place the tip of the pipet beneath the surface of the sample			
6. Draw the sample slowly to the 0.5 mark, using the pipet filler. Do not allow air bubbles to enter, or draw sample past the 0.5 mark			
7. Wipe the outside of the pipet stem with a soft tissue to remove all sample (avoid touching pipet tip)			
8. Select previously opened diluting fluid or water; tilt the container and insert the tip of the pipet beneath the surface of the fluid. Slowly rotate the pipet while aspirating the fluid exactly to the 11 mark. Hold pipet upright to prevent entry of air bubbles (Figure 2–13)			
9. Place the index finger over the tip of the pipet and carefully remove the pipet filler			
10. Hold the pipet horizontally and mix by either method: (a) Place pipet on the automatic pipet shaker and turn the shaker on for at least two minutes or, (b) Mix contents for two to three minutes by rotating in a figure-eight motion while holding pipet with middle finger and thumb over ends			
11. Hold the pipet in a horizontal position when mixing is completed			
12. Place index finger firmly over the end of the pipet which has the 11 mark to control the flow of fluid			
13. Discharge four to five free-falling drops of fluid, one drop at a time, on a gauze pad or paper towel while holding the pipet at a 45° angle or in a nearly vertical position (raise the index finger slightly from the pipet end to allow drops to flow)			

You must:	S	U	Comments
14. Disinfect the pipet by immersing in dilute bleach for 10 minutes			
15. Wash and dry the pipet using (1) detergent, (2) distilled water, and (3) acetone (for drying)			
16. Return pipet and other materials to the proper storage area			
17. Repeat procedure using the RBC pipet (draw diluting fluid to 101 mark in RBC pipet)			
18. Dispose of contaminated materials into biohazard container			
19. Clean equipment and return to proper storage			
20. Clean work area with surface disinfectant			
21. Remove gloves and discard into biohazard container			
22. Wash hands with hand disinfectant			

Comments:

Student/Instructor:

Date:_____ Instructor:_____

LESSON 2–4
The Hemacytometer

LESSON OBJECTIVES

After studying this lesson, you should be able to:
- Identify the parts of a hemacytometer.
- Use the microscope to identify the hemacytometer areas where red cells and white cells are counted.
- Fill the hemacytometer using a blood diluting pipet.
- Clean and dry the hemacytometer and coverglass.
- Write the general formula for calculating cell counts using a hemacytometer.
- List the precautions to observe when using the hemacytometer.
- Define the glossary terms.

GLOSSARY

hemacytometer / a heavy glass slide made to precise specifications and used to count cells microscopically; a counting chamber
hemacytometer coverglass / a special coverglass of uniform thickness used with a hemacytometer

INTRODUCTION

The **hemacytometer** is used to count erythrocytes, leukocytes, and platelets in the blood. It may also be used to count cells in other body fluids. The hemacytometer is a heavy glass slide manufactured to meet the specifications of the National Institute of Standards and Technology (NIST). When viewed from the top, it has two raised platforms surrounded by depressions on three sides (Figure 2–19). Each raised surface contains a ruled counting area which is marked off by precise lines etched into the glass. The depressions surrounding these platforms are sometimes called "moats." The raised areas and the depressions form an "H."

A special coverglass is used with the hemacytometer. Only a **hemacytometer coverglass** of uniform thickness which meets NIST specifica-

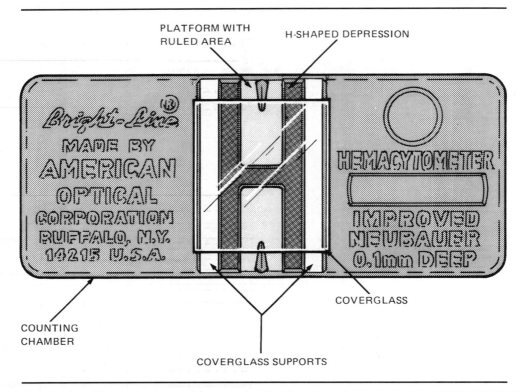

Figure 2–19. Hemacytometer with coverglass in place

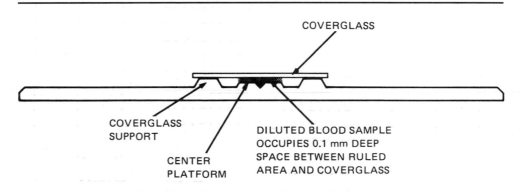

Figure 2–20. Side view of hemacytometer with coverglass in place

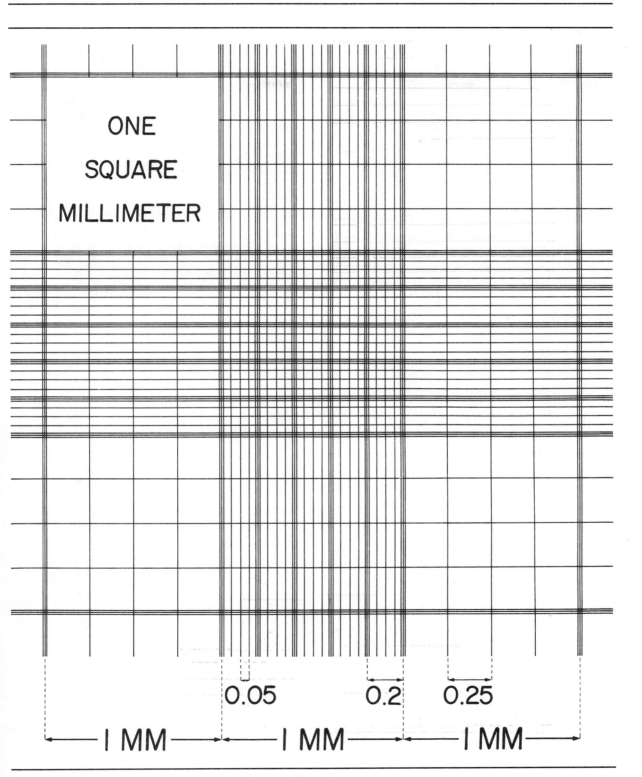

Figure 2–21. Ruled area of hemacytometer showing dimensions

tions should be used. The coverglass is positioned so that it covers both ruled areas of the hemacytometer (Figure 2–19). The coverglass confines the fluid in the chamber and regulates the depth of that fluid. The depth of the fluid in the Neubauer-type hemacytometer is 0.1 mm with the coverglass in place (Figure 2–20, page 108).

Counting Areas

A hemacytometer has two ruled areas. These areas are composed of etched lines which define squares of specific dimensions. The most commonly used hemacytometer is the type with Neubauer ruling. In the Neubauer-type counting chamber, each ruled area consists of a large square, 3 mm × 3 mm. This area of 9 mm^2 is divided into nine equal squares, each of which is 1 mm^2 (Figure 2–21, page 109).

WBC Counting Area. The WBC counting area consists of the four large corner squares labeled "W" in Figure 2–22. Each of these large corner squares is subdivided into sixteen smaller squares. All four large corner squares on both sides of the chamber are used to count WBC.

RBC Counting Area. The center squares on both sides of the chamber are used to count the red blood cells. Each center square is subdivided into twenty-five smaller squares. Only the four corner squares and the center square within the larger center square are used to count RBC (Figure 2–23).

USING THE HEMACYTOMETER

A clean coverglass should be positioned so that it covers both ruled areas of a clean hemacytometer. Then the hemacytometer is filled or charged. This

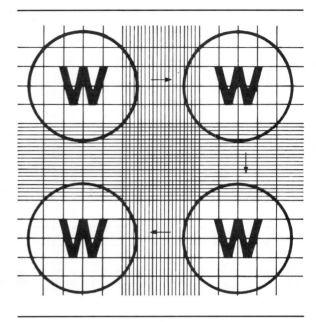

Figure 2–22. WBC counting area

is done by touching the tip of a filled blood diluting pipet to the point where the coverglass and the raised platform on one side meet (Figure 2–24). The fluid from the pipet will flow by capillary action into one side of the hemacytometer, using one-half to one drop of fluid. The opposite side of the chamber is then filled in the same manner. (Some hemacytometers have a V-shaped trough on each raised platform to guide the placement of the pipet tip when filling.)

The fluid should flow into the chamber in a smooth, unbroken stream. It should not be allowed to overflow into the depressions or moats. After the hemacytometer has been correctly filled, it should then stand two minutes to allow the cells to settle.

Viewing the Ruled Areas

The hemacytometer should be placed on the microscope stage with the low power (10×) objec-

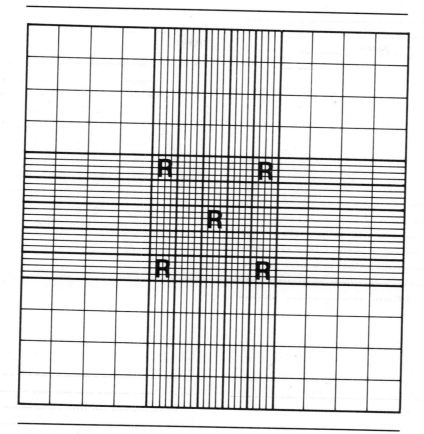

Figure 2–23. RBC counting area. The four corner squares and center square (labeled "R") within the large center square are used to count red blood cells

tive in place so that one of the ruled areas is located over the light source. The coarse adjustment knob should be used to carefully move the hemacytometer and objective closer together. This adjustment is continued until the objective is almost touching the coverglass. Looking into the eyepiece (ocular), the coarse adjustment knob is then used to increase the distance between the objective and the hemacytometer. This is continued until the etched lines come into view. The fine adjustment knob is then used to bring the etched lines into

sharp focus. The etched lines are more easily viewed when the condenser or the light source of the microscope is lowered.

When the ruled area is in sharp focus, the white cell counting areas (four large corner squares) are located by moving the stage (or moving the hemacytometer carefully if the microscope does not have a mechanical stage). After the white cell counting area has been observed, the central square used for the red cell counts should be located. The high power (40×) objective should be carefully

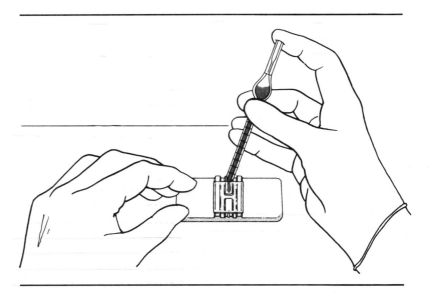

Figure 2–24. Filling the hemacytometer

rotated into place. The five small squares used in a red cell count should be located. (If the microscope is parfocal, the ruled area will be brought into focus with only a slight rotation of the fine adjustment.)

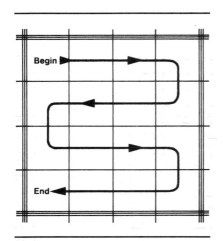

Figure 2–25. Left-to-right, right-to-left counting pattern (shown here in one of the large corner squares)

Once all parts of the ruled area of one side have been located, the hemacytometer should be carefully moved so that the second ruled area can be viewed. When moving the hemacytometer, the low power objective should be in position. The oil immersion objective is never used with a hemacytometer.

Counting Pattern

A counting pattern of left-to-right, right-to-left must be used to insure that cells are counted only one time. The count should begin in the upper left corner of a square and proceed in a serpentine manner (Figure 2–25).

Squares are divided by boundary lines which may be single, double, or triple. When triple lines are present, the center line is considered the boundary. When double lines are present, the outer line is considered the boundary. All cells within a square, cells which touch the left boundary of the square, and cells which touch the top boundary of the square are counted. Cells which touch the

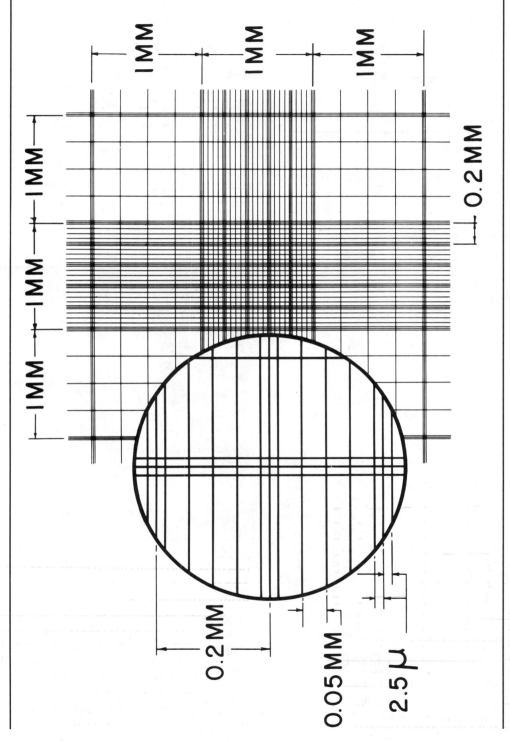

Figure 2–26. Boundaries and dimensions of ruled area (*Photo courtesy of Reichert Scientific Instruments*)

right boundary of a square and cells which touch the lower boundary (Figure 2–26, page 113) of a square should not be counted in that square even though they may lie within the square. The cells in the designated squares should be counted on both sides of the chamber. The results for each side should be recorded. The counts for the two sides are then totaled and the average is calculated.

CALCULATING THE CELL COUNTS

The total number of cells per cubic millimeter (mm^3) of the sample can be calculated from the average number of cells which were counted. This is because the ruled areas of the hemacytometer contain an exact volume of diluted sample. Since only a small volume of diluted sample is counted, a general formula must be used to convert the count into the number of cells/mm^3:

$$C/mm^3 = \frac{Avg \times D\ (mm) \times DF}{A\ (mm^2)}$$

Where:
$$\begin{aligned} C/mm^3 &= \text{Number of cells/}mm^3 \\ Avg &= \text{Average \# of cells counted} \\ D\ (mm) &= \text{Depth factor in mm} \\ DF &= \text{Dilution factor} \\ A\ (mm^2) &= \text{Area counted (}mm^2\text{)} \end{aligned}$$

The dilution factor used in the formula is determined by the dilution obtained with the blood diluting pipet. The depth factor used in the formula is always 10 (the counting chamber is 0.1 mm deep; the depth is converted to 1 mm by multiplying by 10). The area counted will vary for each type of cell count and is calculated using the dimensions of the ruled area.

CARE OF THE HEMACYTOMETER

The hemacytometer is an expensive piece of equipment which must be handled carefully. It should be held by the sides and bottom only, to avoid getting fingerprints on the raised ruled areas. Before each use, the raised surfaces should be wiped with lens paper dipped in 70% alcohol. The hemacytometer should then be immediately dried and polished gently with lens paper. The coverglass should be handled by the edges, and both sides cleaned in the same manner as the hemacytometer. After use, the hemacytometer should be disinfected with weak chlorine bleach. When not in use, the hemacytometer should be stored in a container to keep dirt and dust off the surface and to protect the ruled areas from scratches. When transporting the hemacytometer, one should hold it carefully and place it on a secure surface.

Precautions

■ Disinfect hemacytometer and coverglass after each use.
■ Use care when focusing the microscope on the ruled areas.
■ Be certain that the hemacytometer and coverglass are free from dirt and oil before use.
■ Store and handle the hemacytometer and coverglass carefully to avoid scratches.

LESSON REVIEW

1. List the parts of the hemacytometer.
2. Which squares are counted for a WBC count—for an RBC count?
3. Explain how to fill the hemacytometer using the pipet.
4. What is the proper procedure for cleaning the hemacytometer and coverglass?
5. What is the general formula used to calculate cell counts when using the hemacytometer?
6. List the precautions to be observed when using the hemacytometer.

7. Define hemacytometer and hemacytometer coverglass.

STUDENT ACTIVITIES

1. Re-read the information on the hemacytometer.

2. Review the glossary terms.
3. Practice filling the hemacytometer.
4. Practice locating the WBC counting areas as outlined on the Student Performance Guide.
5. Practice locating the RBC counting areas as outlined on the Student Performance Guide.

Student Performance Guide

NAME _____

DATE _____

LESSON 2–4
THE HEMACYTOMETER

Instructions

1. Practice the procedure for using the hemacytometer.
2. Demonstrate the procedure for using the hemacytometer satisfactorily for the instructor. All steps must be completed as listed on the instructor's Performance Check Sheet.
3. Complete a written examination successfully.

Materials and Equipment

- gloves
- hand disinfectant
- hemacytometer
- chlorine bleach
- hemacytometer coverglass
- lens paper
- 70% ethyl or isopropyl alcohol
- blood (optional)
- blood diluting pipets
- pipet filler
- microscope
- RBC diluting fluid (optional)
- WBC diluting fluid (optional)
- suction apparatus for cleaning pipets (optional)
- paper towels or gauze
- laboratory detergent
- distilled water
- acetone
- pipet shaker (optional)
- soft tissue
- surface disinfectant
- biohazard container

116

Procedure			S = Satisfactory U = Unsatisfactory
You must:	**S**	**U**	**Comments**
1. Assemble equipment and materials			
2. Use lens paper and alcohol to carefully clean hemacytometer and coverglass			
3. Place the coverglass carefully over the ruled areas (chamber) of the hemacytometer			
4. Wash hands with disinfectant and put on gloves			
5. Follow the procedure in the blood diluting pipet lesson and make a cell dilution (or fill pipet with distilled water)			
6. Discharge four to five drops from the pipet onto a paper towel or gauze			
7. Wipe excess fluid from the tip of the pipet using soft tissue			
8. Hold the pipet at a 45° angle and touch the tip to the point where the coverglass and the hemacytometer meet, placing index finger on the short stem of pipet to regulate flow (do not move coverglass)			
9. Allow fluid to flow into one side of the chamber by capillary action (the chamber should fill in one smooth flow without flooding over into the depressions)			
10. Fill the other side of the chamber in the same manner			
11. Position the low power (10×) objective in place			
12. Place the hemacytometer on the microscope stage securely with one ruled area over the light source			
13. Look directly at the hemacytometer and turn the coarse adjustment knob to bring the microscope objective and the hemacytometer close together, continuing until the objective is almost touching the coverglass. *Note:* Use coarse adjustment with care			
14. Look into the eyepiece and slowly turn the coarse adjustment knob in the opposite direction until the etched lines come into view			
15. Rotate the fine adjustment knob until the lines are in clear focus			

You must:	S	U	Comments
16. Find all nine large squares of one side of the chamber by moving the stage or the hemacytometer			
17. Locate four large corner squares used for WBC count (Figure 2–22)			
18. Scan squares using left-to-right, right-to-left counting pattern and observe boundaries			
19. Locate the center square used for the RBC count (Figure 2–23)			
20. Rotate the high power (40×) objective carefully into position and adjust focus using the fine adjustment knob until the etched lines appear distinct			
21. Locate the four small corner squares and the center square used for the RBC count (Figure 2–23)			
22. Scan counting area using left-to-right, right-to-left pattern and observe boundaries			
23. View the second ruled area, repeating steps 16–22			
24. Rotate the low power objective into position			
25. Remove the hemacytometer carefully from the microscope stage. Place hemacytometer and coverglass into chlorine bleach solution to disinfect			
26. Clean the hemacytometer and the coverglass carefully using alcohol and lens paper			
27. Dry the hemacytometer and coverglass with lens paper			
28. Clean and return all equipment to proper storage			
29. Clean work area with surface disinfectant			
30. Remove and discard gloves into appropriate container			
31. Wash hands with hand disinfectant			

Comments:

Student/Instructor:

Date:_____   Instructor:_____

LESSON 2-5

The Red Blood Cell Count

LESSON OBJECTIVES

After studying this lesson, you should be able to:

- Explain the function of red blood cells.
- List the normal red cell counts for males and females.
- Name a condition or disease associated with an increased red cell count.
- Name two conditions or diseases associated with a decreased red cell count.
- State an important property of a red cell diluting fluid.
- Name three red cell diluting fluids.
- Perform a manual red cell count.
- Calculate the results of a red cell count.
- List two precautions to be observed when performing a red cell count.
- Define the glossary terms.

GLOSSARY

anemia / decrease below normal in the red cell count or in the blood hemoglobin level

erythrocytosis / increase above normal in the number of red cells in circulation

hemolysis / the destruction of red blood cells resulting in the liberation of hemoglobin from the cells

isotonic solution / a solution which has the same concentration of dissolved particles as that solution with which it is compared

119

INTRODUCTION

The blood is composed of three groups of cellular elements. These are (1) the erythrocytes or red blood cells (RBC); (2) the leukocytes or white blood cells (WBC); and (3) the platelets or thrombocytes. These cells are vital components of the blood. They are essential for proper functioning of body systems.

Each group of blood cells has a unique function. The red blood cells, the most numerous cells in the blood, transport oxygen to tissues. Red blood cells also carry carbon dioxide to the lungs to be exhaled.

THE RED CELL COUNT

A red cell count is a commonly performed procedure. It is usually a part of a complete blood count (CBC). The red cell count approximates the number of circulating red cells. If the count falls below or above the normal range, an individual may experience a variety of symptoms. A red cell count helps the physician diagnose and treat many diseases.

Normal Values

The normal values for red blood cell counts range from approximately 4 million per cubic millimeter of blood ($4.0 \times 10^6/\text{mm}^3$) to six million per cubic millimeter ($6.0 \times 10^6/\text{mm}^3$). Males usually

Table 2–2. Normal RBC counts in adult males and adult females

Sex	Normal RBC Count
Adult male	4.5–$6.0 \times 10^6/\text{mm}^3$
Adult female	4.0–$5.5 \times 10^6/\text{mm}^3$

have slightly higher RBC counts than females (Table 2–2).

Red cell counts may be reported as the number of cells per cubic millimeter (mm^3), microliter (μl), or liter (L) of blood. For example, a count of $5.6 \times 10^6 \, \text{RBC}/\text{mm}^3$ (or μl) would be reported as $5.6 \times 10^{12} \, \text{RBC}/\text{L}$.

Conditions Associated with Changes in Red Cell Counts

Since the red blood cells carry oxygen, a reduction in their number results in decreased oxygen-carrying capacity. This condition is called **anemia.** The symptoms of anemia include fatigue, weakness, headache, and pallor. Examples of conditions with decreased red cell counts are iron deficiency anemia and sickle cell anemia. Anemias may also be due to deficiencies of vitamins such as B_{12} or folic acid.

An increased red cell count is called **erythrocytosis.** People who live in high altitudes have erythrocytosis because of the lower oxygen content of the air. Polycythemia vera is a disease in which the red cell count is greatly increased.

PERFORMING A MANUAL RED CELL COUNT

Diluting Fluids

There are several fluids which may be used to dilute blood for an RBC count. The diluting fluid used for RBC counts must be an **isotonic solution.** This prevents **hemolysis,** or destruction of the red cells. Commonly used red cell diluting fluids are Hayem's, Gower's, and Dacie's.

Procedure

A capillary sample or a well-mixed anticoagulated blood sample is drawn into the RBC pipet to the 0.5 mark. Red cell diluting fluid is then drawn

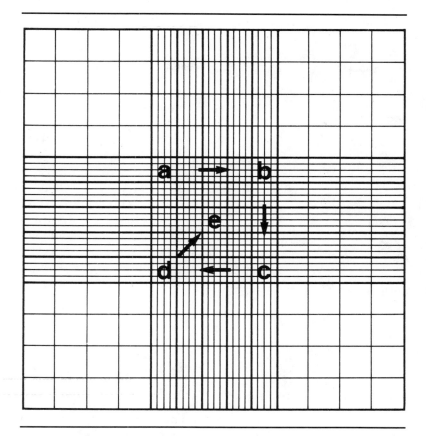

Figure 2–27. RBC counting area

into the pipet to the 101 mark. A second pipet is filled in the same manner. The contents of the pipets are mixed thoroughly. The first 4 to 5 drops are discarded. A coverglass is positioned on the hemacytometer. The tip of the pipet is touched to the edge of the coverglass and one side of the chamber is allowed to fill by capillary action. Using the second pipet, the opposite side is then filled in the same manner. If the fluid overflows into the depression around the platforms, or if air bubbles occur, the chamber should be cleaned and refilled.

After allowing the cells to settle for two to three minutes, the hemacytometer is placed carefully on the microscope stage. The RBC ruled area

is located using the low power (10×) objective. The high power (40×) objective is then rotated into place to perform the count.

The RBC count is performed using the center square of the ruled area as shown in Figure 2–27. Within the center square are twenty-five smaller squares. Of these twenty-five squares, the four corner squares and the center square (marked a, b, c, d, and e) are counted. Each of these five squares in turn contains four rows of squares. All cells within each of the five squares are counted using the left-to-right, right-to-left counting pattern. Be sure to include the cells touching the top and left boundaries of the squares. The cells touching the right boundary and the cells touching the

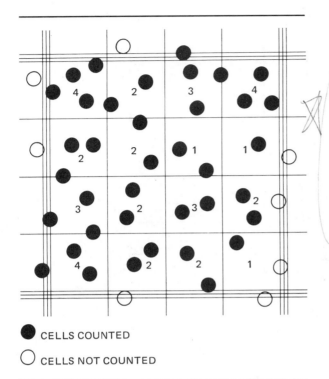

● CELLS COUNTED

○ CELLS NOT COUNTED

Figure 2–28. Sample count in square "a" on one side of chamber. The numbers shown denote the total number of cells counted in each square.

lower boundary of each square are not counted. Cells beyond these boundaries are not counted either (Figure 2–28).

A hand counter is used to tabulate the red cells in the five designated squares. The numbers for each of the five squares are recorded and totaled. If the number of cells in a square varies from any other square on the same side by more than 25 cells, the count must be repeated. A count is then performed in the five squares of the second side of the chamber in the same manner. The two totals are then averaged.

Calculations

The general formula to use for the hemacytometer was given on page 114. To calculate a red cell count, the formula is used in the following manner:

1. The average number of cells is obtained by totaling the counts for the five squares on each side of the chamber. Then divide by two; this gives you the average.
2. The depth factor (mm) is always ten. (The depth of the chamber is 0.1 mm which when multiplied by ten is one.)
3. The dilution using the RBC pipet is 1:200. Therefore, the dilution factor is 200.
4. The area counted is 0.20 mm². (Each square, a to e, has a length of 0.2 mm and a width of 0.2 mm. This gives each square an area of 0.04 mm². Since five squares are counted, the area is 5×0.04 mm² or 0.20 mm².) Substitute these numbers into the formula as shown below.

$$C/mm^3 = \frac{Avg \times 10 \times 200}{0.20}$$

$$= \text{average \# cells} \times 10{,}000$$

When an RBC count is performed this way, the count/mm³ may be calculated by simply adding four zeroes to the average number of cells counted (or multiplying by 10,000). A sample calculation is shown in Figure 2–29.

Precautions

■ All precautions for using blood-diluting pipets and the hemacytometer must be followed.
■ The hemacytometer and coverglass must be free of dirt and oil.
■ Proper counting methods should be carefully followed.
■ The count from one small square (a to e) to another should not vary by more than twenty-five. Any greater variation indicates an uneven distribution of cells. In such cases, the chamber should be cleaned and refilled.
■ Clean any spills with surface disinfectant.
■ Wash hands after procedure is completed.

1. Count the cells:

	Side 1			Side 2	
Square	Cells counted		Square	Cells counted	
a	100		a	105	
b	95		b	115	
c	90		c	100	
d	90		d	106	
e	105		e	94	
Total	480		Total	520	

2. Compute the average:
   A. 480 + 520 = 1000 cells
   B. 1000 ÷ 2 = 500 average

3. Calculate the count:

$$RBC/mm^3 = \frac{average \ \# \ cells \ counted \times depth \ factor \ (mm) \times dilution \ factor}{area \ counted \ (mm^2)}$$

$$RBC/mm^3 = \frac{500 \times 10 \ (mm) \times 200}{0.2 \ mm^2}$$

$$RBC/mm^3 = 500 \times 10000 \ mm^3$$

$$RBC/mm^3 = 5,000,000 \ or \ 5.0 \times 10^6/mm^3$$

Figure 2–29. Sample calculation of an RBC count

UNOPETTE® MICROCOLLECTION SYSTEM

The most acceptable manual method of counting red cells is the use of self-filling, self-diluting systems such as Unopette®. Such a system provides greater accuracy than the pipet method, and the components are disposable (Figure 2–18).

Unopette® systems consist of a reservoir, a capillary pipet, and a pipet shield. The reservoir contains a pre-measured volume of diluting fluid. The capillary pipet is made to contain a specific volume. The shield protects the pipet and is used to puncture the diaphragm which seals the reservoir. The Unopette® system used for red cell counts contains 1.99 ml of diluting fluid in the reservoir. A 10 μl capillary pipet is used to measure the sample. When the sample is diluted in the reservoir, the resulting dilution is 1:200. This blood dilution is then loaded into a hemacytometer and the red cells are counted as in the manual pipet method.

AUTOMATED CELL COUNTS

Although blood cell counts may be performed manually, the majority are performed by automation (Figure 2–30). The instruments used may range from relatively simple inexpensive counters, to very elaborate and expensive instruments. Simple counters may be used in a physician's office or a small hospital. More elaborate equipment may be found in large hospitals and reference laboratories. Some instruments count only erythrocytes and leukocytes. Others count erythrocytes, leukocytes, and platelets.

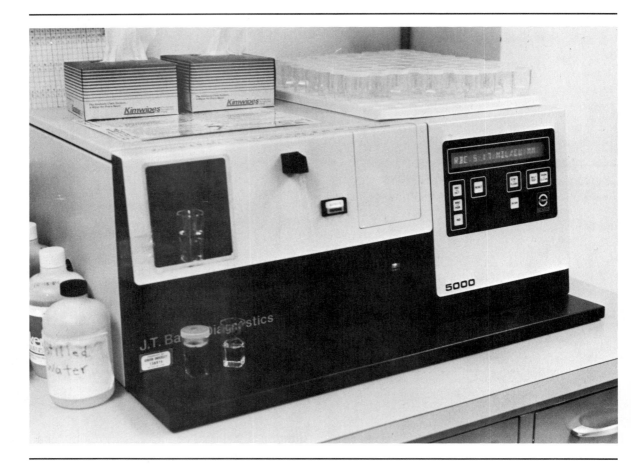

Figure 2–30. Automated cell counters *(Photos courtesy of Auburn University [above], and East Alabama Medical Center [page 125], photographer John Estridge).*

Most automated cell counters operate on one of two principles. In some instruments, the cells to be counted are diluted in a fluid which conducts an electrical current. The cells are aspirated through a special narrow opening called an aperture. As the cells are aspirated, they interrupt the flow of the current across the opening. Each interruption is recorded and counted as a cell. In other instruments, the diluted blood sample is aspirated into a special channel which is so narrow that only one cell can pass through at a time. As the cells pass through the channel, they interrupt a laser beam. The interruptions of the beam are counted as cells. Most automated instruments complete a cell count in less than one minute.

Use of automated cell counters has improved the accuracy of cell counts and the efficiency of laboratories. However, despite the widespread use of these instruments, every laboratory needs to maintain the equipment and trained personnel necessary to perform manual counts.

LESSON REVIEW

1. What is the function of the red blood cell?
2. What is the normal red blood cell count for a male; for a female?

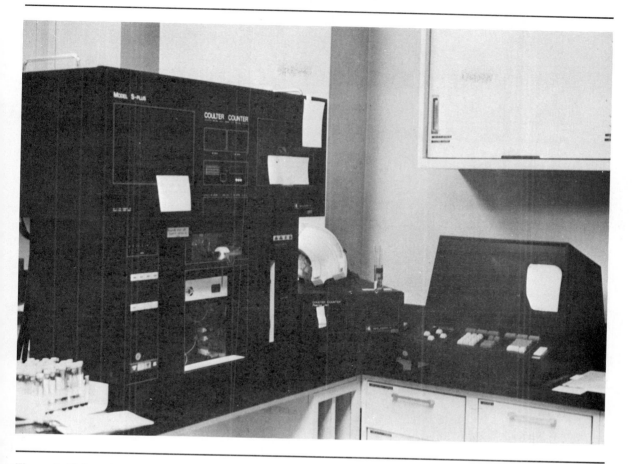

Figure 2–30 *(cont.)*

3. Name three diseases or conditions in which the red cell count is usually abnormal.
4. Name three common red cell diluting fluids and state one requirement of a red cell diluting fluid.
5. Which squares of the counting chamber are used in performing a red cell count?
6. How is a red cell count calculated?
7. What precautions should be observed when performing an RBC count?
8. Define anemia, erythrocytosis, hemolysis, and isotonic solution.

STUDENT ACTIVITIES

1. Re-read the information on red cell counts.
2. Review the glossary terms.
3. Practice making different dilutions with the RBC pipet by varying the mark to which the blood is drawn. Calculate the resulting dilutions.
4. Experiment to see what happens when red cells are exposed to 0.1N Hydrochloric acid (0.1N HCl) or to water.
5. Practice performing and calculating a red cell count as outlined on the Student Performance Guide, using the worksheet.

Student Performance Guide

NAME _____

DATE _____

LESSON 2–5
THE RED BLOOD CELL COUNT

Instructions

1. Practice performing and calculating a red cell count.
2. Demonstrate the red cell count procedure satisfactorily for the instructor. All steps must be completed as listed on the instructor's Performance Check Sheet.
3. Complete a written examination successfully.

Materials and Equipment

- gloves
- hand disinfectant
- RBC pipet
- chlorine bleach
- red blood cell diluting fluid
- hemacytometer with coverglass
- microscope
- hand counter
- pipet washer (optional)
- automatic pipet shaker (optional)
- gauze
- lens paper
- soft tissue
- detergent
- 70% ethyl or isopropyl alcohol
- capillary or EDTA anticoagulated blood specimen
- worksheet
- materials for capillary puncture
- surface disinfectant
- biohazard container
- pipet filler

Procedure

S = Satisfactory
U = Unsatisfactory

You must:	S	U	Comments
1. Assemble equipment and materials			
2. Attach pipet filler to RBC pipet (short stem)			
3. Wash hands with disinfectant and put on gloves			
4. Tilt well-mixed tube of blood (invert tube twenty to thirty times to mix) and insert pipet tip			
5. Draw blood up to the 0.5 mark on the pipet. *Note:* Do not allow blood to pass the 0.5 mark			
6. Wipe excess blood from pipet exterior with tissue to avoid the transfer of cells to the diluting fluid			
7. Insert pipet tip into diluting fluid being careful not to allow cells to flow into diluting fluid			
8. Draw the diluting fluid up to the 101 mark on the pipet. *Note:* Do not fill the pipet past the 101 mark			
9. Place finger over the tip of pipet and remove the rubber tubing from stem			
10. Fill a second pipet in the same manner			

11. Mix contents of pipets manually or by automatic shaker:
A. Manual Method
   (1) Hold pipet horizontally with thumb and middle finger over the ends of pipet
   (2) Mix for two to three minutes by rotating the pipet gently in a figure-eight motion
B. Automatic Shaker
   (1) Place pipets securely on automatic shaker and turn shaker on
   (2) Allow shaker to complete the cycle (usually two minutes) and come to a full stop
   (3) Remove pipets from shaker			

12. Fill the hemacytometer: a. Position a clean hemacytometer coverglass over the counting chamber b. Place the index finger over the tip of the short stem of pipet to control the flow of fluid c. Discard the first four to five drops of fluid from the long stem of the pipet			

You must:	S	U	Comments
d. Touch the tip of the pipet to the edge of the cover-glass and counting chamber			
e. Allow the fluid to flow under the coverglass until one side of the counting chamber is completely full (usually one half to one drop). Do not overfill			
f. Fill the opposite side in the same manner using the second pipet			
g. Allow the cells to settle about two minutes			
13. Place hemacytometer on the microscope stage and secure			
14. Locate the central square of the ruled area using low power (10×) magnification			
15. Switch to high power (40×) and focus with fine adjustment			
16. Count the red cells: a. Count the RBCs in the four corner squares and center square (a, b, c, d, and e) of the large central square using the left-to-right and right-to-left counting pattern			
b. Count the RBCs lying within each square, including the cells touching the top boundary, and the cells touching the left boundary. Do not count the cells touching the right or lower boundary			
17. Record results from side 1 on the worksheet			
18. Count side 2 in the same manner			
19. Record results from side 2 on the worksheet			
20. Average the counts from sides 1 and 2			

21. Calculate the RBC count:
   a. Multiply the average number of cells counted times the depth factor, times the dilution factor. Divide this by the area counted, or
   b. Multiply the average number of cells by 10,000			

22. Record RBC count on worksheet			
23. Disinfect pipets, hemacytometer and coverglass			
24. Clean pipets carefully			
25. Clean hemacytometer and coverglass carefully using 70% alcohol and lens paper			

You must:	S	U	Comments
26. Discard specimen and contaminated materials into biohazard container			
27. Clean and return equipment to proper storage			
28. Clean work area with surface disinfectant			
29. Remove and discard gloves appropriately			
30. Wash hands with hand disinfectant			

Comments:

Student/Instructor:

Date:_____ Instructor:_____

Student Performance Guide

NAME _____

DATE _____

LESSON 2–5
THE RED BLOOD CELL COUNT
(UNOPETTE® METHOD)

Instructions

1. Practice performing and calculating a red cell count using the Unopette®.
2. Perform the red cell count procedure satisfactorily for the instructor. All steps must be completed as listed on the instructor's Performance Check Sheet.
3. Complete a written examination successfully.

Materials and Equipment

- gloves
- hand disinfectant
- blood sample, anticoagulated with EDTA
- hemacytometer with coverglass
- test tube rack or beaker to hold blood sample
- Unopette® for red cell count (reservoir and pipet assembly)
- microscope
- lens paper
- alcohol (70% ethanol)
- hand tally counter
- surface disinfectant
- biohazard container

Note: The following is a general procedure for the use of the Unopette® system. Consult the package insert for specific instructions.

Procedure			S = Satisfactory U = Unsatisfactory
You must:	**S**	**U**	**Comments**
1. Assemble equipment and materials			
2. Place a clean hemacytometer coverglass over a clean hemacytometer			
3. Wash hands with disinfectant and put on gloves			
4. Puncture the diaphragm of the Unopette® reservoir. Hold the reservoir firmly on a flat surface with one hand and use the tip of the pipet shield to puncture the diaphragm. *Note:* The opening must be made large enough to easily accommodate the pipet			
5. Remove the shield from the pipet assembly			
6. Fill the capillary pipet from a capillary puncture or from a tube of well-mixed EDTA anticoagulated blood. The pipet will fill by capillary action and will stop filling automatically. *Note:* Keep pipet horizontal or at a slight (5°) angle to avoid overfilling			
7. Wipe excess blood from the outside of the capillary pipet with soft laboratory tissue. *Note:* Do not allow tissue to touch pipet tip			
8. Squeeze the reservoir slightly, being careful not to expel any of the liquid			
9. Maintain the pressure on the reservoir and insert the capillary pipet into the reservoir, seating the pipet firmly into the neck of the reservoir. Do not expel any of the liquid			
10. Release the pressure on the reservoir, drawing the blood out of the capillary pipet into the diluent			
11. Squeeze the reservoir gently three to four times to rinse the remaining blood from the capillary pipet. *Note:* Do not allow the blood-diluent mixture to flow out the top			
12. Mix the contents of the reservoir thoroughly by gently swirling the reservoir and/or turning it side to side			
13. Withdraw the capillary pipet from the reservoir and place into the neck of the reservoir in reverse position (the pipet tip should now project upward from the reservoir)			

You must:	S	U	Comments
14. Mix the contents of the reservoir thoroughly. Invert the reservoir and gently squeeze to discard 4–5 drops onto gauze or paper towel			
15. Fill both sides of the hemacytometer			
16. Place the hemacytometer on the microscope stage carefully and secure			
17. Use the low power (10×) objective to bring the ruled area into focus			
18. Locate the large central square (Figure 2–27)			
19. Rotate the high power (45×) objective into position carefully and focus with the fine adjustment knob until lines are clear			
20. Adjust the light so that red cells are visible			
21. Count the cells in the four corner squares and one center square within the large center square of the counting area, using the left-to-right, right-to-left counting pattern			
22. Record the results for each of the five squares (4 corner and 1 center)			
23. Repeat the count using the other side of the hemacytometer			
24. Use the worksheet to calculate the red cell count			
25. Record the result			
26. Disinfect the hemacytometer and coverglass			
27. Discard specimen and disposable materials appropriately			
28. Return equipment to proper storage			
29. Clean work area with disinfectant			
30. Remove and discard gloves and wash hands with hand disinfectant			

Comments:

Student/Instructor:

Date:_____ Instructor:_____

Worksheet

NAME_____ DATE _____

LESSON 2–5 THE RED BLOOD CELL COUNT

Side 1	Number of cells counted
Square a	_____
Square b	_____
Square c	_____
Square d	_____
Square e	_____
Total cells counted side 1 =	_____

Side 2	Number of cells counted
Square a	_____
Square b	_____
Square c	_____
Square d	_____
Square e	_____
Total cells counted side 2 =	_____

Total of sides 1 and 2 = _____

Average of two sides (total divided by two) = _____

Multiply average number of cells $\times$ 10 $\times$ 200 and divide by 0.2 = _____ = RBC/mm^3

or

Add four zeroes to the average number of cells = _____ = RBC/mm^3

LESSON 2–6

The White Blood Cell Count

LESSON OBJECTIVES

After studying this lesson, you should be able to:
- List the normal white cell count for adults, children, and newborn infants.
- Name a condition that causes leukocytosis and one that causes leukopenia.
- Perform a manual white blood cell count.
- Calculate the results of a white blood cell count.
- List the precautions to observe when performing a white blood cell count.
- List two white blood cell diluting fluids and state the function of each.
- Define the glossary terms.

GLOSSARY

immunity / resistance to disease or infection

leukocytosis / increase above normal in the number of leukocytes in the blood

leukopenia / decrease below normal in the number of leukocytes in the blood

INTRODUCTION

Five types of white blood cells (WBC) or leukocytes are present in the blood. These are neutrophils, eosinophils, basophils, monocytes, and lymphocytes. The white cells play an important role in providing **immunity,** resistance to infection.

The white blood cell count or leukocyte count is a routine part of a complete blood count (CBC). The white blood cell count gives an approxima-tion of the total number of leukocytes in circulating blood.

Normal Values

The normal white cell count varies with age (Table 2–3). Newborn infants usually have a WBC count of 9,000–30,000/mm^3. The count drops rapidly with age and children have a normal count ranging from 4,500–14,000/mm^3. By adulthood the normal WBC count is 4,500–11,000/mm^3.

Table 2–3. Normal leukocyte counts

| Age | Leukocyte Count (cells/mm³) | |
	Average	Range
Newborn	18,000	9,000–30,000
One year	11,000	6,000–14,000
Six years	8,000	4,500–12,000
Adult	7,400	4,500–11,000

Factors that Influence White Cell Counts

Once adulthood is reached, the WBC count remains stable unless an individual experiences a physical, emotional, or pathological condition that influences the count. Many factors may affect the white cell count. The changes in WBC counts due to factors such as stress, exercise, and anesthesia are temporary while changes due to disease may last until the disease is under control. Most commonly, any increase or decrease in leukocytes is produced by a change in concentration of only one cell type.

An elevated white cell count, **leukocytosis,** may be related to physiologic conditions such as exercise, exposure to sunlight, obstetric labor, and anesthesia. Leukocytosis can also be due to pathologic conditions such as bacterial infections or leukemia.

A decrease below the normal number of leukocytes is called **leukopenia.** This condition may be caused by some viral infections or by exposure to ionizing radiation, some chemicals, and the drugs used in chemotherapy.

PERFORMING A MANUAL WBC COUNT

Diluting Fluids

A white cell count is performed similarly to an RBC count. The diluting fluids used for WBC counts should be solutions which will not damage the leukocytes but will destroy the erythrocytes in the sample. The red blood cells must be destroyed because they are present in such large numbers that they will interfere with the count. Two common WBC diluting fluids are 2% acetic acid and 0.1 N Hydrochloric acid.

Diluting the Sample

The sample is diluted by filling a WBC pipet to the 0.5 mark with blood. The WBC diluting fluid is then drawn into the pipet to the 11 mark. The contents of the pipet are mixed to assure even distribution of cells. Four to five drops of fluid are discarded. The two sides of a clean hemacytometer are filled by touching the pipet to the edge of the coverglass on each side and allowing fluid to flow under the coverglass. If the fluid overflows into the moat or depression, the chamber should be cleaned and refilled.

Counting the Cells

The cells should be allowed to settle for about two minutes before counting. Then the hemacy-

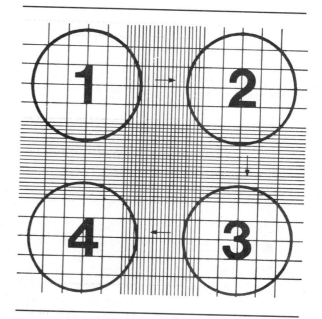

Figure 2–31. WBC counting area

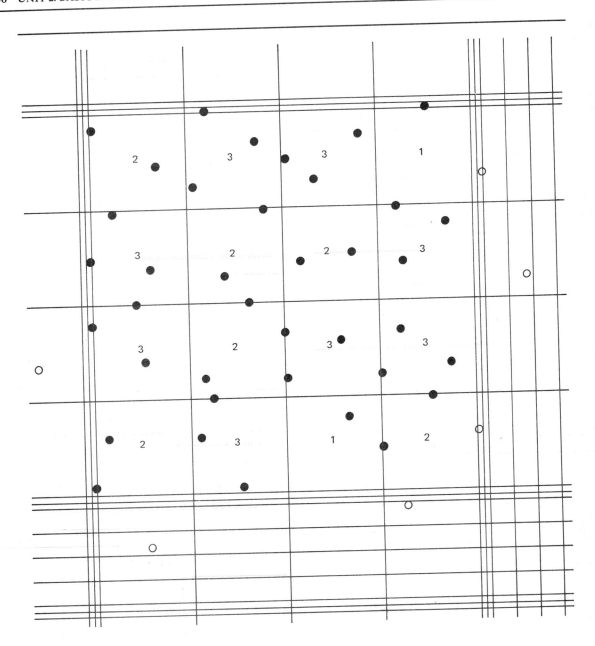

● CELLS COUNTED

○ CELLS NOT COUNTED

Figure 2–32. Sample count in square one (1) of WBC counting area. The numbers shown denote the total number of cells counted in each square.

1. Count the cells:

Side 1			Side 2	
Square	Cells counted		Square	Cells counted
1	30		1	30
2	25		2	26
3	27		3	35
4	33		4	34
Total	115		Total	125

2. Compute the average:
    A. 115 + 125 = 240 cells
    B. 240 ÷ 2 = 120 average

3. Calculate the count:

$$\text{WBC/mm}^3 = \frac{\text{average \# cells counted} \times \text{depth factor (mm)} \times \text{dilution factor}}{\text{area counted (mm}^2)}$$

$$\text{WBC/mm}^3 = \frac{120 \times 10 \text{ mm} \times 20}{4 \text{ mm}^2}$$

$$\text{WBC/mm}^3 = 120 \times 50 \text{ mm}^3$$

$$\text{WBC/mm}^3 = 6{,}000 \text{ (or } 6.0 \times 10^3)/\text{mm}^3$$

Figure 2–33. Sample calculation of a WBC count

tometer is placed securely on the microscope stage and the ruled grid is located using the low power (10×) objective. The cells are more distinct if the microscope light level is reduced. The four large corner squares are used to count the WBC, as shown in Figure 2–31, page 135. The white cells lying within each of the four corner squares are counted using the left-to-right, right-to-left pattern. All cells touching the upper boundary or the left boundary of the square are counted. Cells touching the lower boundary or the right boundary of the square are not counted (Figure 2–32). The results from the four squares of side 1 are recorded and the procedure is repeated using side 2.

Calculations

The formula for calculating cell counts (as discussed in Lesson 2–4, page 114) is:

$$C/\text{mm}^3 = \frac{\text{Avg} \times D \text{ (mm)} \times DF}{A \text{ (mm}^2)}$$

For the WBC count, the dilution factor is 20 and the area counted is 4 mm². To calculate a WBC count, the number of cells counted on each side of the chamber is totaled. The average of the two sides is calculated. The numbers are then substituted into the formula:

$$\text{WBC/mm}^3 = \frac{\text{Average \# cells} \times 10 \times 20}{4 \text{ mm}^2}$$

$$= \text{Average \# cells} \times 50$$

A sample calculation for a WBC count is shown in Figure 2–33.

> *Precautions*
>
> ■ Observe all precautions for using blood diluting pipets and the hemacytometer.
> ■ If the number of cells in a large square varies from any other square on the same side by more than ten cells, repeat the count after cleaning and refillng the chamber.

UNOPETTE® MICROCOLLECTION SYSTEM

The most acceptable manual method of counting white cells is the use of self-filling, self-diluting systems such as Unopette®. Such a system provides greater accuracy than the pipet method, and the components are disposable (Figure 2–18).

Unopette® systems consist of a reservoir, a capillary pipet, and a pipet shield. The reservoir contains a pre-measured volume of diluting fluid. The capillary pipet is made to contain a specific volume. The shield protects the pipet and is used to puncture the diaphragm which seals the reservoir. The Unopette® system used for white cell counts contains 1.98 ml of diluting fluid in the reservoir. A 20 µl capillary pipet is used to measure the sample. When the sample is diluted in the reservoir, the resulting dilution is 1:100. This blood dilution is then loaded into a hemacytometer and the white cells are counted as in the manual pipet method.

Note: The dilution for Unopette® method is different from the dilution of white cells using the blood diluting pipet. The dilution factor which should be used for calculating the Unopette® white cell count is 100. The WBC count may also be performed and calculated as directed in the Unopette® package insert.

AUTOMATED WHITE CELL COUNTS

Almost all laboratories which perform hematology procedures have some type of automatic cell counter. The exceptions are specialty areas, where only one test is performed routinely. An example of this is an OB-Gyn practice, where only a hematocrit may be run to determine whether a patient is anemic. Many types of cell counters are available. Some of these are sophisticated, having the capability to perform the complete blood count, while others may perform only certain parts of the CBC. Two basic types of automatic cell counters are described briefly in Lesson 2–5.

Although automated cell counters aid in the efficiency of laboratories, manual counts are still performed in some circumstances. Therefore, laboratory personnel should be trained in performing manual WBC counts.

LESSON REVIEW

1. Give the normal WBC count for newborns, children, and adults.
2. Name three factors that may cause leukocytosis.
3. Name three factors that may cause leukopenia.
4. Describe the procedure for performing a WBC count.
5. What areas of the hemacytometer are used for a WBC count?
6. What dilution is made?
7. Write a formula for calculating the WBC count.
8. Name two WBC diluting fluids.
9. What is the function of a WBC diluting fluid?
10. Define immunity, leukocytosis, and leukopenia.

STUDENT ACTIVITIES

1. Re-read the information on the white blood cell count.
2. Review the glossary terms.
3. Practice performing WBC counts as outlined in the Student Performance Guide, using the worksheet.
4. Calculate the WBC counts when the average number of cells counted is 100; 125; and 175.

Student Performance Guide

NAME _____

DATE _____

LESSON 2–6
THE WHITE BLOOD CELL COUNT

Instructions

1. Practice performing and calculating a white cell count.
2. Demonstrate the white cell count satisfactorily for the instructor. All steps must be completed as listed on the instructor's Performance Check Sheet.
3. Complete a written examination successfully.

Materials and Equipment

- gloves
- surface disinfectant
- microscope
- chlorine bleach
- WBC diluting fluid
- WBC diluting pipet
- pipet filler
- hemacytometer with coverglass
- hand counter
- 70% alcohol
- lens paper
- soft tissue
- EDTA anticoagulated blood sample
- automatic pipet shaker (optional)
- pipet washer (optional)
- WBC worksheet
- hand disinfectant
- biohazard container

Procedure	S = Satisfactory U = Unsatisfactory		
You must:	**S**	**U**	**Comments**
1. Assemble equipment and materials			
2. Place a clean hemacytometer coverglass over a clean hemacytometer			
3. Attach pipet filler to WBC pipet			
4. Wash hands with disinfectant and put on gloves			
5. Tilt well-mixed tube of blood and insert pipet tip			
6. Draw blood up to the 0.5 mark on the pipet. *Note:* Do not allow blood to pass the 0.5 mark			
7. Wipe the excess blood from the outside of the pipet stem to avoid the transfer of cells to the diluting fluid (avoid touching the pipet with tissue)			
8. Draw the WBC diluting fluid up to the 11 mark on the pipet. *Note:* Do not fill the pipet past the 11 mark			
9. Place finger over the tip of pipet and remove the pipet filler			
10. Mix the contents of the pipet using the manual method or an automatic pipet shaker (see Lesson 2–3)			
11. Place the index finger over the top of the pipet to control the flow of fluid			
12. Discard the first 4 or 5 drops of fluid from the pipet			
13. Touch the tip of the pipet to the edge of the coverglass and counting chamber			
14. Allow the fluid to flow under the coverglass until one side of the chamber is completely full (usually one-half to one drop)			
15. Fill the opposite side of the chamber in the same manner			
16. Allow the cells to settle about two minutes			
17. Place hemacytometer on the microscope stage and secure			
18. Locate the ruled area of the chamber using the low power (10×) objective			

You must:	S	U	Comments
19. Locate the correct area for counting WBC (four large corner squares)			
20. Count all the WBCs lying within the four large corner squares (1, 2, 3, and 4) using the boundary rule			
21. Record results on worksheet			
22. Repeat steps 19–20 using side 2			
23. Record results from side 2 on the worksheet			
24. Average the total cells counted on the two sides of the chamber			
25. Use the formula to calculate the WBC count and record on worksheet			
26. Disinfect pipets, hemacytometer and coverglass with chlorine bleach			
27. Clean WBC pipet carefully			
28. Clean hemacytometer and coverglass carefully			
29. Return equipment to proper storage			
30. Discard contaminated materials into biohazard container			
31. Clean work area with surface disinfectant			
32. Remove and discard gloves and wash hands with hand disinfectant			

Comments:

Student/Instructor:

Date:_____ Instructor:_____

Student Performance Guide

NAME _____

DATE _____

LESSON 2–6
WHITE BLOOD CELL COUNT
(UNOPETTE® METHOD)

Instructions

1. Practice performing and calculating a white cell count using the Unopette®.
2. Perform the white cell count procedure satisfactorily for the instructor. All steps must be completed as listed on the instructor's Performance Check Sheet.
3. Complete a written examination successfully.

Materials and Equipment

- gloves
- hand disinfectant
- blood sample, anticoagulated with EDTA
- hemacytometer with coverglass
- test tube rack or beaker to hold blood sample
- Unopette® for WBC count (reservoir and pipet assembly)
- microscope
- lens paper
- alcohol (70% ethanol)
- hand tally counter
- surface disinfectant
- biohazard container

Note: The following is a general procedure for the use of the Unopette® system. Consult the package insert for specific instructions. An alternate method of performing and calculating a WBC count is also given in the package insert.

Procedure

S = Satisfactory
U = Unsatisfactory

You must:	S	U	Comments
1. Assemble equipment and materials			
2. Place a clean hemacytometer coverglass over a clean hemacytometer			
3. Wash hands with disinfectant and put on gloves			
4. Puncture the diaphragm of the Unopette® reservoir. Hold the reservoir firmly on a flat surface with one hand and use the tip of the pipet shield to puncture the diaphragm. *Note:* The opening must be made large enough to easily accommodate the pipet			
5. Remove the shield from the pipet assembly			
6. Fill the capillary pipet from a capillary puncture or from a tube of well-mixed EDTA anticoagulated blood. The pipet will fill by capillary action and will stop filling automatically. *Note:* Keep pipet horizontal or at a slight (5°) angle to avoid overfilling			
7. Wipe excess blood from the outside of the capillary pipet with soft laboratory tissue. *Note:* Do not allow tissue to touch pipet tip			
8. Squeeze the reservoir slightly, being careful not to expel any of the liquid			
9. Maintain the pressure on the reservoir and insert the capillary pipet into the reservoir, seating the pipet firmly into the neck of the reservoir. Do not expel any of the liquid			
10. Release the pressure on the reservoir, drawing the blood out of the capillary pipet into the diluent			
11. Squeeze the reservoir gently three to four times to rinse the remaining blood from the capillary pipet. *Note:* Do not allow the blood-diluent mixture to flow out the top			
12. Mix the contents of the reservoir thoroughly by gently swirling the reservoir and/or turning it side to side			
13. Let the reservoir sit 5 to 10 minutes until red cells are completely destroyed. Do not allow it to stand longer than 1 hour			

You must:	S	U	Comments
14. Withdraw the capillary pipet from the reservoir and place into the neck of the reservoir in reverse position (the pipet tip should now project upward from the reservoir)			
15. Mix the contents of the reservoir thoroughly. Invert the reservoir and gently squeeze to discard 4–5 drops onto gauze or paper towel			
16. Fill both sides of the hemacytometer			
17. Place the hemacytometer on the microscope stage carefully and secure			
18. Use the low power (10×) objective to bring the ruled area into focus			
19. Locate the WBC counting area (four large corner squares)			
20. Count the WBCs lying within the four large corner squares using the boundary rule			
21. Record the results			
22. Repeat the count using the other side of the hemacytometer			
23. Record the results			
24. Use the formula to calculate the WBC count. *Note:* The Unopette® dilution is 1:100. This differs from the dilution used when using the WBC pipet $$C/mm^3 \ = \ \frac{Avg \times D\ (mm) \times DF}{A\ (mm^2)}$$			
25. Disinfect hemacytometer and coverglass			
26. Discard specimen and disposable materials appropriately			
27. Return equipment to proper storage			
28. Clean work area with disinfectant			
29. Remove and discard gloves appropriately and wash hands with hand disinfectant			

Comments:

Student/Instructor:

Date:_____   Instructor:_____

Worksheet

NAME_____ DATE_____

LESSON 2–6 THE WHITE BLOOD CELL COUNT

Side 1	WBC Pipet Method Number of cells counted	Unopette® Method Number of cells counted
Square 1	_____	_____
Square 2	_____	_____
Square 3	_____	_____
Square 4	_____	_____
Total cells counted side 1 =	_____	_____

Side 2	Number of cells counted	Number of cells counted
Square 1	_____	_____
Square 2	_____	_____
Square 3	_____	_____
Square 4	_____	_____
Total cells counted side 2 =	_____	_____
Total of sides 1 and 2 =	_____	
Average of two sides (divide by 2) =	_____	_____

	WBC Pipet Method		Unopette® Method	
Multiply average number of cells × 10 × 20 and divide by 4 =	_____	Multiply average × 10 × 100 and divide by 4 =	_____
or		or	
Multiply average number of cells by 50 =	_____	Multiply average by 250 =	_____
WBC/mm^3 =	_____	WBC/mm^3 =	_____

LESSON 2–7
Hemoglobin Determination

LESSON OBJECTIVES

After studying this lesson, you should be able to:
- List the two main components of hemoglobin.
- State the function of hemoglobin.
- List the manual and automated methods for determining hemoglobin and explain them.
- List the normal hemoglobin values for children and adults.
- Perform a hemoglobin determination using a cyanmethemoglobin method.
- List the precautions to be observed when performing the hemoglobin determination.
- Define the glossary terms.

GLOSSARY

cyanmethemoglobin / a stable compound formed when hemoglobin is combined with Drabkin's reagent

Drabkin's reagent / a diluting reagent used for hemoglobin determination which contains iron, potassium, cyanide, and sodium bicarbonate

globin / the portion of the hemoglobin molecule composed of protein

heme / the portion of the hemoglobin molecule containing iron

hemoglobin / a red blood cell constituent which is composed of heme and globin and which carries oxygen to the tissues of the body; abbreviated "Hb" or "Hgb"

Sahli pipet / a pipet with a volume of 0.02 ml which was formerly widely used for manual hemoglobin determinations

synthesis / combination of parts or elements into a whole

THE HEMOGLOBIN MOLECULE

Hemoglobin is the main constituent of red blood cells. This molecule gives the characteristic red color to erythrocytes and to the blood because of the large number of red blood cells. The main function of hemoglobin is to transport oxygen (O_2) to the tissue cells of the body and to carry the carbon dioxide (CO_2) from the tissues to the lungs to be expelled.

The hemoglobin molecule is composed of two substances, **heme** and **globin.** The heme portion of the molecule requires iron for its **synthesis.** If the diet is deficient in iron-containing foods, the red cells will not contain enough hemoglobin. When the red cells contain less than the normal amount of hemoglobin, their oxygen-carrying capacity is decreased and the patient suffers symptoms of anemia.

NORMAL HEMOGLOBIN VALUES

The hemoglobin value at birth is normally in the range of 16–23 g/dl. In the early childhood years the value declines and 10–14 g/dl is considered normal. When children begin the rapid growth period associated with adolescence, the hemoglobin values increase until adult levels are reached. Adult males usually have a value in the range of 13.5–17.5 g/dl and females have values of 12.5–15.5 g/dl. The normal hemoglobin values are listed in Table 2–4.

Factors Affecting Hemoglobin Levels

There are several factors which influence the amount of hemoglobin. The diet must contain adequate amounts of iron in order for the red cells to synthesize the hemoglobin molecule. Certain foods are higher in iron content than others; for example, red meat has more iron than cow's milk. If the diet is deficient in iron, the condition of iron deficiency anemia will develop.

The hemoglobin value is affected by the age and gender of the patient. Normally, males have

Table 2–4. Normal hemoglobin values

Age/Sex	Hemoglobin Range (g/dl)
newborn	16.0-23.0
children	10.0-14.0
adult males	13.5-17.5
adult females	12.5-15.5

higher hemoglobin values than females in the child-bearing years. Newborns have higher values than both children and adults.

People who live at high altitudes have hemoglobin values which are higher than those of people who live at lower altitudes. The reason for this is that more red cells are required to carry sufficient oxygen since the air pressure is lower (thinner) than it is at sea level.

DETERMINING HEMOGLOBIN LEVELS

The hemoglobin test is used to indirectly evaluate the oxygen-carrying capacity of the blood. Hemoglobin determination may be performed on either capillary or venous blood. It may be requested as an individual test or as part of a CBC.

Various methods of determining hemoglobin have been used through the years. Early methods utilized the addition of acid or alkali to a blood sample. Newer procedures based on various principles have been developed. Some of the most commonly used ones are the specific gravity technique, traditional cyanmethemoglobin method, and methods that utilize the technology of discrete analyzers. (These analyzers are described in Lesson 7–4.)

Methods of Determining Hemoglobin

Specific Gravity Technique. This method gives only an estimate of hemoglobin concentration and requires no special instrument. A drop of blood is dropped into a pre-prepared copper

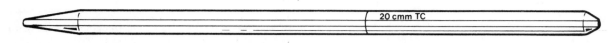

Figure 2–34. Sahli pipet

sulfate ($CuSO_4$) solution of a particular density or specific gravity. If the drop falls to the bottom of the container rapidly, the specific gravity of the blood is greater than the specific gravity of the copper sulfate. Blood with the normal amount of hemoglobin falls rapidly; blood with a low hemoglobin concentration does not fall rapidly. This test is not routinely performed in the United States except as a method of screening blood donors. However, many blood centers now estimate hemoglobin indirectly by determining the hematocrit.

Cyanmethemoglobin. This is the most widely-used method of determining hemoglobin concentration in blood. In this method, blood is reacted with **Drabkin's reagent** which contains iron, potassium, cyanide, and sodium bicarbonate. The Drabkin's and the hemoglobin combine to form a very stable end product, **cyanmethemoglobin.**

The use of Drabkin's and the formation of a stable compound such as cyanmethemoglobin was an advancement in hematology because for the first time stable hemoglobin standards were available. A standard solution of hemoglobin made with Drabkin's is accurate for at least six months. This means that laboratories have a stable, reliable material to use to standardize their hemoglobin assays.

Manual Methods

The concentration of hemoglobin can be determined by any of several manual methods. One method used for years involves adding 20 µl (0.02 ml) of blood measured in a Sahli-Helige pipette (Figure 2–34) to 4.98 ml of Drabkin's solution in a test tube or cuvette. A **Sahli** pipet is a glass pipet which will dispense 20 µl. The solution is mixed thoroughly and allowed to stand for 10 minutes. At the end of the reaction period, the absorbance of the cyanmethemoglobin is read in a spectrophotometer at 540 nm. This absorbance is compared to the absorbance of a standard of known concentration, usually 15 or 20 g/dl, read at 540 nm. The concentration of the unknown (patient) sample is calculated by using the formula:

$$\frac{C_u}{C_s} = \frac{A_u}{A_s}$$

Where: A_u = absorbance of unknown
A_s = absorbance of standard
C_u = concentration of unknown
C_s = concentration of standard

Therefore:

$$C_u = \frac{A_u}{A_s} \times C_s$$

Another manual method involves the use of a Unopette® system. For hemoglobin determination, the blood is drawn up into the Unopette® capillary (20 µl) and added to 4.98 ml of a modified Drabkin's solution in the reservoir. After ten minutes, the absorbance is read at 540 nm and compared to a standard as in the Sahli method (Figure 2–35).

Both the Sahli and the Unopette® methods require the use of a spectrophotometer, which is discussed in Lesson 7–3. If the student is not familiar with the operation of the spectrophotometer, Lesson 7–3 should be completed before attempting to make a hemoglobin determination.

Recently, another method has been marketed by ISOLAB, Inc. This method, called Hb-Direct™, is noteworthy because of its unique method of collecting the sample and reading the results

Given the following values, use the absorbance formula to find the hemoglobin concentration of the unknown:

$$A_s = 0.600$$
$$A_u = 0.300$$
$$C_s = 20 \text{ g/dl}$$

Use the absorbance formula:

$$\frac{C_u(\text{g/dl})}{C_s(\text{g/dl})} = \frac{A_u}{A_s}$$

Substitute the values given:

$$\frac{C_u(\text{g/dl})}{20 \text{ g/dl}} = \frac{0.300}{0.600}$$

$C_u = 10.0$ g/dl. Therefore, the unknown hemoglobin = 10.0 g/dl.

Figure 2–35. Sample calculation of hemoglobin using the absorbance formula

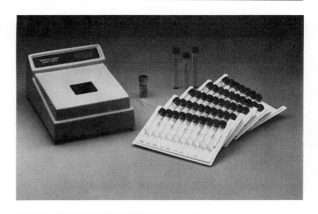

Figure 2–36. The Hb-Direct™ system. The Hemoglobin Analyzer, cuvettes, and collecting tubes. (*Photo courtesy of ISOLAB, Inc.*)

(Figure 2–36). The Hb-Direct™ also uses 20 µl of blood added to Drabkin's. The difference in this and other manual methods is in the collection of the sample and its addition to the Drabkin's. The kit supplies capillary tubes into which 20 µl of blood can be drawn directly from a capillary puncture. The capillary tube, containing the sample, is dropped into a pre-measured quantity of Drabkin's reagent. The Drabkin's is supplied in tubes which are used as cuvettes in the Hemoglobin Analyzer, a special spectrophotometer. After five minutes, the tubes are placed into the spectrophotometer. This spectrophotometer, called a dedicated spectrophotometer, is pre-set to read the absorbance of the methemoglobin. The hemoglobin concentration is displayed in g/dl. There are no calculations required. To assure quality control, both a calibrator and standard set are available.

Automated Methods

Many varieties of instruments used for other hematology analyses also perform hemoglobin determinations. Many of these offer convenience

and safety for the worker because the sample is aspirated from the capped tube by a probe which penetrates the stopper. One example of this type of instrument is the Cellect 8 Hematology Analyzer manufactured by Instrumentation Laboratory. New methods for hemoglobin determination are constantly being developed. The manufacturers of several analyzers which are used for clinical chemistry either already offer hemoglobin assays for their instruments or plan to do so. Some of these involve the technology of solid-phase or centrifugal analysis using the principles described in Lesson 7–4. (The mention of instruments in this lesson does not constitute endorsement of the instrument, just as omission of an instrument(s) does not imply lack of endorsement.)

LESSON REVIEW

1. What are the two main components of hemoglobin?
2. Discuss the function of hemoglobin.

3. What is the importance of the development of cyanmethemoglobin standards?
4. List three methods of hemoglobin determination.
5. Give the normal hemoglobin values for children and adults.
6. List some precautions to be observed when making a hemoglobin determination using Drabkin's.
7. Define cyanmethemoglobin, Drabkin's reagent, globin, heme, hemoglobin, Sahli pipet, spectrophotometer, and synthesis.

STUDENT ACTIVITIES

1. Re-read the information on hemoglobin.
2. Review the glossary terms.
3. Practice the procedure for determining hemoglobin as listed on the Student Performance Guide.
4. Inquire at physicians' offices or anemia screening clinics in the community to find out what methods of hemoglobin determination are in use.

Student Performance Guide

NAME _____

DATE _____

LESSON 2–7
HEMOGLOBIN DETERMINATION
HB-DIRECT™ METHOD

Instructions

1. Practice performing a hemoglobin determination.
2. Demonstrate the hemoglobin procedure satisfactorily for the instructor. All steps must be completed as listed on the instructor's Performance Check Sheet.
3. Complete a written examination successfully.

Materials and Equipment

- gloves
- capillary puncture equipment
- biohazard container
- Hb-Direct™ system (obtain supplies specified by manufacturer)
- hand disinfectant
- surface disinfectant
- puncture-proof container for sharp objects

Note: Consult manufacturer's instructions for specific procedure.

Procedure			S = Satisfactory U = Unsatisfactory
You must:	**S**	**U**	**Comments**
1. Wash hands with disinfectant and put on gloves			
2. Assemble equipment and materials for Hb-Direct™ method			
3. Perform capillary puncture using aseptic techniques. Wipe away first drop of blood with a tissue or sterile cotton ball.			
4. Put end of 20 µl pipet, supplied by manufacturer, into second drop of blood and fill by capillary action			

You must:	S	U	Comments
5. Wipe excess blood from outside of tube with a clean laboratory tissue, being careful not to touch the open end of pipet			
6. Insert a filled capillary tube into one cyanmethemoglobin vial. Place cap tightly on vial and invert gently 5–10 times until capillary tube is completely evacuated of blood. (The light red reaction color is stable for 5 days at room temperature, 20–25°C)			
7. Let stand at room temperature for 5 minutes			
8. Insert vial into the Hemoglobin Analyzer, using the following procedure (these steps should be followed closely to insure that the capillary tube does not obstruct the Analyzer light path): a. Invert the vial slowly, then hold it horizontally for three seconds. As the vial is slowly returned to its upright position, the capillary tube should adhere to the upper side of the vial b. Position the vial so that the capillary tube is at the BACK of the vial c. Wipe fingerprints from sides of vial with tissue d. Check that reagent vial is tightly capped e. Insert vial into Hemoglobin Analyzer with capillary tube positioned to back of vial f. Wait five seconds. Read Analyzer display. Check to insure that the capillary tube has remained in the upper half of the vial			
9. Read hemoglobin concentration directly off the display in g/dl and record			
10. Return all equipment to proper storage			
11. Dispose of all contaminated materials in biohazard container			
12. Wipe counters with surface disinfectant			
13. Remove and discard gloves into appropriate container			
14. Wash hands with hand disinfectant			

Comments:

Student/Instructor:

Date:_____ Instructor:_____

Student Performance Guide

NAME _____

DATE _____

LESSON 2–7
HEMOGLOBIN DETERMINATION USING THE SAHLI PIPET

Instructions

1. Practice the procedure for determining hemoglobin concentration.
2. Demonstrate the procedure for hemoglobin determination satisfactorily for the instructor. All steps must be completed as listed on the instructor's Performance Check Sheet.
3. Complete a written examination successfully.

Materials and Equipment

- gloves
- hand disinfectant
- spectrophotometer
- graduated pipet, 5 ml
- cuvette
- blood sample
- Sahli pipet
- Drabkin's reagent
- pipet filler
- test tubes
- standard hemoglobin solution (20 g/dl)
- safety bulb for pipet or automatic pipetter
- parafilm
- surface disinfectant
- biohazard container

Note: Consult operating manual for specific instructions for spectrophotometer.

Procedure			S = Satisfactory U = Unsatisfactory
You must:	**S**	**U**	**Comments**
1. Wash hands with disinfectant and put on gloves			
2. Assemble equipment and materials			
3. Turn on spectrophotometer			
4. Set wavelength at 540 nm			
5. Label two test tubes: blank and unknown			
6. Dispense 5.0 ml of Drabkin's reagent into each test tube using a safety bulb and a 5 ml pipet			
7. Attach pipet filler to Sahli pipet			
8. Draw blood up to 0.02 ml (20 µl) mark on the pipet			
9. Wipe excess blood from exterior of pipet with tissue			
10. Dispense blood sample into the unknown tube			
11. Rinse the pipet at least 3 times with the solution in the tube by alternately aspirating the solution into the pipet and gently dispensing it			
12. Mix contents of test tube thoroughly and let it stand for at least ten minutes (tubes can be mixed by inverting after placing parafilm over the top of the tube)			
13. Transfer contents of the blank tube to a cuvette; place cuvette in the well of spectrophotometer; set absorbance to zero following manufacturer's instructions			
14. Transfer contents of unknown tube to a cuvette; place cuvette in the well of spectrophotometer			
15. Read the absorbance and record results			
16. Pipet 5.0 ml of 20 gm/dl hemoglobin standard into a cuvette; read the absorbance and record			
17. Use the following formula to calculate hemoglobin concentration and record results $$\frac{A_{unk}}{A_{std}} \times conc_{std} = Conc_{unk} \ (g/dl)$$			

You must:	S	U	Comments
18. Discard all specimens into biohazard container			
19. Clean equipment and return to proper storage		.	
20. Clean work area with surface disinfectant			
21. Remove and discard gloves into appropriate container and wash hands with hand disinfectant			

Comments:

Student/Instructor:

Date:_____   Instructor:_____

LESSON 2-8

Preparation of a Blood Smear

LESSON OBJECTIVES

After studying this lesson, you should be able to:
- Discuss the purpose and importance of the blood smear.
- List the components that may normally be observed in a blood smear.
- Prepare a blood smear.
- Preserve a blood smear.
- List the precautions to observe when preparing a blood smear.
- Define the glossary terms.

GLOSSARY

CBC / complete blood count; a commonly performed group of hematological tests

fixative / preservative; chemical which prevents deterioration of cells or tissues

morphology / study of form and structure of cells, tissues, organs

INTRODUCTION

Examining a stained blood smear is a routine part of the **CBC,** or complete blood count. A blood smear is prepared by spreading blood on a microscope slide. The smear is dried and stained. The blood components may then be viewed microscopically, identified, and evaluated, as in the white cell differential count. Careful examination of a well-prepared blood smear can provide valuable information to the physician in the diagnosis and treatment of many diseases such as leukemia, sickle cell anemia, and malaria.

A blood smear enables the technologist to view the cellular components of blood in as natural a state as possible. The **morphology,** or structure, of the cellular components can then be studied. The erythrocytes, leukocytes, and platelets are viewed to evaluate relative numbers, size, structure, and maturity. It is important that the cell morphology and relative distribution of cells are altered as little as possible while preparing the smear.

PREPARING A BLOOD SMEAR

The best specimen for a blood smear is capillary blood which has had no anticoagulant added. However, a satisfactory smear may be made from venous blood which has the anticoagulant EDTA

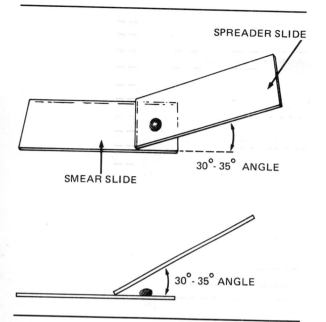

Figure 2–37. Positioning the spreader slide in front of the drop of blood

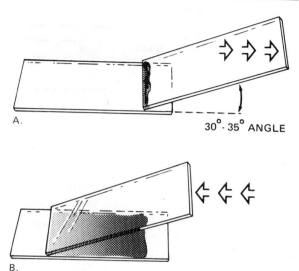

Figure 2–38. Spreading the blood with a spreader slide

added to it, provided the smear is made within two hours of collection. Other anticoagulants should not be used since they may alter the morphology or staining characteristics of the cells.

Cleaning the Slides

The slides that are used to make a blood smear must be entirely free of grease and dust. Slides may be purchased pre-cleaned. Or, slides may be washed with soap and water, rinsed thoroughly in hot water and then distilled water, dipped in 95% ethyl alcohol, and polished with a clean, lint-free cloth. Clean slides may be stored in 95% ethyl alcohol and should be handled by the edges only.

Making the Smear

There are several methods of spreading the blood on a slide which result in good smears. Each individual needs to find the technique that is least awkward and that provides good results. The blood smear can be prepared by placing one-half drop of blood about one-half to three-fourths inch from the right end (left end for left-handed) of a pre-cleaned slide which has been placed on a flat surface. The end of a second "spreader" slide is brought to rest at a 30–35° angle in front of the drop of blood (Figure 2–37). The spreader is then brought back into the drop of blood until the drop spreads along 3/4 of the edge of the spreader slide. This should be performed in a smooth, quick sliding motion. As soon as the blood spreads along the edge of the spreader, the spreader is pushed to the left (right for left-handed) with a quick, steady motion (avoiding pressure on the slide) to spread the blood (Figure 2–38). Each end of the spreader slide should be used only one time unless the slide is cleaned and kept unchipped. The smear is allowed to air dry as quickly as possible. It is then ready for staining or preserving.

FEATURES OF A GOOD SMEAR

A well-prepared smear is illustrated in Figure 2–39. The smear should cover about one-half to three-fourths of the slide and should show a

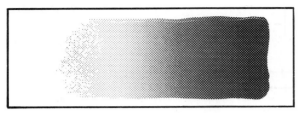

A.

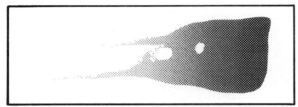

B.

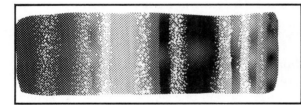

C.

Figure 2–39. Properly prepared smear A) vs improper smears B) and C)

gradual transition from thick to thin. It should have a smooth appearance with no holes or ridges and should have a feathered edge (about 1.5 cm long) at the thin end. When the smear is examined microscopically, the cells should be distributed evenly.

FACTORS AFFECTING SMEAR QUALITY

The length and thickness of the smear are affected by the size of the drop of blood and the angle at which the spreader slide is held. Thick smears occur when the angle of the spreader is too high or the drop of blood is too large. Thin smears occur when the drop is too small or the angle is too low. Thin, uneven smears may also occur when too much pressure is applied to the spreader. The faster the spreading procedure, the thinner the smear.

Drying time may affect the appearance of the cellular elements. If high humidity causes slow drying, the cells may appear abnormal. For example, the red blood cells may appear moth-eaten.

PRESERVING AND STAINING THE SMEAR

Dried smears should be stained immediately. If this is not possible, however, the slide may be immersed in methanol in a Coplin jar for thirty to sixty seconds and allowed to air dry. It may then be stained at a later date. The methanol is a **fixative** or preservative that prevents changes or deterioration of cellular components.

Precautions

■ Methanol is poisonous; do not inhale fumes; wash hands thoroughly.

■ The spreader slide should have a clean, polished end to prevent holes and streaks in the smear.

■ The drop of blood should not be too small or too large.

■ Delay between applying the drop and spreading the drop may cause uneven cell distribution.

■ Hesitation or jerky motion when spreading the blood will cause uneven cell distribution.

■ Smears should be stained within one to two hours after preparation or should be preserved.

■ Smears should be dried as quickly as possible (do not blow on slides to dry them).

■ To prevent clotting of the blood, capillary blood must be spread immediately.

LESSON REVIEW

1. What is the purpose of a blood smear?
2. What components in the blood can be viewed on a smear?
3. What specimen(s) may be used for blood smears?
4. Explain the two-slide method for making a blood smear.
5. What are some of the errors to avoid when making a blood smear?
6. Describe and diagram the appearance of a properly prepared blood smear.
7. How may unstained blood smears be preserved?
8. Define CBC, fixative, and morphology.

STUDENT ACTIVITIES

1. Re-read the information on preparing a blood smear.
2. Review the glossary terms.
3. Practice preparing blood smears by the two-slide method as outlined on the Student Performance Guide.

Student Performance Guide

NAME _____

DATE _____

LESSON 2–8
PREPARATION OF A
BLOOD SMEAR

Instructions

1. Practice preparing a blood smear.
2. Demonstrate the procedure for preparation of a blood smear satisfactorily for the instructor. All steps must be completed as listed on the instructor's Performance Check Sheet.
3. Complete a written examination successfully.

Materials and Equipment

- gloves
- hand disinfectant
- microscope slides
- 95% ethyl alcohol
- laboratory tissue
- capillary tubes (plain and heparinized)
- slide rack
- hot water
- detergent
- distilled water
- methanol in covered staining (Coplin) jar
- EDTA anticoagulated blood specimen (fresh)
- materials for capillary puncture
- surface disinfectant
- biohazard container
- puncture-proof container for sharp objects

Procedure

S = Satisfactory
U = Unsatisfactory

You must:	S	U	Comments
1. Assemble equipment and materials			
2. Prepare several clean slides: A. Use pre-cleaned slides, or B. Clean slides with soap, rinse with hot water followed by distilled water, dip in 95% ethyl alcohol, and polish dry with clean lint-free cloth			
3. Place a clean slide on a flat surface (be sure to touch only the edges of the slide with fingers)			
4. Wash hands with disinfectant and put on gloves			
5. Obtain an anticoagulated blood sample (provided by the instructor)			
6. Mix blood well and fill a plain capillary tube with blood			
7. Dispense a small drop of blood from the capillary tube onto the slide about one-half to three-fourths inch from the right end (if left-handed, reverse instructions)			
8. Place the end of a clean, polished unchipped spreader slide in front of the drop of blood at a 30–35° angle. Spreader should be lightly balanced with fingertips			
9. Pull the spreader slide back into the drop of blood by sliding gently along the slide until the blood spreads along three-fourths of the width of the spreader			
10. Push the spreader slide forward with a quick steady motion (use other hand to keep slide from moving while spreader is pushed)			
11. Examine the smear to see if it is satisfactory			
12. Repeat the procedure until two satisfactory smears are obtained			
13. Allow the smear to air dry quickly (slide may be waved gently to accelerate drying) and label the slide			
14. Place the dried smear in absolute methanol for thirty to sixty seconds to preserve the smear			
15. Remove the slide from methanol and allow to air dry			

You must:	S	U	Comments
16. Store slide for staining			
17. Perform a capillary puncture, wipe away the first drop of blood, and fill one or two heparinized capillary tubes			
18. Prepare two blood smears from capillary blood, repeating steps 7–16			
19. Discard blood specimens and contaminated materials into biohazard container			
20. Clean equipment and return to proper storage			
21. Clean work area with surface disinfectant			
22 Remove and discard gloves appropriately and wash hands with hand disinfectant			

Comments:

Student/Instructor:

Date:_____ Instructor:_____

LESSON 2–9
Staining a Blood Smear

LESSON OBJECTIVES

After studying this lesson, you should be able to:
- Discuss the purpose of staining blood smears.
- Explain what information may be obtained from a stained blood smear.
- Stain a blood smear.
- List precautions to be observed for proper staining of a blood smear.
- Define the glossary terms.

GLOSSARY

buffer / a substance which prevents changes in the pH of solutions when additional acid or base is added

cytoplasm / the fluid portion of the cell outside the nucleus

eosin / a dye that produces a red stain

methylene blue / a dye that produces a blue stain

nucleus, nuclei / the central structure of a cell which contains DNA and controls cell growth and function

polychromatic / multicolored

INTRODUCTION

Stains are applied to blood smears so that the formed elements may be more easily viewed and evaluated. A stained blood smear can provide important information regarding a patient's health. The evaluation of a blood smear often leads to the diagnosis or verification of disease.

A stained blood smear is evaluated in a procedure called the leukocyte differential count. Stained smears may also be examined to identify blood parasites such as those that cause malaria. Bone marrow smears may be examined to evaluate blood cell production.

TYPES OF STAINS

The stains commonly used for the routine microscopic examination of blood are called **polychromatic.** These stains are thus named because they contain dyes that will stain various components of cells different colors. Most polychromatic blood stains contain combinations of **methylene blue,** a blue stain; **eosin,** a red-orange stain; and methyl alcohol, a fixative. The different dyes are attracted to the different cell structures. The cells and structures are thus more easily visualized and differentiated (hence the name diferential count). The two most commonly used blood stains are Wright's and Giemsa's.

SPECIAL STAINS

Information gained during routine blood smear evaluation may cause the physician to order special blood stains for further study. These special stains may be used to identify specific components of cells such as iron granules or nucleic acids.

STAINING PROCEDURES

Blood smears should be stained as soon as they have been thoroughly air-dried. If more than one or two hours will pass before staining, the smears should be preserved. Smears may be stained by a two-step method, quick-stain method, or by an automatic stainer. A quick-stain is adequate for most routine work, but the two-step method (or automatic stainer) should be used to evaluate cell abnormalities and bone marrow cells.

Two-Step Method

In a two-step method, a stain such as Wright's stain is applied to the slide for approximately 1–3 minutes (Figure 2–40). Fixation occurs in this step because of the methyl alcohol in the stain. A **buffer** is then added to the stain until the buffer volume is about equal to the stain volume (Figure 2–41). Buffers are substances which prevent changes in the pH of solutions when additional acid or base is added. The stain is gently blown until a green metallic sheen appears (this occurs when the solutions mix), usually two to four minutes (Figure 2–42). Times may vary according to the stain and buffer used. The slide is rinsed gently, allowed to air dry, and can then be examined using the microscope.

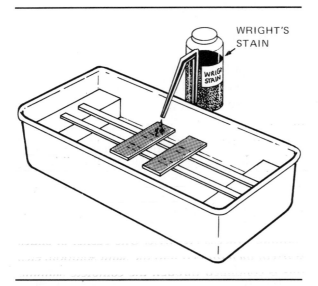

Figure 2–40. Applying Wright's stain to a blood smear

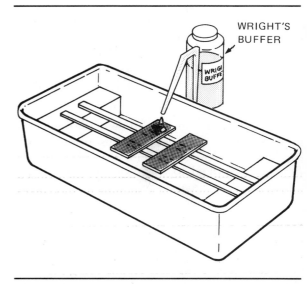

Figure 2–41. Applying buffer to Wright's stain

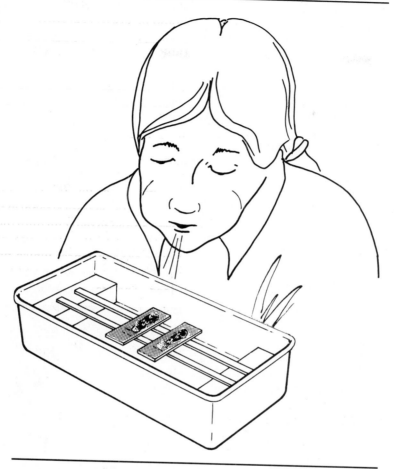

Figure 2–42. Mixing buffer and stain

Quick Stains

Quick stains, which are variations of the polychromatic stains, are available in kits from several companies. In these quick stains, the slide is dipped into two or three solutions quickly, then rinsed and dried. The entire quick-staining method takes less than a minute whereas the two-step method requires 4–6 minutes. It may be easier for the inexperienced technician to obtain an adequate stain with quick methods, but experienced technicians can achieve superior results using the two-step method.

Automatic Stainers

Blood smears may also be stained by use of automatic stainers. There are two basic types of stainers. In one type of stainer, the slides are placed on a moving belt which carries them through the various staining reagents. The other type of stainer is the "basket" or "batch" type in which baskets of slides are taken through the staining process stepwise. One basket of slides is fixed, then dipped into the stain solution, etc.; this is continued through the complete staining process.

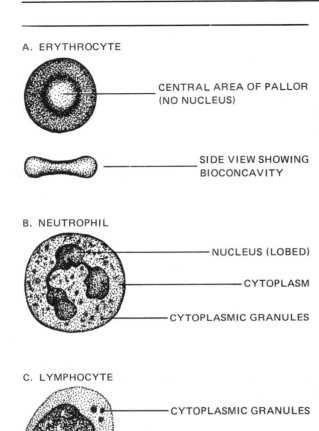

A. ERYTHROCYTE

CENTRAL AREA OF PALLOR (NO NUCLEUS)

SIDE VIEW SHOWING BIOCONCAVITY

B. NEUTROPHIL

NUCLEUS (LOBED)

CYTOPLASM

CYTOPLASMIC GRANULES

C. LYMPHOCYTE

CYTOPLASMIC GRANULES

CYTOPLASM

NUCLEUS

Figure 2–43. Parts of a A) stained erythrocyte, B) segmented neutrophil, and C) lymphocyte

Automatic stainers are an advantage when large numbers of slides must be stained or staining must be performed frequently during a workday. A disadvantage of automatic stainers is that if the stain is bad, the worker may not know until many slides have been processed.

EVALUATING STAIN QUALITY

A properly stained smear should appear pinkish-purple to the naked eye. When viewed microscopically, the red cells should appear pinkish-tan. The **nucleus**, or central structure, of the leukocytes should appear purple. The leukocyte **cytoplasm,** or area surrounding the nucleus, may vary from pink to blue or blue-gray, depending on the cell type (Figure 2–43). Variations in color intensities may be due to pH, timing, or characteristics of the stain and/or buffer. Colors are best evaluated using the oil immersion objective. Some hints for correcting poor stains are given in the Precautions section.

STORAGE OF STAINED SMEARS

Stained smears should be stored in the dark in a dust-free slide box or container. If protected from light when not in use, the stains will last for years with little fading. Surfaces may be protected from scratches by mounting a permanent coverglass over the smear. For routine work, however, this is not necessary.

Precautions

■ Handle methyl alcohol with care; it is poisonous.
■ Store stains tightly capped to prevent absorption of moisture.
■ Stains may precipitate and should be filtered often.
■ Stains should not be allowed to dry on the slide before rinsing.
■ Slides should be rinsed thoroughly after staining.
■ Proper staining and buffering times should be observed for best staining results.
■ Slides that are too pink may be due to (1) pH of stain or buffer too acidic, (2) wash time too long, or (3) stain time too short.
■ Slides that are too blue may be due to (1) overstaining, (2) wash time or buffering time too short, or (3) pH of stain or buffer too alkaline.
■ To avoid getting stain on hands and clothing, wear gloves and lab coats and handle slides with forceps.

LESSON REVIEW

1. What is the purpose of staining blood smears?
2. What observations can be made from a stained blood smear?
3. Explain what is meant by polychromatic stains.
4. What two dyes are usually components of polychromatic blood stains?
5. Name two types of commonly used blood stains.
6. Which provides the most satisfactory stain, the two-step method or the quick stains?
7. How should a properly stained smear appear?
8. What is the proper method of storing slides?
9. Name four precautions that must be observed to achieve good staining results.
10. Define buffer, cytoplasm, eosin, methylene blue, nucleus, and polychromatic.

STUDENT ACTIVITIES

1. Re-read the information on staining a blood smear.
2. Review the glossary terms.
3. Practice staining blood smears by the two-step method as outlined on the Student Performance Guide.
4. Practice staining blood smears by a quick method.
5. Compare smears stained by the two-step and quick methods. Observe the most desired effect.
6. Experiment with variations in the staining and buffering times using the two-step method. Explain the results.

Student Performance Guide

NAME _____

DATE _____

LESSON 2–9
STAINING A BLOOD SMEAR

Instructions

1. Practice staining a blood smear.
2. Demonstrate the procedure for staining a blood smear satisfactorily for the instructor. All steps must be completed as listed on the instructor's Performance Check Sheet.
3. Complete a written examination successfully.

Materials and Equipment

- gloves
- hand disinfectant
- blood smears, freshly prepared or preserved
- Wright's stain and buffer
- staining rack
- immersion oil
- microscope
- lens paper
- forceps
- laboratory tissue
- lab apron or lab coat
- quick stain (optional)
- staining jars (optional)
- surface disinfectant
- biohazard container
- puncture-proof container for sharp objects

Note: Stain characteristics may vary with stain lot. Follow manufacturer's instructions for best results.

Procedure

S = Satisfactory
U = Unsatisfactory

You must:	S	U	Comments
1. Wash hands with disinfectant and put on gloves			
2. Assemble equipment and materials			
3. Obtain a dried blood smear			
4. Stain a blood smear by one of the following methods: A. Two-step method			
(1) Place the dried smear on the staining rack or on a flat surface, blood side up			
(2) Flood the smear with Wright's stain but do not let stain overflow the sides of the slide			
(3) Leave stain on slide 1–3 minutes (get exact time from instructor)			
(4) Add buffer, dropwise, to the stain until the buffer volume is about equal to the stain			
(5) Blow gently on the surface of the fluid to mix the solutions. A green metallic sheen should appear on the surface			
(6) Allow buffer to remain on slide for 2–4 minutes (do not allow mixture to run off slide); get exact time from instructor			
(7) Rinse thoroughly and continuously with a gentle stream of tap or distilled water			
(8) Drain water from slide			
(9) Wipe the back of the slide with a wet gauze to remove excess stain			
(10) Stand smear on end to dry or			
B. Quick stain			
(1) Dip dry smear into solutions as directed by manufacturer's instructions (do not allow slide to dry between solutions)			
(2) Rinse slide (if instructed to do so)			
(3) Remove excess stain from the back of the slide with wet gauze			
(4) Allow slide to air dry by standing on end			
5. Place thoroughly-dried slide on microscope stage, stain side up			
6. Focus with low power (10×) objective			

You must:	S	U	Comments
7. Scan slide to find area where cells are barely touching each other (in feathered edge of smear)			
8. Place a drop of immersion oil on the slide			
9. Rotate oil immersion lens carefully into position			
10. Focus with fine adjustment knob only			
11. Observe erythrocytes; color should be pinkish-tan			
12. Observe leukocytes; nuclei should be purple			
13. Observe platelets; they should appear purple and granular			
14. Rotate 10× objective into position			
15. Remove slide from microscope stage			
16. Clean oil objective thoroughly with lens paper			
17. Wipe oil from slide gently with soft tissue			
18. Clean equipment and return to proper storage			
19. Discard slides as instructed			
20. Clean work area with surface disinfectant			
21. Remove and discard gloves appropriately and wash hands with hand disinfectant			

Comments:

Student/Instructor:

Date:_____ Instructor:_____

HEMATOLOGY

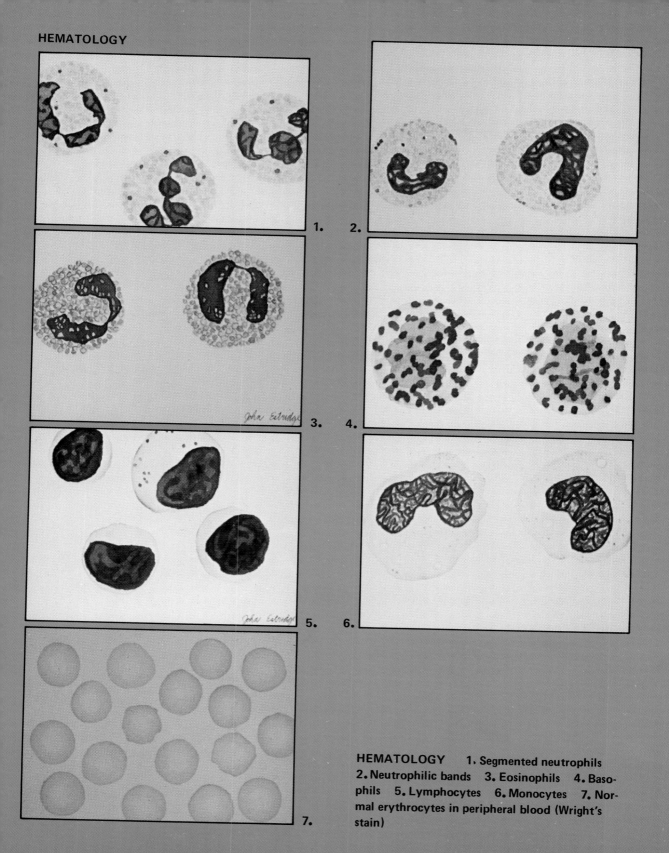

HEMATOLOGY 1. Segmented neutrophils
2. Neutrophilic bands 3. Eosinophils 4. Basophils 5. Lymphocytes 6. Monocytes 7. Normal erythrocytes in peripheral blood (Wright's stain)

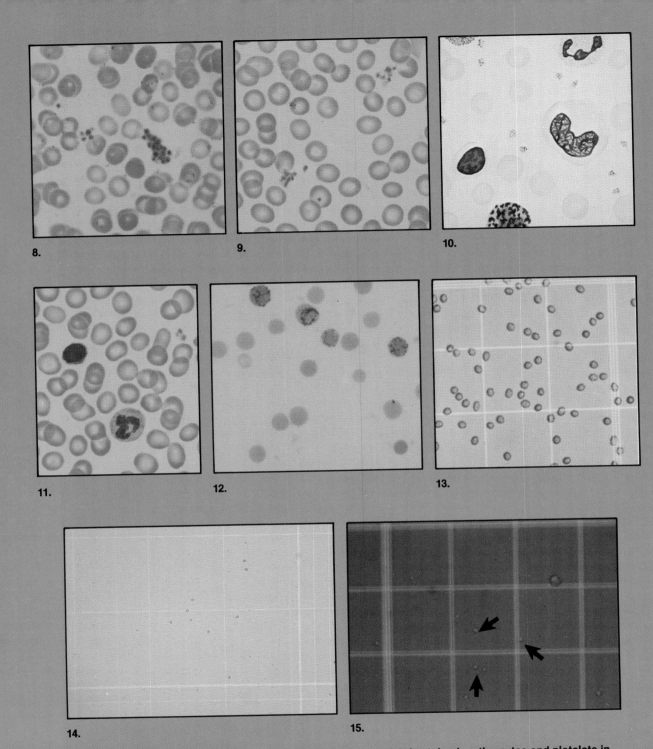

8. Platelets in peripheral blood (1000X)   **9.** Photomicrograph of Wright's stained erythrocytes and platelets in peripheral blood (1000X)   **10.** Examples of blood cells seen in peripheral blood smear from normal individual   **11.** Photomicrograph of lymphocyte and segmented neutrophil (1000X)   **12.** Photomicrograph of reticulocytes stained with New Methylene Blue (1000X)   **13.** Photomicrograph of erythrocytes as they appear in an RBC count (400X)   **14.** Photomicrograph of leukocytes as they appear in a hemacytometer (100X)   **15.** Photomicrograph of platelets (arrows) as they appear in a platelet count (400X)

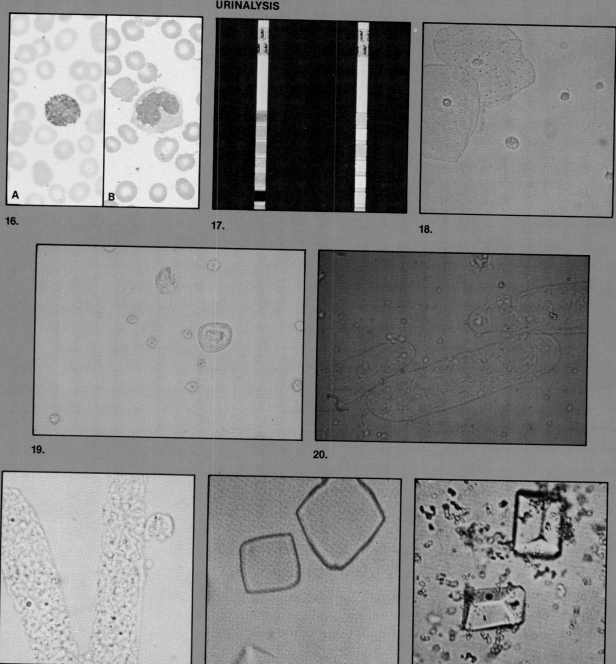

URINALYSIS

16.

17.

18.

19.

20.

21.

22.

23.

16. Normal peripheral blood. A. basophil B. monocyte   URINALYSIS   17. Reagent strips used for chemical analysis of urine (positive reactions, Left)   18. Squamous epithelial cells, red blood cells, leukocyte   19. Renal epithelial cell and erythrocytes   20. Hyaline casts   21. Granular casts and a leukocyte   22. Two uric acid crystals   23. Two ammonium magnesium phosphate crystals (triple phosphate) with amorphous phosphate granules

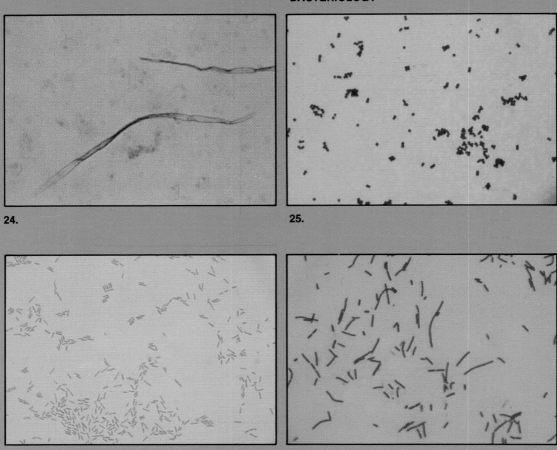

24.

25.

26.

27.

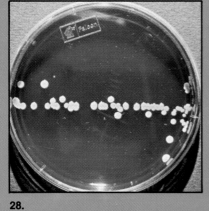

28.

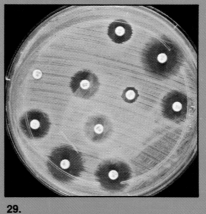

29.

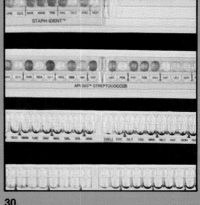

30.

24. Fibers in urine BACTERIOLOGY **25. Gram positive coccus from a pure culture** **26. Gram negative rod from a pure culture** **27. Gram positive bacillus from a pure culture** **28. A blood agar plate showing isolated colonies of bacteria** **29. Antibiotic susceptibility test plate** **30. Biochemical strip tests for bacterial identification**

LESSON 2–10
Identification of Normal Blood Cells

LESSON OBJECTIVES

After studying this lesson, you should be able to:
- State the importance of blood cell identification.
- List three features of cells which are evaluated in blood cell identification.
- Use the microscope to identify five types of leukocytes from a stained, normal blood smear.
- Identify platelets microscopically.
- Identify erythrocytes microscopically.
- List precautions to be observed in identifying cellular components of blood.
- Define the glossary terms.

GLOSSARY

band cell / an immature neutrophil with a non-segmented nucleus; a stab cell

basophil / a leukocyte containing basophilic-staining granules

basophilic / blue in color; having affinity for the basic stain

eosinophil / a leukocyte containing acid- or eosin-staining granules

lymphocyte / a small basophilic staining leukocyte having a round or oval nucleus and which is important in the immune process

megakaryocyte / a large bone marrow cell which releases platelets into the blood stream

monocyte / a large leukocyte which usually has a convoluted or horse-shoe shaped nucleus

neutrophil / a neutral staining leukocyte; first line of defense against infection

platelet / thrombocyte; a small, disc-shaped fragment of cytoplasm from a megakaryocyte which plays an important role in blood coagulation

vacuole / a clear space in cytoplasm filled with fluid or air

171

INTRODUCTION

Useful information can be gained from the microscopic identification and evaluation of blood cells from a stained smear. Many situations arise in medical practice in which the physician needs to know more concerning the blood cells than is provided by the cell counts alone. By microscopically viewing a blood smear, the technologist or physician can identify blood cells and evaluate any abnormalities present. Many hematologists say that more information is gained from a blood smear than from any other laboratory test.

The features of blood cells which must be observed and evaluated are: (1) cell size, (2) nuclear characteristics, and (3) cytoplasmic characteristics. The size of cells can be estimated by comparing them with red cells. The nucleus must be observed for shape, size, structure, and color. The cytoplasm is evaluated by noting the color, amount, and type of inclusions. When the information from these three observations is combined, the identification of most cells is possible. Beginners will find it necessary to consciously consider each of the properties of the cells. As experience is gained, the process becomes almost automatic for normal cells. Much practice is required to be able to recognize and classify the cells that may be seen in various disease states.

BLOOD CELLS IN A NORMAL BLOOD SMEAR

The cells usually seen in a normal blood smear are described below. The descriptions are for cells as they would appear in Wright's stained smears. A leukocyte identification guide with abbreviated descriptions is given in Table 2–5, and Color Plates 1–10 depict typical appearances of stained cells.

Erythrocytes

Red cells are the most numerous of the blood cells. Normal mature red cells stain pink-tan, have no nuclei, and are 6–8 micrometers in diameter. The pink-tan color is due to the staining of hemoglobin within the cells. Red cells are shaped like biconcave discs. Because they are thin in the center, the central area of the cell is paler than the margins. This is called the "central area of pallor."

Platelets

Platelets, or thrombocytes, are the smallest of the stained blood elements. They are usually two to three micrometers in diameter, or one-third the diameter of a red cell. No nucleus is present because the platelet is simply a fragment of cytoplasm from a large bone marrow cell called a **megakaryocyte.** The cytoplasm stains bluish and usually contains small reddish-purple granules. Platelets may be round, oval, or have spiny projections.

Leukocytes

The leukocytes are the largest of the normal blood components. Their sizes range from slightly larger than a red cell to more than twice the diameter of a red cell. Each of the five types of leukocytes has a characteristic appearance. The granular leukocytes —neutrophil, eosinophil, and basophil—contain many distinctive cytoplasmic granules, and may have segmented nuclei. The lymphocyte and monocyte have few, if any, easily visible cytoplasmic granules and have nonsegmented nuclei.

Neutrophil. The granular leukocyte which takes up the neutral portion of the stain is called the **neutrophil.** The neutrophil nucleus is usually segmented into two to five lobes, each connected by a strand or filament. The nucleus stains a dark purple and has a coarse appearance. The cytoplasm is pale pink to tan and contains fine pink or lilac granules. The neutrophil is about twice the diameter of an erythrocyte and is the most numerous of the white cells in normal adult blood. Other names for the neutrophil are PMN (polymorphonuclear neutrophil), "poly," or "seg." The

Table 2–5. Leukocyte identification guide

	Neutrophilic Series		Eosinophil	Basophil	Lymphocyte	Monocyte
	Segmented (mature)	Band or Stab (immature)				
Cell Size (µm)	10–15	10–15	10–15	10–15	8–15	12–20
Nucleus						
shape	2–5 lobes	sausage or U-shaped	bilobed	segmented	round, oval	horseshoe
structure	coarse	coarse	coarse	difficult to see	smudged (smoothly stained)	folded, convoluted
Cytoplasm						
amount	abundant	abundant	abundant	abundant	scant	abundant
color	pink-tan	pink-tan	pink-tan	pink-tan	clear blue	opaque, blue-gray
inclusions	small, lilac granules	small, lilac granules	coarse, orange-red granules	coarse, blue-black granules	occasional red-purple granules	ground-glass appearance

band cell is a younger (more immature) stage of the neutrophil. The staining characteristics are like the neutrophil, but the nucleus is not segmented.

Eosinophil. The **eosinophil** is the granular leukocyte which has granules that have an affinity for the eosin portion of the stain. The nucleus of the eosinophil is usually divided into two or three lobes and stains purple. The cytoplasm is pink-tan but may be difficult to see because it is filled with large red-orange (eosinophilic) granules. Eosinophils are approximately the size of neutrophils but are much less numerous.

Basophil. The **basophil** is the granular leukocyte with granules that have an affinity for the basic portion of the stain. The nucleus of the basophil is segmented and stains light purple. However, the nuclear shape is often difficult to see. This is because numerous coarse blue-black granules often obscure the nucleus and cytoplasm. Basophils are seen only occasionally in normal smears.

Lymphocyte. The **lymphocytes** are the smallest of the leukocytes. Most lymphocytes are only slightly larger than an RBC. The nucleus is usually rather smooth, has a round or oval shape, and stains purple. The cytoplasm is **basophilic** or sky-blue and varies in amount. Occasionally, a few red-purple granules may be present in the cytoplasm.

Monocyte. The **monocyte** is the largest circulating leukocyte. The nucleus may be oval, indented, or horseshoe-shaped and may have brain-like convolutions or folds. The cytoplasm is a dull gray-blue and may have an irregular outline. Very fine granules are distributed throughout the cytoplasm, giving the cytoplasm a ground-glass appearance. **Vacuoles** may be present. These appear as a clear space in the cytoplasm which is filled with fluid or air.

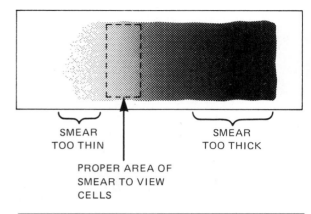

SMEAR
TOO THIN

SMEAR
TOO THICK

PROPER AREA OF
SMEAR TO VIEW
CELLS

Figure 2–44. Proper area of slide to view

METHOD OF OBSERVING A STAINED SMEAR

A well-prepared Wright's stained blood smear is used to learn cell identification. The smear should always be examined using immersion oil on the slide and the oil immersion objective. The light should be bright so that colors and small structures may be readily seen. The slide should be examined near the feathered edge of the smear. This is where the red cells are barely touching and do not overlap (Figure 2–44). In this area of the slide, the cells are easiest to identify because of their slightly flattened shape and large appearance.

Precautions

■ Oil immersion objective must be used for cell identification. If the field appears hazy, clean the objective and add an additional drop of oil to slide.
■ Cell identification may be difficult, inaccurate, or impossible with an improperly stained smear.
■ Much practice is required before cells can be identified with confidence.

LESSON REVIEW

1. List three features of cells which must be considered in cell identification.
2. Describe the appearance of a stained red blood cell.
3. What is the largest circulating leukocyte?
4. What is the stab or band cell?
5. Describe the appearance of a stained platelet.
6. What color granules are present in neutrophils —eosinophils—basophils?
7. What is the smallest leukocyte?
8. State the importance of blood cell identification.
9. What are the precautions to observe in identification of blood cells?
10. Define band cell, basophil, basophilic, eosinophil, lymphocyte, megakaryocyte, monocyte, neutrophil, platelet, and vacuole.

STUDENT ACTIVITIES

1. Re-read the information on blood cell identification.
2. Review the glossary terms.
3. Practice cell identification as outlined on the Student Performance Guide.
4. Practice identifying cells in additional stained smears or from unlabeled colored illustrations of cells.
5. Make simple drawings of each type of cell and label the parts.

Student Performance Guide

NAME _____

DATE _____

LESSON 2–10
IDENTIFICATION OF NORMAL BLOOD CELLS

Instructions

1. Practice identifying erythrocytes, leukocytes, and platelets from a stained blood smear.
2. Identify erythrocytes, the five classes of leukocytes, and platelets satisfactorily for the instructor. All steps must be completed as listed on the instructor's Performance Check Sheet.
3. Complete a written examination successfully.

Materials and Equipment

- hand disinfectant
- stained normal blood smear
- microscope
- lens paper
- immersion oil
- drawings (or photographs) and descriptions of stained blood cells
- soft laboratory tissue
- surface disinfectant

Procedure			S = Satisfactory U = Unsatisfactory
You must:	**S**	**U**	**Comments**
1. Wash hands with disinfectant			
2. Assemble equipment and materials			
3. Place stained smear on microscope stage and secure it with clips			
4. Bring cells into focus using low power (10×) objective and coarse adjustment knob			

You must:	S	U	Comments
5. Scan slide to find area of slide where cells are barely touching each other			
6. Place one drop of immersion oil on slide			
7. Rotate oil immersion objective carefully into position			
8. Focus with fine adjustment knob until cells can be seen clearly			
9. Raise the condenser and open the diaphragm to allow maximum light into objective			
10. Scan slide to observe leukocytes			
11. Study the smear and identify all leukocytes seen			
12. Scan the slide to observe erythrocytes			
13. Scan the slide to observe platelets			
14. Rotate low power objective into position			
15. Remove slide from microscope stage			
16. Clean oil objective thoroughly			
17. Clean oil from slide gently			
18. Repeat steps 3–17 with another stained smear			
19. Wipe any oil from the microscope stage and condenser with soft laboratory tissue			
20. Discard blood smears as instructed			
21. Return equipment to proper storage			
22. Clean work area with surface disinfectant			
23. Wash hands with hand disinfectant			

Comments:

Student/Instructor:

Date:_____ Instructor:_____

LESSON 2–11
Differential Leukocyte Count

LESSON OBJECTIVES

After studying this lesson, you should be able to:
- Explain the purpose of a differential leukocyte count.
- List the normal values for a differential leukocyte count.
- Perform a differential leukocyte count.
- Report the results of a differential leukocyte count.
- Evaluate and report the morphology of the red cells.
- Evaluate platelets and estimate their numbers.
- List the precautions that should be observed when performing a differential leukocyte count.
- Define the glossary terms.

GLOSSARY

anisocytosis / marked variation in the size of erythrocytes
differential leukocyte count / determination of the relative numbers of each type of leukocyte in a blood smear
hypochromic / having reduced color or hemoglobin content
macrocytic / having a larger than normal cell size
microcytic / having a smaller than normal cell size
normochromic / having normal color
normocytic / having a normal cell size and shape
poikilocytosis / significant variation in the shape of erythrocytes

INTRODUCTION

The **differential leukocyte count** is part of a complete blood count. It is often referred to simply as a "diff." The purpose of the count is to obtain the percentage of each of the five types of leukocytes. The procedure involves counting either 100 or 200 white cells from a stained smear and recording each type observed. Information is also obtained from the smear concerning the erythrocytes and platelets. The red cells are evaluated for morphology and hemoglobin content. The platelets are evaluated for morphology and an estimation is made of the number of platelets in circulation. Leukemias, anemias, and other diseases can often be diagnosed and monitored by the differential leukocyte count. For example, the viral infection causing infectious mononucleosis produces a characteristic white cell differential and iron deficiency anemia produces small red cells with little hemoglobin.

PERFORMING THE DIFFERENTIAL COUNT

A specific area of the stained smear must be examined when doing the differential count and observing the red cells and platelets (Figure 2–45).

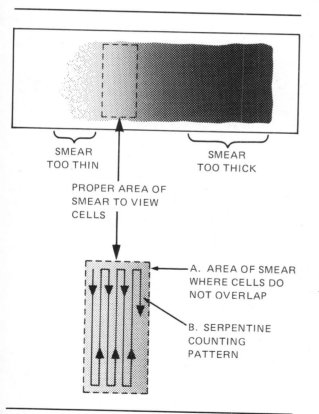

SMEAR TOO THIN

SMEAR TOO THICK

PROPER AREA OF SMEAR TO VIEW CELLS

A. AREA OF SMEAR WHERE CELLS DO NOT OVERLAP

B. SERPENTINE COUNTING PATTERN

Figure 2–45. Proper area of slide to be viewed for differential count: A) closeup of proper area and B) counting pattern

The best area for observation is where the red cells are just touching but not overlapping when viewed microscopically. After a good observation area has been located using the low power objective (10×), the count is performed using the oil immersion objective (97×).

When an area of the slide has been located in which the stain appears satisfactory and the cells are not crowded or distorted, 100 leukocytes are counted. A definite pattern, such as the one shown in Figure 2–45, must be followed to avoid counting the same cells twice. The numbers of each type of white cell observed are recorded using a differential counter (Figure 2–46) or a tally counter. Any abnormalities of the cells are also noted.

After the leukocyte differential has been completed, the stained red cells and platelets are observed and evaluated. With some experience, one may estimate the red cell size as **normocytic** (normal size), **microcytic** (small), or **macrocytic** (large). The condition in which markedly different sizes of red cells are present in a smear is called **anisocytosis**. The hemoglobin content of the red cells can also be estimated. A red cell with the normal amount of hemoglobin is called **normochromic**. It stains evenly with only a small pale area in the center of the cell. A **hypochromic** red cell is one which has less than the normal amount of hemoglobin. It has only a ring of hemoglobin around the outer edge of the cell and a large pale area in the center. Normal red cells are round or slightly oval. The condition in which there is a significant variation in the shape of erythrocytes is called **poikilocytosis**. The platelets are also observed for any abnormalities in their morphology. The total number of platelets counted in 10 oil immersion fields is divided by 10 to give the average number per field. (The total platelet count per mm³ can be estimated by multiplying this number by 20,000.)

NORMAL VALUES

The normal values of the differential count will vary with age. Normal values for adults and

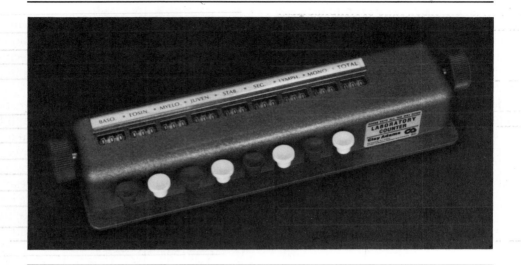

Figure 2–46. Differential counter *(Photo courtesy of Clay Adams Division of Becton Dickinson & Co.)*

children are listed in Table 2–6. In a normal differential count, neutrophils and lymphocytes comprise 85–95% of cells with monocytes, eosinophils and basophils making up the remaining 5–15%. Children normally have a higher percentage of lymphocytes than adults.

Factors Affecting the Leukocyte Ratios

Many disease states can change the ratios of the different types of leukocytes. Bacterial infections usually cause an increase in the bands and segmented neutrophils. Viral infections can increase the number of lymphocytes and/or change their morphology, causing them to appear atypical. The number of eosinophils is increased in parasitic infections and allergies. The number of monocytes is usually not affected by infections, but occasionally will increase in tuberculosis. In the leukemias, there is usually an increase and abnormality in one type of cell. The leukemia is named according to the predominant cell present.

Table 2–6. Normal values for differential count

Type of cell	Normal Values			
White cell	1 month	six-year-old	12-year-old	adult
neutrophil (seg)	15–35%	45–50%	45–50%	50–65%
neutrophil (band)	7–13%	0–7%	6–8%	0–7%
eosinophil	1–3%	1–3%	1–3%	1–3%
basophil	0–1%	0–1%	0–1%	0–1%
monocyte	5–8%	4–8%	3–8%	3–9%
lymphocyte	40–70%	40–45%	35–40%	25–40%
Platelets	An average of 5–15 platelets per oil immersion field is considered normal			

For example, an increased ratio of lymphocytes is found in the lymphocytic leukemias.

Factors Affecting the Red Cells

Normal production and development of red blood cells requires certain factors such as vitamins and minerals. Iron deficiency is one cause of microcytic, hypochromic red cells. Deficiencies of vitamins such as B_{12} and folic acid cause the cells to be macrocytic.

Factors Affecting the Platelets

The platelets can be affected by several factors. In some leukemias, the number of platelets is below normal. Exposure to chemicals, radiation, or drugs used in cancer therapy can also cause a reduction of platelets. If there is a delay in making a smear from a capillary puncture, the platelet distribution may be uneven; this will cause the platelet number to appear reduced.

AUTOMATION

Automated instruments for differential leukocyte counts are used in many medical laboratories, especially those in larger hospitals. The instruments may operate either on the principle of enzyme staining characteristics or pattern recognition. In the enzyme staining method, 10,000 white cells are counted and differentiated in each sample according to the enzymes present in the cells. The pattern recognition method compares the morphology pattern of 100 to 200 white cells in the sample with hundreds of normal morphology patterns which are stored in the computer. Whichever method is used, a technologist must check all cells which have been designated as abnormal by the instrument.

Precautions

■ The condenser of the microscope should be raised until it is almost touching the bottom surface of the slide.
■ The diaphragm of the microscope must be fully opened to allow maximum light.
■ The differential count must be performed in a good area of the slide, following a definite pattern.
■ The oil immersion objective should be rotated carefully into place to avoid breaking the slide or lens.
■ The area being counted should be checked occasionally to insure that it is not near the edge of the smear where cells may be distorted.
■ A more experienced technologist or a pathologist should be consulted if there is any difficulty in identifying cells.

LESSON REVIEW

1. What is the purpose of the differential leukocyte count?
2. A differential is performed as a part of what hematological procedure?
3. What red cell information can be obtained from the smear?
4. Name some diseases which can be diagnosed or monitored by examining the smear.
5. What area of the smear should be used to perform the differential?
6. What method is used to avoid counting the same cells twice?
7. Which microscope objective is used to perform the differential?
8. What is the normal percentage of segmented neutrophils for an adult—for a child?
9. State the normal adult values for eosinophils, basophils, lymphocytes, and monocytes.

10. What information about platelets can be obtained from the smear?
11. Bacterial infections usually increase the percentage of which cells?
12. What precautions should be observed when performing a differential leukocyte count?
13. Define anisocytosis, differential leukocyte count, hypochromic, macrocytic, microcytic, normochromic, normocytic, and poikilocytosis.

STUDENT ACTIVITIES

1. Re-read the information on the differential leukocyte count.
2. Review the glossary terms.
3. Practice performing a differential count as outlined on the Student Performance Guide, using the worksheet.
4. Perform differential counts on additional smears provided by the instructor.

Student Performance Guide

NAME _____

DATE _____

LESSON 2–11
DIFFERENTIAL LEUKOCYTE COUNT

Instructions

1. Practice the procedure for performing the leukocyte differential count.
2. Demonstrate the procedure for performing the leukocyte differential count satisfactorily for the instructor. All steps must be completed as listed on the instructor's Performance Check Sheet.
3. Complete a written examination successfully.

Materials and Equipment

- hand disinfectant
- microscope with oil immersion lens
- immersion oil
- lens paper
- soft tissue or soft paper towels
- stained blood smears
- blood atlas
- tally counter or differential counter
- worksheet
- surface disinfectant
- puncture-proof container for sharp objects

Procedure			S = Satisfactory U = Unsatisfactory
You must:	**S**	**U**	**Comments**
1. Wash hands with disinfectant			
2. Assemble equipment and materials.			
3. Place stained blood smear on microscope stage and secure it with clips			
4. Use the 10× objective to locate an area of the smear which is not near the edges and in which the red cells just touch			

You must:	S	U	Comments
5. Place a drop of immersion oil on the area of the smear to be viewed			
6. Rotate the oil immersion objective (97×) carefully into place			
7. Insure that the area is one in which the stain is correct and the red cells just touch			
8. Count 100 consecutive leukocytes moving the slide or mechanical stage so that consecutive microscopic fields are viewed. Use the counting pattern illustrated in Figure 2–45			
9. Record on worksheet how many of each type of leukocyte are seen and note any abnormalities			

10. Observe the red cells in at least ten fields:
  a. Note the hemoglobin content; record as normochromic or hypochromic
  b. Note the red cell size; record as normocytic, microcytic, or macrocytic. An approximation of the number of cells affected may be recorded using a plus system (1+ to 4+) or using terms such as small, moderate, large			

11. Observe platelets in at least ten fields:
  a. Note morphology
  b. Estimate the number per oil immersion field; record as adequate, decreased, or increased using the guide on the worksheet			

12. Rotate low power (10×) objective into position			
13. Remove slide from microscope stage			
14. Clean oil immersion objective thoroughly			
15. Check microscope stage and condenser for oil and clean if necessary			
16. Blot smear gently with lens paper or soft tissue			
17. Discard or store slides as instructed			
18. Clean equipment and return to proper storage			
19. Wash hands with hand disinfectant			
Comments:			
Student/Instructor:			

Date:_____ Instructor:_____

Worksheet

NAME_____ DATE _____

SPECIMEN NO. _____

LESSON 2–11 DIFFERENTIAL LEUKOCYTE COUNT

		Normal Values (Adult)
Segmented Neutrophils _____%		50–65%
Lymphocytes _____%		25–40%
Monocytes _____%		3–9%
Eosinophils _____%		1–3%
Basophils _____%		0–1%
Bands _____%		0–7%

Other   _____

Platelet Estimate: ☐ appear adequate   5–15/oil immersion field
                        ☐ appear decreased   <4/oil immersion field
                        ☐ appear increased   >16/oil immersion field

RBC Morphology: Normal
    Cell size: ☐ normocytic
                   ☐ microcytic   normocytic (6–8 micrometers)
                   ☐ macrocytic
    Cell color: ☐ normochromic   normochromic
                   ☐ hypochromic

Comments: _____

           _____

UNIT 3
Advanced Hematology

UNIT OBJECTIVES

After studying this unit, you should be able to:
- Perform a venipuncture.
- Perform an erythrocyte sedimentation rate test.
- Perform a reticulocyte count.
- Perform a platelet count.
- Perform a prothrombin time test.
- Calculate erythrocyte indices.
- Perform a bleeding time test.
- Perform a capillary coagulation test.

OVERVIEW

The hematology procedures in this unit are ones which, for the most part, are not considered routine. These procedures give the physician additional information beyond that provided by the procedures in Unit 2. The lessons in this unit are generally ones which take more technical skill. They also require the worker to use judgment and to make use of principles learned earlier.

Venipuncture is presented as another method of obtaining a blood sample. This method is used routinely when the blood sample required is too large to be obtained by capillary puncture. Venipuncture also takes more skill than a capillary puncture. Since veins are used to administer drugs or other treatment, care must be taken not to damage the veins. An improperly performed venipuncture could have serious consequences for the patient. However, a properly performed venipuncture is a safe, convenient means of obtaining a blood sample.

The erythrocyte sedimentation rate (sed rate) is used to follow the progress of some inflammatory disease processes. The results of the procedure can be used with other laboratory results to aid the physician in diagnosis.

The reticulocyte count tells the physician if the patient is producing a sufficient number of new red blood cells. The results can be used to evaluate the treatment and progress of anemia patients.

The platelet count is frequently requested. It is included in advanced hematology because of technical difficulties in counting platelets. Since platelets are very small, any dirt or debris present in the sample could be confused with platelets. For this reason, all equipment and reagents must be very clean.

The calculation of the erythrocyte indices uses the red blood cell count, the hemoglobin value and the hematocrit. The physician can use these indices values to classify anemias and to evaluate anemia treatment.

The bleeding time test and the capillary coagulation test are both screening procedures which can detect blood clotting disorders. The tests are not specific for any certain deficiency. They are presented as an introduction to the principles involved in hemostasis, the blood clotting process. The prothrombin time is a frequently ordered coagulation screening test, and is also included in this unit.

With the completion of units 2 and 3 many of the hematology procedures performed in medical laboratories will have been covered. However, these are actually only a few of a large number of tests available and are meant as illustrations of some basic laboratory principles.

LESSON 3–1
Venipuncture

LESSON OBJECTIVES

After studying this lesson, you should be able to:
- Explain the venipuncture procedure to a patient.
- Select the equipment necessary to perform a venipuncture.
- Apply a tourniquet.
- Select a proper venipuncture site.
- Prepare a venipuncture site.
- Perform a venipuncture.
- Care for a puncture site after venipuncture.
- List the precautions to be observed when performing a venipuncture.
- Explain the use of vacuum tubes.
- Name three common anticoagulants and state when they are used.
- Define the glossary terms.

GLOSSARY

artery / a blood vessel that carries oxygenated blood from the heart to the tissues

gauge / a measure of the diameter of a needle

hematoma / the swelling of tissue around a vessel due to leakage of the blood into the tissue

hypodermic needle / a hollow needle used for injections or for obtaining fluid specimens

lumen / the open space within a tubular organ or tissue

median cephalic vein / a vein located in the bend of the elbow and frequently used for venipuncture

phlebotomy / venipuncture; entry of a vein with a needle

syringe / a hollow, tube-like container with a plunger, used for injecting or withdrawing fluids

tourniquet / a band used to constrict the blood flow in the vein from which blood is to be drawn

vein / a blood vessel that carries deoxygenated blood to the heart
venipuncture / entry of a vein with a needle; a phlebotomy

INTRODUCTION

The most common method of obtaining blood for laboratory examination is by venipuncture. In a **venipuncture,** sometimes called a **phlebotomy,** the blood is taken directly from a superficial **vein.** The vein is punctured with a needle and blood is collected in a syringe or tube. The venipuncture is a quick way to obtain a large sample of blood from which many different analyses can be made.

The venipuncture is a safe procedure when performed correctly by a skilled worker. The procedure should be performed with care. Every effort should be made to preserve the condition of the vein. Much observation and practice is required to become skilled and self-confident in the art of venipuncture.

VENIPUNCTURE BY SYRINGE METHOD

Performing a venipuncture with a syringe involves several important steps. It is necessary that these steps be thoroughly understood before the procedure is attempted. The steps are (1) selecting proper equipment, (2) preparing the patient for

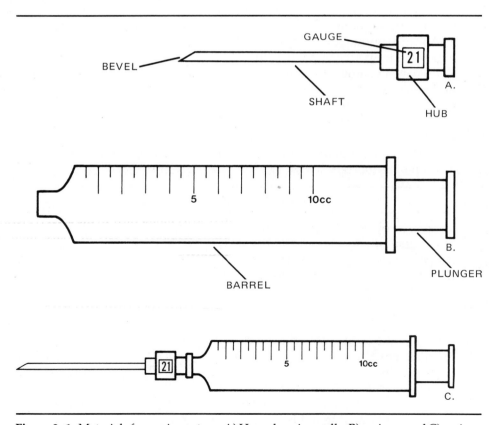

Figure 3–1. Materials for venipuncture: A) Hypodermic needle, B) syringe, and C) syringe and needle assembled

venipuncture, (3) applying the tourniquet, (4) preparing the puncture site, (5) obtaining the blood, and (6) care of the puncture site. When performing a venipuncture, the student must be supervised by a qualified instructor. Gloves must be worn by the phlebotomist when performing venipunctures. It is best to use gloves without talc to avoid contaminating collection tubes.

Selecting the Equipment

The equipment required for venipuncture by syringe includes a sterile **syringe** and **hypodermic needle** (Figure 3–1), 70% alcohol, sterile gauze, tourniquet, and a blood collecting tube. Most laboratories use disposable syringes and needles. To maintain sterility, the syringe and needle should be assembled carefully. The tip of the syringe or the needle must not be touched. The needle should remain capped until ready to use. Needles of 20 to 22 **gauge** are usually used for venipuncture. (The higher the gauge, the smaller the needle.) The plunger of the syringe should be pushed up and down to see that it moves freely. It should then be left pushed completely into the barrel so that no air remains in the syringe. The needle should be positioned firmly on the syringe so that the bevel and the graduations of the syringe face in the same direction. The needle should be inspected carefully to see that the point is sharp and smooth. The needle should then be capped until used. All materials should be placed within easy reach of the venipuncturist. Gloves must be worn while performing venipuncture. It is important that gloves fit well so that veins may be located easily.

Preparation of Patient

The venipuncturist should always identify the patient by name and by checking the laboratory request form. If the patient is hospitalized, patient identification wristband should be checked. The procedure should be explained to the patient to minimize apprehension. The patient should be lying down or seated in a chair which has arms. The venipuncturist should always be prepared for the occasional patient who may faint and should be trained to administer current first aid techniques should this occur. The patient's arm needs to be fully extended and firmly supported during the venipuncture procedure.

Application of Tourniquet

A **tourniquet** is applied to the arm to slow the blood flow and make the veins more prominent. A small piece of rubber tubing may be used for this purpose. The tourniquet must be applied correctly. To do so, the tourniquet is placed under the arm above the elbow and the two ends are stretched and crossed over the top of the arm. While maintaining tension on the ends, one side should be looped and pulled halfway through in a slipknot (Figure 3–2). If the tourniquet is tied in this manner, it will release easily with a gentle pull on one end (Figure 3–3). The tourniquet should be applied to select the puncture site. It should then be released while the site is cleansed, and retied before the puncture is performed. *The tourniquet is always released before the needle is withdrawn from the vein* after the puncture has been completed. A tourniquet should never be tied tight enough to restrict blood flow in the **artery**. Neither should the tourniquet be left in place more than two minutes.

Selection of Puncture Site

The puncture site should be carefully selected after inspecting both arms to locate the best vein. The vein most frequently used is the **median cephalic vein** of the forearm (Figure 3–4). The fingertips should be used to gently press on the veins to determine the direction of the vein and to estimate the size and depth of the vein (Figure 3–5). The vein will feel like an elastic tube.

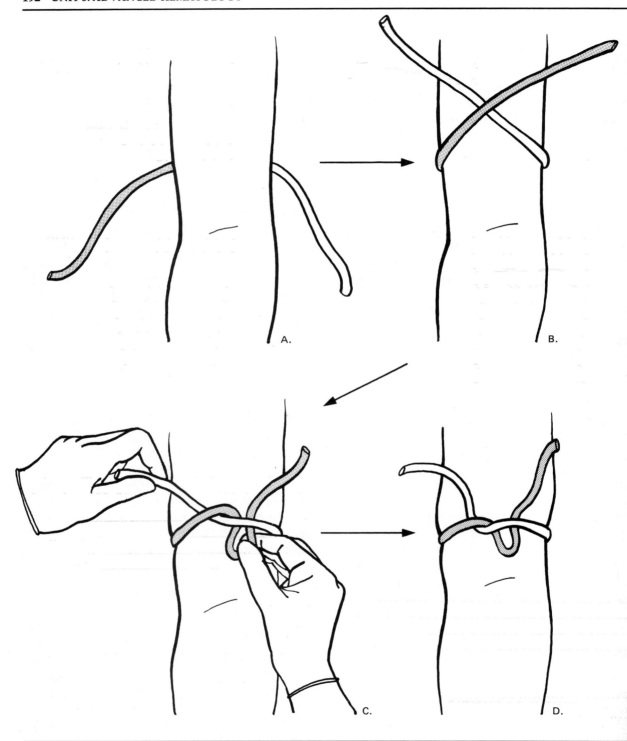

Figure 3–2. Tying a tourniquet

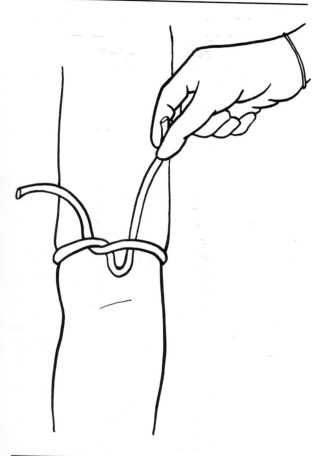

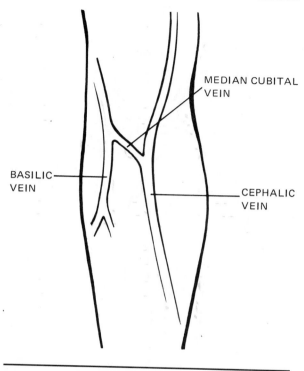

Figure 3–4. Veins most commonly used for venipuncture (left arm)

Figure 3–3. Releasing the tourniquet

Preparation of the Puncture Site

The area around the puncture site should be cleansed thoroughly with 70% alcohol and a sterile gauze. The site may then be dried using dry sterile gauze, or it may be allowed to air dry. Once the site is cleansed, it should not be touched again except to enter the vein with the needle.

Performing the Puncture

When the puncture site has been cleansed, the tourniquet should be reapplied to the arm; it should not touch the cleansed area. The syringe should be held in one hand at a 15–30° angle to the arm. The bevel should be up, and the needle should point in the same direction as the vein. Penetrating the vein at the proper angle will prevent penetrating both blood vessel walls. (The thumb may be placed about one inch below the point of entry, and the skin pressed and pulled toward the venipuncturist, to anchor the vein and lessen the pull of the needle on the skin.) The skin and vein should be entered in one smooth motion until the needle is in the **lumen** of the vein (Figure 3–6). The syringe and needle should then be held motionless while the plunger is gently pulled back with the other hand to draw blood into the syringe. The needle should be observed while the syringe is filling to be sure it is not pulled out of

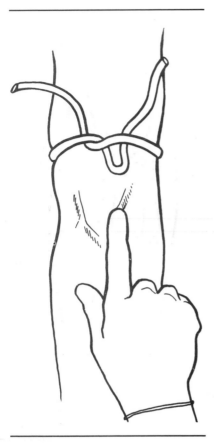

Figure 3–5. Palpating a vein with fingertip

the vein. When the proper amount of blood has been obtained, the tourniquet should be released. The needle can then be withdrawn from the vein while gauze is placed over the puncture site (Figure 3–7). Used needles should not be recapped but should be carefully discarded using a needle disposal container. Several types are available commercially. The blood should then be transferred to the appropriate blood collecting tube using only light pressure on the plunger. The tube should be labeled with the patient's name, identification number, date, time of collection, and initials of the venipuncturist. (Tubes should not be prelabeled; this will prevent possibility of using an empty labeled tube for the wrong patient.)

Care of the Puncture Site

The patient should be instructed to press the gauze on the puncture site for two to five minutes with arm extended to insure that bleeding stops and that a swelling of tissue, or a **hematoma,** does not form. The venipuncturist should check the site to see that it has stopped bleeding before leaving the patient and should apply a bandage if necessary.

VENIPUNCTURE BY VACUUM TUBE SYSTEM

Blood may also be collected from a vein using a vacuum tube system such as VACUTAINER®. This system consists of a special disposable needle, a reusable needle holder or adapter, and blood collecting tubes which have had most of the air evacuated (Figure 3–8). This is the most widely used method of collecting blood. The needle used has two sharp ends; the short end is fitted into the adapter, and the longer end is used to puncture the vein. After the vein is entered, the collecting tube is pushed onto the needle in the adapter and blood is drawn into the tube by vacuum. When the tube is filled, it can be removed from the needle and replaced with another tube. In this manner, several tubes of blood can be collected, using a variety of types of vacuum tubes.

VACUUM TUBES AND ANTICOAGULANTS

Vacuum tubes are available in a variety of sizes and with or without anticoagulants added. Tubes are color-coded so that the color of the stopper denotes which, if any, anticoagulant is present in the tube (see Appendix L and Table 3–1). Laboratory procedures performed on plasma usually require that blood be collected with a specific anticoagulant. For example, tubes with lavender stoppers contain EDTA, which is the anticoagulant used for most hematology studies such as cell

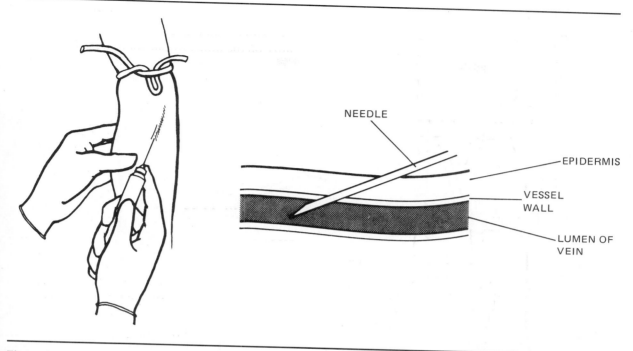

Figure 3–6. Performing the puncture (left). Expanded view of needle positioned in lumen of vein (right).

counts and differential counts. For coagulation tests such as prothrombin time, a blue-stoppered tube containing sodium citrate is commonly used. Tubes with green stoppers contain heparin which is used for some special tests in chemistry and hematology. Heparin should not be used for stained blood smears. Gray-stoppered tubes contain potassium oxalate and sodium fluoride and are used for certain glucose methods. Red-stoppered tubes contain no anticoagulant and are used for tests which require serum, such as most blood chemistries.

Tubes are available in a variety of sizes; each size draws a specific volume of blood. The tubes contain the proper amount of anticoagulant for the volume of blood that the tube will draw. It is important that tubes be filled to their stated capacity since an improper ratio of anticoagulant to blood may alter cell morphology and interfere with test results.

Precautions

■ Wear gloves when performing venipuncture.
■ Students should only perform a venipuncture under the supervision of a qualified instructor.
■ Be sure that the patient is lying down or sitting with the arm firmly supported. Be prepared for the patient who might faint.
■ Do not allow the tourniquet to remain on the arm for more than two minutes.
■ Check the pulse to be sure that arterial circulation is not hindered.
■ Before performing the puncture, push the plunger all the way to the bottom of the syringe barrel to expel all air from the syringe.
■ Always remove the tourniquet before taking the needle out of the vein to prevent the formation of a hematoma.

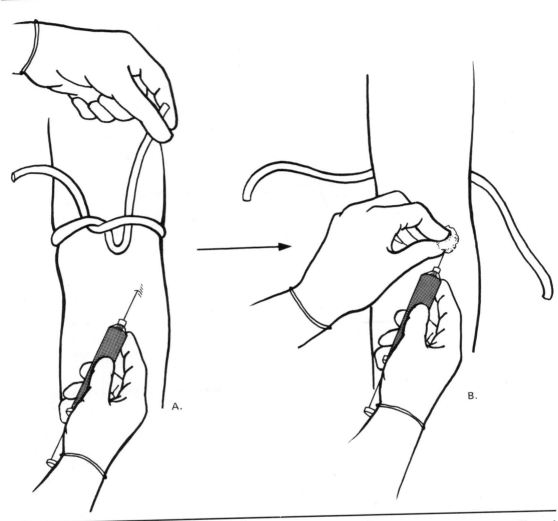

Figure 3–7. Withdrawing needle from puncture. A) Remove tourniquet and B) withdraw needle and apply pressure with sterile cotton

■ If difficulty is encountered when entering the vein or if a hematoma or swelling begins to form, release the tourniquet immediately, quickly withdraw the needle, and apply pressure to the puncture site with gauze.

■ Do not reuse needles or syringes; this prevents possible transmission of disease.
■ Used needles must be discarded into a needle disposal container.

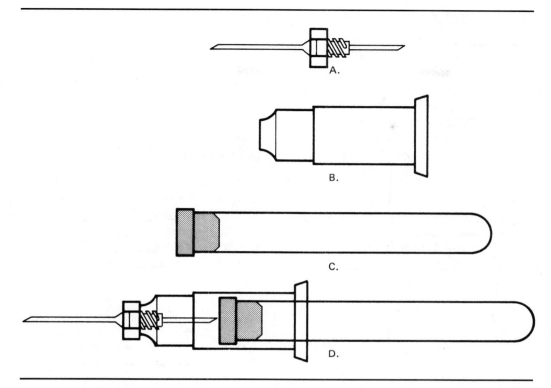

Figure 3–8. Vacuum tube blood collecting system. A) needle, B) holder, C), vacuum tube, and D) assembled unit

Table 3–1. Guide for selection of vacuum tubes

Stopper Color	Anticoagulant in Tube	Examples of Use
red	none	tests which require serum, such as most blood chemistries and serology tests
lavender	EDTA	most hematological tests, blood typing
green	heparin	some special chemistry tests, certain lymphocyte studies, LE test
blue	sodium citrate	most coagulation studies
gray	sodium fluoride	certain glucose methods

LESSON REVIEW

1. Why is a venipuncture performed?
2. What is the purpose of a tourniquet?
3. Name five precautions which must be observed when performing a venipuncture.
4. What are the steps in performing a venipuncture?
5. Where is the most common venipuncture site?
6. Why must the tourniquet be removed before taking the needle out of the vein?
7. How should the puncture site be treated after the needle is removed?
8. Explain briefly the vacuum system of obtaining venous blood.
9. Name three anticoagulants used in collecting blood. Which one is most commonly used in hematology?
10. Define artery, gauge, hematoma, hypodermic needle, lumen, median cephalic vein, phlebotomy, syringe, tourniquet, vein, and venipuncture.

STUDENT ACTIVITIES

1. Re-read the information on venipuncture.
2. Review the glossary terms.
3. Practice applying a tourniquet and locating suitable veins for venipuncture.
4. Practice performing a venipuncture as outlined on the Student Performance Guide.

Student Performance Guide

NAME _____

DATE _____

LESSON 3–1
VENIPUNCTURE

Instructions

1. Practice performing a venipuncture.
2. Demonstrate the procedure for performing a venipuncture satisfactorily for the instructor. All steps must be completed as listed on the instructor's Performance Check Sheet.
3. Complete a written examination successfully.

Materials and Equipment

- gloves
- hand disinfectant
- tourniquet
- sterile gauze or cotton
- 70% alcohol or alcohol swabs
- sterile disposable hypodermic needle, 20–22 gauge
- sterile syringe
- collection tubes
- container for needle disposal
- surface disinfectant
- biohazard container

Procedure			S = Satisfactory U = Unsatisfactory
You must:	**S**	**U**	**Comments**
1. Wash hands with disinfectant and put on gloves			
2. Assemble equipment and materials			
3. Place venipuncture equipment and clean gauze within easy reach			
4. Identify patient properly			

You must:	S	U	Comments
5. Explain venipuncture procedure to patient and position patient			
6. Attach the sterile capped needle to the sterile syringe, maintaining sterility (if packed separately)			
7. Remove cap and position needle so that the bevel faces in the same direction as the graduations on the syringe			
8. Inspect the needle to see that the point is smooth and sharp			
9. Replace needle cap to maintain sterility			
10. Slide the plunger up and down in the barrel of the syringe to be sure that it moves freely			
11. Push the plunger to the bottom of the barrel so that no air remains in the syringe			
12. Place the tourniquet around the patient's arm above the elbow; it should be just tight enough so that the venous circulation is restricted, but not so tight that the arterial circulation is stopped. CAUTION: Do not allow the tourniquet to remain on for more than two minutes			
13. Instruct the patient to open and close the fist a few times in order to increase circulation and to make the veins more noticeable			
14. Inspect the bend of the elbow to locate a suitable vein			
15. Palpate the vein with the fingertip(s) to determine the direction of the vein, and to estimate its size and depth. *Note:* The vein most frequently used is the median cephalic vein of the forearm			
16. Release the tourniquet			
17. Cleanse the skin of the puncture site using an alcohol-soaked gauze			
18. Allow alcohol to dry			
19. Retie the tourniquet, being careful not to touch the sterile puncture site			
20. Instruct the patient to straighten the arm and make a fist			
21. Uncap needle and hold the syringe so that the graduations on the syringe and the bevel of the needle are in full view			

You must:	S	U	Comments
(facing toward ceiling). With thumb of other hand, hold skin taut			
22. Hold the needle at a 30° angle to the arm and insert the needle into the vein. Watch for blood flow into the syringe			
23. Instruct the patient to open the fist as soon as the vein has been entered			
24. Pull the plunger back slowly with the other hand to withdraw the blood while steadying the syringe and needle with the right hand			
25. Release the tourniquet when the desired amount of blood is obtained			
26. Place a dry, sterile gauze over the puncture site and withdraw the needle from the vein (do not press down on the needle)			
27. Instruct the patient to press the sterile gauze over the wound for three to five minutes with the arm extended			
28. Discard needle into needle disposal container (do not recap)			
29. Fill the collecting tube with blood from the syringe and label the tube properly			
30. Discard used syringe as instructed by the teacher			
31. Check patient to be sure that bleeding has stopped; apply bandage if necessary			
32. Clean and return equipment to storage			
33. Clean work area with surface disinfectant			
34. Remove and discard gloves appropriately			
35. Wash hands with hand disinfectant			

Comments:

Student/Instructor:

Date:_____ Instructor:_____

LESSON 3–2

Erythrocyte Sedimentation Rate

LESSON OBJECTIVES

After studying this lesson, you should be able to:

- List four properties of blood which affect the erythrocyte sedimentation rate and explain how the rate is affected by each factor.
- Perform a test to measure the erythrocyte sedimentation rate.
- State the normal values for the erythrocyte sedimentation rate.
- List technical factors which may affect the erythrocyte sedimentation rate.
- Define the glossary terms.

GLOSSARY

aggregate / total substances making up a mass; a clustering of particles

inflammation / a tissue reaction to injury

rouleau(x) / a group of red cells arranged like a roll of coins

sedimentation / the process of solid particles settling at the bottom of a liquid

Wintrobe tube / a slender thick-walled tube marked from 0-100 mm; used in Wintrobe method of macrohematocrit and erythrocyte sedimentation rate

INTRODUCTION

The erythrocyte sedimentation rate (ESR) is a simple, frequently performed hematology test. The test is not specific for a particular disease but is used as a general indication of **inflammation** or to follow the course of inflammatory disease.

In a sample of anticoagulated whole blood, the erythrocytes will gradually separate from the plasma and settle to the bottom of the container. The rate at which the erythrocytes fall is known as the erythrocyte sedimentation rate. In the blood of most healthy persons, **sedimentation** takes place slowly. In many diseases, however, the rate is rapid. In some cases, the rate is proportional to the severity of the disease. Measurement of the ESR may be helpful in confirming or following the course of certain diseases.

WINTROBE METHOD OF MEASURING THE ESR

The Wintrobe method is a common method of measuring the ESR. A **Wintrobe tube** graduated from 0–100 millimeters and with a capacity of one milliliter of blood is used for this method (Figure 3–9). The use of disposable Wintrobe tubes is recommended because of the difficulty in disinfecting and cleaning the reusable type. A special rack which holds the tube vertically is also re-

quired (Figure 3–10). The sample tested is venous blood with the anticoagulant, EDTA, added.

A long-tipped Pasteur pipet is used to fill the Wintrobe tube to the zero mark with blood (Figure 3–10). The tube is then placed in the sedimentation rack for one hour. At the end of the hour, the total distance which the erythrocytes have fallen is measured. The rate is recorded in mm/hour (Figure 3–11).

Normal Values for the Wintrobe Method

Normal values for the ESR vary slightly with age and sex (Table 3–2). Only increased rates are significant. Children usually have a lower ESR than middle-aged adults. Elderly people tend to have a higher ESR. Females have a higher rate than males.

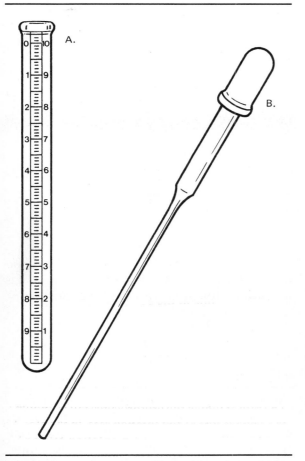

Figure 3–9. Materials for erythrocyte sedimentation rate. A) Wintrobe sedimentation tube and B) long-stemmed Pasteur-type pipet used for filling Wintrobe tube

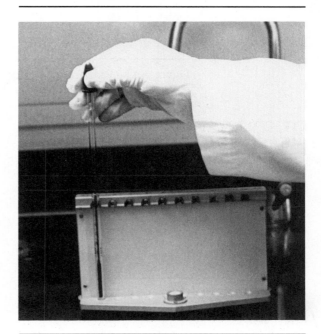

Figure 3–10. Erythrocyte sedimentation rate. Filling a Wintrobe sedimentation tube. *(Photo courtesy of John Estridge)*

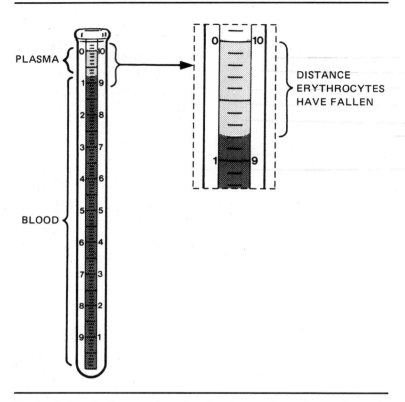

Figure 3–11. Sedimentation tube showing settling of cells. Example shown illustrates a sedimentation of 8 mm

OTHER METHODS OF MEASURING THE ESR

Other methods of measuring the erythrocyte sedimentation rate are Westergren and Landau-Adams. These methods are based on the same principle as the Wintrobe method but they differ in the amount of sample needed and the size and design of the tubes used for the tests. Each method has its own set of normal values. Therefore, it is necessary to follow instructions which are specific to each method used.

RELATIONSHIP OF ESR TO DISEASE

Conditions in which the erythrocyte sedimentation rate is increased include tuberculosis, acute and chronic infections, acute viral hepatitis, cancer, multiple myeloma, lupus erythematosus, and inflammatory processes such as rheumatic fever and rheumatoid arthritis. Pregnant females also have an increased ESR. In polycythemia and sickle cell anemia, the ESR is low or zero.

Table 3–2. Normal values for Wintrobe method of erythrocyte sedimentation rate

Age/Sex	Normal rate
Males	0–9 mm/hour
Females	0–20 mm/hour
Children	0–13 mm/hour

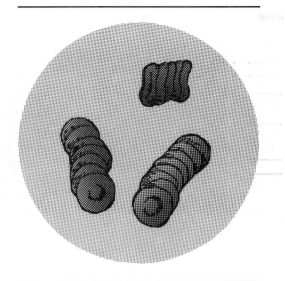

Figure 3–12. Erythrocytes forming rouleau

FACTORS AFFECTING THE RATE OF SEDIMENTATION

Three factors which affect the ESR are: (1) properties of the erythrocytes, (2) properties of the plasma, and (3) mechanical or technical factors.

Properties of Erythrocytes

The rate of sedimentation is affected by the size, shape, and number of erythrocytes. In normal blood, erythrocytes suspended in the plasma form few, if any, **aggregates.** The mass of the falling erythrocytes is small and the ESR tends to be low. In abnormal blood, the erythrocytes sometimes aggregate to form what is called **rouleau.** This phenomenon is called rouleau because the cells form aggregates that look like rolls or stacks of coins (Figure 3–12). This causes an increase in the mass and an increased rate of sedimentation. Changes in the shape of the erythrocytes can also

affect the ESR. For example, in sickle cell anemia the irregularly shaped erythrocytes cannot form rouleau and the ESR may be slow. The sedimentation rate may be rapid in other anemias because there are fewer erythrocytes to interfere with settling. When erythrocytes are increased, as in polycythemia, the erythrocytes settle slowly.

Properties of the Plasma

The amount and type of plasma proteins present in a blood sample may affect the ESR. If protein levels are elevated, the sedimentation rate may be increased.

Mechanical or Technical Factors

Mechanical and technical factors such as temperature, time, size of tube, and tilting or vibration of tube during incubation will affect the sedimentation rate. The points listed below should be heeded if the test results are to be correct:

1. The sedimentation tube must be kept exactly vertical; even minor degrees of tilting may greatly increase the ESR.
2. The test should be set up on a counter free from vibration, such as that from a centrifuge, to avoid a falsely increased rate of settling.
3. The temperature in the room should be kept constant while the test is being performed. Low temperatures cause erythrocytes to settle more slowly.
4. The test should be set up within two hours after the blood sample is collected.
5. The length and diameter of the sedimentation tube affect the rate of sedimentation. Therefore, standard tubes should be used in the test.
6. The test must be timed carefully. The ESR increases with time.

LESSON REVIEW

1. Why would an ESR be performed?
2. What four properties of blood affect the ESR? Explain how the ESR is affected by each of these factors.
3. Name five conditions in which the ESR would be increased.
4. What two conditions would have a low ESR?
5. What are the normal values for the ESR using the Wintrobe method?
6. List four technical factors that affect the ESR, and explain what effect each has.
7. Define aggregate, inflammation, rouleau, sedimentation, and Wintrobe tube.

STUDENT ACTIVITIES

1. Re-read the information on erythrocyte sedimentation rate.
2. Review the glossary terms.
3. Practice performing the erythrocyte sedimentation rate test as outlined on the Student Performance Guide.
4. Evaluate the effect of technical factors on the ESR: set up three ESR tests on a blood sample. Treat one tube correctly, place one in the refrigerator, and place one at an angle at room temperature. Compare the results and explain them.

Student Performance Guide

NAME _____

DATE _____

LESSON 3–2
ERYTHROCYTE
SEDIMENTATION RATE

Instructions

1. Practice performing the procedure to measure the erythrocyte sedimentation rate.
2. Demonstrate the procedure for measuring the erythrocyte sedimentation rate satisfactorily for the instructor. All steps must be completed as listed on the instructor's Performance Check Sheet.
3. Complete a written examination successfully.

Materials and Equipment

- gloves
- hand disinfectant
- sample of venous, anticoagulated blood
- long-stem Pasteur pipet with rubber bulb
- Wintrobe sedimentation tube (disposable or reusable)
- sedimentation rack
- timer
- surface disinfectant
- biohazard container

Procedure			S = Satisfactory U = Unsatisfactory
You must:	**S**	**U**	**Comments**
1. Wash hands with disinfectant and put on gloves			
2. Assemble equipment and materials			
3. Check the leveling bubble to insure that the rack is level			
4. Obtain anticoagulated blood sample			
5. Mix blood well and fill Pasteur pipet			

You must:	S	U	Comments
6. Fill Wintrobe tube to the "0" mark using the Pasteur pipet, being careful not to overfill. *Note:* Tube must be filled from bottom to avoid getting air bubbles in the tube			
7. Place tube in sedimentation rack and set timer for one hour. Be certain the tube is vertical			
8. Measure the distance the erythrocytes have fallen (in mm): after one hour, use the scale on the tube to measure the distance from the top of the plasma to the top of the red cells			
9. Record the sedimentation rate in mm/hour			
10. Disinfect and clean equipment and return to storage. *Note:* If disposable equipment is used, dispose of in biohazard container			
11. Clean work area with surface disinfectant			
12. Remove and discard gloves appropriately			
13. Wash hands with hand disinfectant			

Comments:

Student/Instructor:

Date:_____ Instructor:_____

LESSON 3–3
Reticulocyte Count

LESSON OBJECTIVES

After studying this lesson, you should be able to:
- Explain why a reticulocyte count is performed.
- Prepare a reticulocyte smear.
- Perform a reticulocyte count.
- Calculate a reticulocyte percentage.
- Name three dyes commonly used in the reticulocyte procedure.
- Name two conditions in which the reticulocyte count would be low.
- Name two conditions in which the reticulocyte count would be elevated.
- List the normal reticulocyte count for an adult and a newborn.
- List the precautions that should be observed when performing a reticulocyte count.
- Define the glossary terms.

GLOSSARY

reticulocyte / an immature erythrocyte which has retained basophilic substance in the cytoplasm

reticulocytopenia / a decrease below the normal number of reticulocytes

reticulocytosis / an increase above the normal number of reticulocytes in the circulating blood

reticulum / a network

supravital stain / a stain which will color living cells or tissues

INTRODUCTION

A reticulocyte count is a method of estimating the number of immature erythrocytes in the circulating blood. The test is most commonly used to determine the cause of a decreased red cell count, or anemia. It is also used in following the course of treatment for anemia.

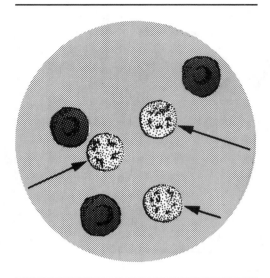

Figure 3–13.   Reticulocytes showing stained reticulum

Erythrocytes are produced in the bone marrow. After a maturation process, the erythrocytes then enter the blood circulation. For the first twenty-four hours after red cells enter the circulation, they are still immature as evidenced by the presence of basophilic substance in the cytoplasm. If the cell is exposed to certain stains, the basophilic substance forms granular aggregates or filaments called a **reticulum,** and the cell is called a **reticulocyte** (Figure 3–13). The staining technique is called **supravital** staining, a procedure in which the cell is stained while it is still living. The three most common dyes used for supravital stains are: New Methylene Blue, Brilliant Cresyl Blue, and Nile Blue Sulfate. Reticulocytes appear as blue-tinged erythrocytes with dark bluish-purple granules or filaments. Mature red cells simply appear bluish (see Color Plate 12).

In a healthy adult, approximately 1% of the erythrocytes will stain as reticulocytes when a supravital stain is applied to a blood sample. Reticulocyte counts above 3% in an adult indicate that erythrocytes are being produced at an in-

creased rate. **Reticulocytosis,** an increased number of reticulocytes, may be due to acute blood loss due to hemorrhage, chronic blood loss such as from a bleeding ulcer, or response to treatment of anemia.

Reticulocyte values below 0.5% indicate that the rate of erythrocyte production is decreased. A decrease in reticulocytes, **reticulocytopenia,** may be seen in iron deficiency anemia, vitamin B_{12} or folic acid deficiencies, or aplastic anemia.

PERFORMING THE RETICULOCYTE COUNT

A reticulocyte count may be performed using capillary or venous blood. A few drops of blood are mixed with equal parts of New Methylene Blue stain in a small test tube and allowed to stand for fifteen minutes. The blood-stain mixture is then used to prepare blood smears. After the blood smears air dry, they are examined microscopically using the oil immersion objective. A total of 1000 erythrocytes are counted (500 counted per slide) and the number of reticulocytes seen per 1000 erythrocytes is recorded. (A reticulocyte is counted as a red cell.) The percentage of reticulocytes is then calculated.

Calculating the Reticulocyte Percentage

A reticulocyte count is reported as the percentage of erythrocytes that are reticulocytes. This count is not a quantitative count but is only an estimate. The percentage of reticulocytes is calculated using the formula:

$$\frac{\text{\# reticulocytes counted}}{\text{\# erythrocytes counted}} \times 100 = \% \text{ reticulocytes}$$

or

$$\frac{\text{\# reticulocytes}}{1000} \times 100 = \% \text{ reticulocytes}$$

or

$$\frac{\text{\# reticulocytes}}{10} = \% \text{ reticulocytes}$$

A sample calculation is shown in Figure 3–14.

I. Count the reticulocytes using two smears:

	Erythrocytes counted	Reticulocytes seen
Smear 1	500	7
Smear 2	500	5
Total	1000	12

II. Calculate the percentage of reticulocytes:

$$\% \text{ retics } = \frac{\# \text{ Reticulocytes counted}}{\# \text{ RBC counted}} \times 100$$

$$\% \text{ retics } = \frac{12}{1000} \times 100$$

$$\% \text{ retics } = \frac{12}{10}$$

$$\% \text{ retics } = 1.2$$

Figure 3–14. Sample calculation of reticulocyte percentage

NORMAL VALUES

The normal reticulocyte count varies with age (Table 3–3). Newborn infants have high counts which decrease to the adult level by 2 weeks of age.

Precautions

■ The reticulum may be easily overlooked; cells should be examined thoroughly.
■ Use care to avoid confusing artifacts with reticulum.
■ Use a definite counting pattern to insure that cells are not counted twice.
■ Fresh blood must be used to perform the reticulocyte count.
■ The stain must be filtered frequently to prevent stain precipitate from forming on smear and being confused with reticulum.

Table 3-3. Normal reticulocyte percentages

	Normal Reticulocyte Count	Upper Limit of Normal
Adults	0.5–1.5%	3%
Newborns	2.5–6.5%	10%

LESSON REVIEW

1. What is a reticulocyte?
2. Why would a reticulocyte count be performed?
3. What is the normal reticulocyte count for adults; for newborns?
4. What are three of the dyes used to stain reticulocytes?
5. What conditions can cause a high reticulocyte count?
6. What conditions can cause a low reticulocyte count?
7. State the formula for calculating a reticulocyte count.
8. List the precautions to be observed when performing a reticulocyte count.
9. Define reticulocyte, reticulocytopenia, reticulocytosis, reticulum, and supravital stain.

STUDENT ACTIVITIES

1. Re-read the information on reticulocyte counts.
2. Review the glossary terms.
3. Practice performing reticulocyte counts and calculating reticulocyte percentages as outlined on the Student Performance Guide.

Student Performance Guide

NAME _____

DATE _____

LESSON 3–3
RETICULOCYTE COUNT

Instructions

1. Practice performing a reticulocyte count.
2. Demonstrate the procedure for performing a reticulocyte count satisfactorily for the instructor. All steps must be completed as listed on the instructor's Performance Check Sheet.
3. Complete a written examination successfully.

Materials and Equipment

- gloves
- hand disinfectant
- microscope
- microscope slides
- lens paper
- immersion oil
- Pasteur pipet with bulb
- New Methylene Blue stain, freshly filtered
- 70% alcohol or alcohol swabs
- sterile cotton or gauze
- sterile lancet
- capillary tubes, heparinized and plain
- test tube 10×75 mm
- tally counter
- surface disinfectant
- biohazard container
- puncture-proof container for sharp objects
- commercially available stained reticulocyte slides (optional)

Procedure			S = Satisfactory
			U = Unsatisfactory

You must:	S	U	Comments
1. Wash hands with disinfectant and put on gloves			
2. Assemble equipment and materials			
3. Perform a capillary puncture and wipe away the first drop of blood with dry sterile cotton or gauze (or use fresh, well-mixed venous anticoagulated blood to perform the test)			
4. Fill one or two heparinized capillary tubes with blood (use plain capillary tubes if using anticoagulated blood)			
5. Dispense two to three drops of blood into the bottom of a small test tube			
6. Add an equal amount of New Methylene Blue stain to the test tube and mix			
7. Allow mixture to stand for fifteen minutes at room temperature			
8. Remix contents of test tube and fill a plain capillary tube with blood-stain mixture			
9. Prepare two blood smears from blood-stain mixture and allow to air dry			
10. Place one slide on microscope stage and secure			
11. Use low power (10×) objective to find a good area of the smear			
12. Place one drop of immersion oil on the slide and carefully rotate oil immersion objective into position			
13. Count all erythrocytes in one oil immersion field and record the number of reticulocytes in the field. *Note:* A reticulocyte is counted as a red cell			
14. Move slide to an adjacent microscopic field			
15. Count all erythrocytes in the (adjacent) field and record the number of reticulocytes in the field			
16. Continue steps 14–15 until 500 erythrocytes have been counted			
17. Repeat steps 10–16 using the second slide			

You must:	S	U	Comments
18. Calculate the reticulocyte percentage using the formula: $$\frac{\#\ of\ retics\ counted}{1000\ rbcs} \times 100 = \%\ reticulocytes$$			
19. Record the results			
20. Clean oil immersion objective carefully and thoroughly with lens paper			
21. Clean any oil from microscope stage with laboratory tissue			
22. Return equipment to proper storage			
23. Store or discard slides as instructed			
24. Clean work area with surface disinfectant			
25. Remove and discard gloves appropriately			
26. Wash hands with hand disinfectant			

Comments:

Student/Instructor:

Date:_____ Instructor:_____

LESSON 3–4
Platelet Count

LESSON OBJECTIVES

After studying this lesson, you should be able to:
- Discuss the functions of platelets.
- Name two pathological conditions in which the platelet counts may be abnormal.
- Perform a blood dilution for a platelet count.
- Perform a platelet count.
- Calculate the results of a platelet count.
- List three precautions which must be observed when performing a platelet count.
- Define the glossary terms.

GLOSSARY

hemostasis / process of stopping blood flow
petri dish / a shallow, covered dish made of plastic or glass
platelet / a formed element in the blood which plays an important part in blood clotting; a thrombocyte
thrombocytopenia / a decrease below the normal number of platelets in the blood
thrombocytosis / an increase above the normal number of platelets in the blood

INTRODUCTION

Platelets, the smallest of the formed elements in the blood, play an important role in the clotting of blood and in **hemostasis,** the process of stopping bleeding. They help stop bleeding by forming a sticky plug to seal vessel walls and also help initi-ate a series of enzymatic reactions which result in the formation of the blood clot.

The platelet count is one important test used to investigate bleeding disorders, to assess clotting ability, or to monitor drug treatments. Platelets are difficult to count accurately because of their small size and their tendency to clump.

The normal platelet count is 150,000 to 400,000 platelets per cubic millimeter (cu mm or mm³) of blood. An increase in platelets, **thrombocytosis,** may occur in conditions such as polycythemia or after a splenectomy. **Thrombocytopenia,** a decrease in platelets, may occur in some anemias, some leukemias, and following chemotherapy and radiation therapy.

PROCEDURE FOR PLATELET COUNT

Diluting the Sample

A platelet count is performed by mixing a blood sample with a diluting fluid of 1% ammonium oxalate in a RBC diluting pipet. Capillary blood may be used but venous anticoagulated blood

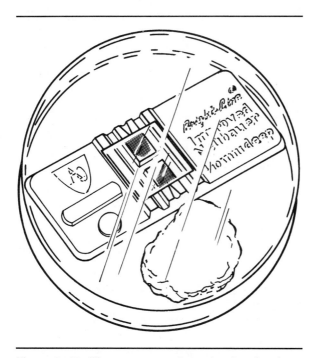

Figure 3–15. Hemacytometer in moist chamber (covered petri dish containing moistened cotton)

gives better results. This is because platelets tend to clump rapidly in a capillary sample. The blood is drawn to the 1.0 mark, and the diluting fluid is then drawn to the 101 mark. The resulting dilution for the platelet count is 1:100. The pipet is then shaken for three minutes to mix the sample.

Filling the Chamber

After mixing, four to five drops are discarded from the stem of the pipet. Both sides of a clean hemacytometer are loaded. Since platelets are so small, they move around easily in the counting chamber. This makes it difficult to count them accurately. To allow time for the platelets to settle and to prevent evaporation of the solution in the counting chamber, the filled hemacytometer is placed in a **petri dish** containing a moist cotton ball for ten minutes (Figure 3–15).

Counting the Platelets

To perform the platelet count, the hemacytometer is removed from the moist chamber and placed on the microscope stage. The low power (10×) objective is used to locate the counting area. In a platelet count, the entire center square (1 mm²) is counted (Figure 3–16) using the high power (45×) objective. The platelets may be seen more clearly if the microscope condenser is lowered and the light is decreased (by adjusting the diaphragm). The platelets will appear as shiny refractile objects which darken when the fine adjustment knob is rotated (see Color Plate 15). The platelets in all 25 small squares of the large central square are counted. The count is performed using both sides of the chamber and the average of the two sides is calculated.

Calculating the Platelet Count

The number of platelets per mm³ of blood is calculated using the general formula:

$$C/mm^3 = \frac{Avg \times D\ (mm) \times DF}{A\ (mm)^2}$$

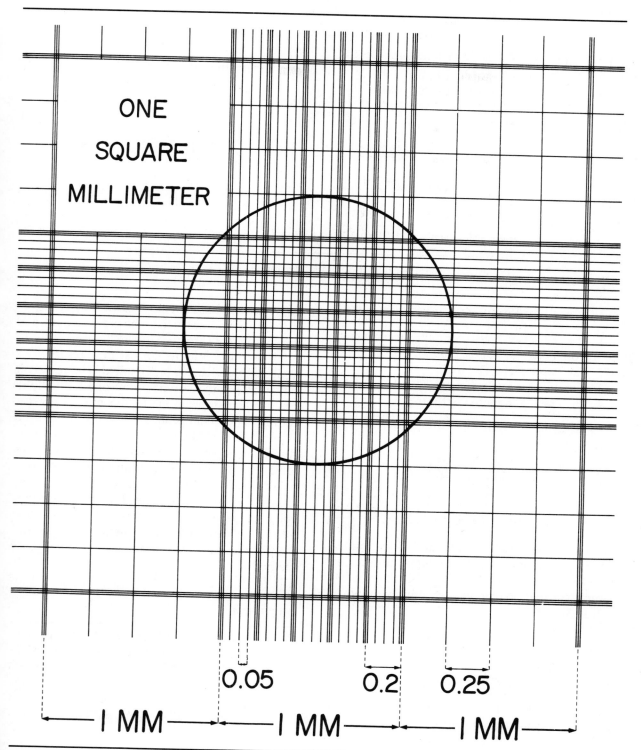

Figure 3–16. Platelet counting area (circled)

1. Count the platelets in the entire large center square (1 mm^2):

   Side 1 = 156   Side 2 = 180

2. Compute the average:
   A. 156 + 180 = 336 platelets
   B. 336 ÷ 2 = 168 average

3. Calculate the count:

$$\text{platelets/mm}^3 = \frac{\text{average \# platelets} \times \text{depth factor (mm)} \times \text{dilution factor}}{\text{area counted (mm}^2)}$$

$$\text{platelets/mm}^3 = \frac{168 \times 10 \times 100}{1}$$

$$\text{platelets/mm}^3 = 168 \times 1000$$

$$\text{platelets/mm}^3 = 168,000 \text{ (or } 1.68 \times 10^5)/\text{mm}^3$$

Figure 3-17. Sample calculation of platelet count

To simplify, use the following figures:

1. The platelet average is computed using counts from both sides of the chamber.
2. The depth factor (D) is 10.
3. The dilution factor (DF) is 100.
4. The area (A) counted is 1 mm^2.

These numbers are substituted into the formula as follows:

$$\frac{\text{Average \# of platelets} \times 10 \times 100}{1}$$

$$= \text{average \# platelets} \times 1000 = \frac{\text{platelets}}{\text{mm}^3}$$

Therefore, the platelet count can be determined by simply multiplying the average number of platelets by 1000 (or by adding three zeroes). A sample calculation of a platelet count is shown in Figure 3–17.

UNOPETTE® MICROCOLLECTION SYSTEM

The most acceptable manual method of counting platelets is the use of self-filling, self-diluting systems such as Unopette®. Such a system provides greater accuracy than the pipet method, and the components are disposable (Figure 3–18).

Unopette® systems consist of a reservoir, a capillary pipet, and a pipet shield. The reservoir contains a pre-measured volume of diluting fluid. The capillary pipet is made to contain a specific volume. The shield protects the pipet and is used to puncture the diaphragm which seals the reservoir. The Unopette® system used for platelet counts contains 1.98 ml of diluting fluid in the reservoir. A 20 µl capillary pipet is used to measure the sample. When the sample is diluted in the reservoir, the resulting dilution is 1:100. This blood dilution is then loaded into a hemacytometer and the platelets are counted as in the manual pipet method.

AUTOMATION

Platelet counts are still performed by hand in many laboratories. However, there are instruments which have been used for several years which have the ability to perform platelet counts. The platelet counter may be a part of a system which performs several other procedures, such as

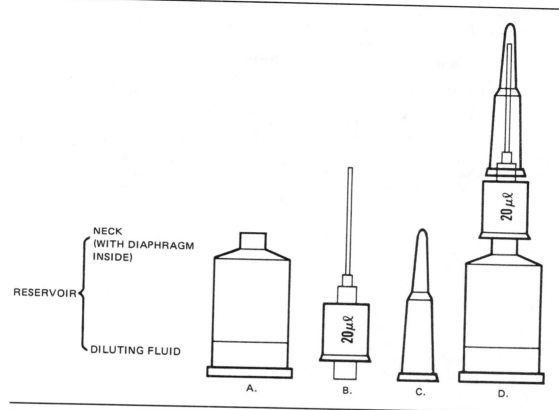

NECK
(WITH DIAPHRAGM
INSIDE)

RESERVOIR

DILUTING FLUID

20 μℓ

20 μℓ

A.   B.   C.   D.

Figure 3–18. Unopette® microcollection system

cell counts and hemoglobin measurements, or it may perform only platelet counts.

Precautions

■ The hemacytometer must be free of dirt and debris which might be confused with platelets.
■ The platelet count must be performed within 30 minutes of dilution of the sample.
■ Platelets clump easily; therefore, counts performed from capillary blood are usually lower than those performed on an anticoagulated sample.
■ The microscope light must be decreased to provide good contrast and to enable platelets to be seen.

■ If platelets are clumped or are distributed unevenly in the counting chamber, the chamber should be cleaned and refilled (after remixing pipet contents). If clumps are still present, a new sample should be obtained.
■ The moist cotton ball must not come into contact with the coverglass or the fluid in the hemacytometer.

LESSON REVIEW

1. Explain the function of platelets.
2. Name a condition in which thrombocytosis may occur.

3. Name a cause of thrombocytopenia.
4. Why is it important to thoroughly clean the coverglass and hemacytometer before performing the platelet count?
5. What is the purpose of the moist chamber?
6. What area of the hemacytometer is used to count platelets?
7. State the formula for calculating a platelet count.
8. How is a blood dilution performed for a platelet count?
9. Define hemostasis, petri dish, platelet, thrombocytopenia, and thrombocytosis.

STUDENT ACTIVITIES

1. Re-read the information on platelet counts.
2. Review the glossary terms.
3. Practice performing a platelet count as outlined on the Student Performance Guide, using the worksheet.
4. Prepare a stained blood smear from the blood sample used for the platelet count. Compare the number of platelets in the stained smear with the number counted.

Student Performance Guide

NAME _____

DATE _____

LESSON 3–4
PLATELET COUNT
(PIPET METHOD)

Instructions

1. Practice performing and calculating a platelet count.
2. Perform the platelet count procedure satisfactorily for the instructor. All steps must be completed as listed on the instructor's Performance Check Sheet.
3. Complete a written examination successfully.

Materials and Equipment

- gloves
- hand disinfectant
- RBC pipet
- pipet filler
- EDTA blood sample
- hemacytometer with coverglass
- test tube rack or beaker to hold blood sample
- platelet diluting fluid: 1% ammonium oxalate (store in refrigerator and filter before using)
- microscope
- petri dish
- cotton ball (slightly moistened with water)
- lens paper
- alcohol (70% ethanol)
- pipet shaker (optional)
- hand tally counter
- surface disinfectant
- biohazard container
- chlorine bleach

Procedure			S = Satisfactory U = Unsatisfactory
You must:	**S**	**U**	**Comments**
1. Wash hands with disinfectant and put on gloves			
2. Assemble equipment and materials			
3. Clean and polish the hemacytometer and coverglass carefully with alcohol and lens paper			

You must:	S	U	Comments
4. Attach pipet filler to the end of the RBC pipet which has the 101 mark			
5. Mix the tube of blood by inverting tube thirty times (if anticoagulated blood is unavailable, obtain blood by capillary puncture)			
6. Tilt the sample so that the blood flows near the lip of the tube and insert the pipet tip into the tube			
7. Draw the blood exactly to the 1.0 mark on the pipet			
8. Replace the blood sample tube into test tube rack			
9. Wipe the blood from the outside of the pipet stem with soft tissue			
10. Aspirate platelet diluting fluid to the 101 mark			
11. Mix the pipet contents for three minutes gently (or place on pipet shaker)			
12. Prepare a moist chamber: Place a slightly moist cotton ball into a petri dish leaving enough space for the hemacytometer			
13. Discard four to five drops from the pipet and wipe the stem			
14. Fill both sides of the hemacytometer			
15. Place the hemacytometer into the petri dish. Do not allow the cotton ball to touch the hemacytometer			
16. Place the cover on the petri dish and allow the preparation to stand ten minutes (this permits the platelets to settle in the chamber)			
17. Place the hemacytometer on the microscope stage carefully and secure. Do not wait longer than thirty minutes to complete the platelet count			
18. Use the low power (10×) objective to bring the ruled area into focus			
19. Locate the large central square (Figure 3–16)			
20. Rotate the high power objective (45×) into position carefully and focus with the fine adjustment knob until lines are clear			

You must:	S	U	Comments
21. Lower the condenser and reduce the light by partially closing the diaphragm for best contrast. Platelets should appear as round or oval particles which are refractile and are smaller than red blood cells (Color Plate 15)			
22. Count the platelets in the entire center square of the ruled area (all twenty-five small squares) using the left-to-right, right-to-left counting pattern and record results			
23. Repeat the procedure on the other side of the hemacytometer			
24. Average the results from the two sides			
25. Calculate the platelet count: $$\text{platelets/mm}^3 = \frac{\text{Avg} \times D \text{ (mm)} \times DF}{A \text{ (mm}^2)}$$ or $$\text{platelets/mm}^3 = \text{ average \# platelets} \times 1000$$			
26. Record the result			
27. Disinfect hemacytometer, coverglass and pipets			
28. Clean pipets, hemacytometer and coverglass			
29. Return equipment to proper storage			
30. Clean work area with surface disinfectant			
31. Remove and discard gloves appropriately			
32. Wash hands with hand disinfectant			

Comments:

Student/Instructor:

Date:_____ Instructor:_____

Student Performance Guide

NAME _____

DATE _____

LESSON 3–4
PLATELET COUNT
(UNOPETTE® METHOD)

Instructions

1. Practice performing and calculating a platelet count using the Unopette®.
2. Perform the platelet count procedure satisfactorily for the instructor. All steps must be completed as listed on the instructor's Performance Check Sheet.
3. Complete a written examination successfully.

Materials and Equipment

- gloves
- hand disinfectant
- blood sample, anticoagulated with EDTA
- hemacytometer with coverglass
- test tube rack or beaker to hold blood sample
- Unopette® for platelet count (reservoir and pipet assembly)
- microscope
- petri dish
- cotton ball (moistened slightly with water)
- lens paper
- alcohol (70% ethanol)
- hand tally counter
- surface disinfectant
- biohazard container

Note: The following is a general procedure for the use of the Unopette® system. Consult the package insert for specific instructions.

Procedure			S = Satisfactory U = Unsatisfactory
You must:	**S**	**U**	**Comments**
1. Wash hands with disinfectant and put on gloves			
2. Assemble equipment and materials			
3. Place a clean hemacytometer coverglass over a clean hemacytometer			

You must:	S	U	Comments
4. Puncture the diaphragm of the Unopette® reservoir. Hold the reservoir firmly on a flat surface with one hand and use the tip of the pipet shield to puncture the diaphragm. *Note:* The opening must be made large enough to easily accommodate the pipet			
5. Remove the shield from the pipet assembly			
6. Fill the capillary pipet from a capillary puncture or from a tube of well-mixed EDTA anticoagulated blood. The pipet will fill by capillary action and will stop filling automatically. *Note:* Keep pipet horizontal or at a slight (5°) angle to avoid overfilling			
7. Wipe excess blood from the outside of the capillary pipet with soft laboratory tissue. *Note:* Do not allow tissue to touch pipet tip			
8. Squeeze the reservoir slightly, being careful not to expel any of the liquid			
9. Maintain the pressure on the reservoir and insert the capillary pipet into the reservoir, seating the pipet firmly into the neck of the reservoir. Do not expel any of the liquid			
10. Release the pressure on the reservoir, drawing the blood out of the capillary pipet into the diluent			
11. Squeeze the reservoir gently three to four times to rinse the remaining blood from the capillary pipet. *Note:* Do not allow the blood-diluent mixture to flow out the top			
12. Mix the contents of the reservoir thoroughly by gently swirling the reservoir and/or turning it side to side			
13. Let stand at least ten minutes until red cells are completely destroyed. *Note:* Do not allow to stand longer than 2 hours			
14. Prepare a moist chamber: Place a slightly moist cotton ball into a petri dish, leaving enough space for the hemacytometer			
15. Withdraw the capillary pipet from the reservoir and place into the neck of the reservoir in reverse position (the pipet tip should now project upward from the reservoir)			
16. Mix the contents of the reservoir thoroughly. Invert the reservoir and gently squeeze to discard 4–5 drops onto gauze or paper towel			
17. Fill both sides of the hemacytometer			
18. Place the hemacytometer into the petri dish. Do not allow the cotton ball to touch the hemacytometer			

You must:	S	U	Comments
19. Place the cover on the petri dish and allow the preparation to stand ten minutes (this permits the platelets to settle in the chamber)			
20. Place the hemacytometer on the microscope stage carefully and secure. Do not wait longer than 30 minutes to complete the platelet count			
21. Use the low power (10×) objective to bring the ruled area into focus			
22. Locate the large central square (Figure 3–16)			
23. Rotate the high power (45×) objective into position carefully and focus with the fine adjustment knob until lines are clear			
24. Lower the condenser and reduce the light by partially closing the diaphragm for best contrast. Platelets should appear as round or oval particles which are refractile and are smaller than red blood cells			
25. Count the platelets in the entire center square of the ruled area (all twenty-five small squares) using the left-to-right, right-to-left counting pattern and record results			
26. Repeat the procedure on the other side of the hemacytometer			
27. Average the results from the two sides			
28. Calculate the platelet count: $$\text{platelets/mm}^3 = \frac{\text{Avg} \times \text{D (mm)} \times \text{DF}}{\text{A (mm}^2)}$$ or $$\text{platelets/mm}^3 = \text{average \# platelets} \times 1000$$			
29. Record the results			
30. Disinfect hemacytometer and coverglass and clean			
31. Discard specimen and disposable materials properly			
32. Return equipment to proper storage			
33. Clean work area with surface disinfectant			
34. Remove and discard gloves appropriately			
35. Wash hands with hand disinfectant			
Comments: Student/Instructor:			

Date:_____ Instructor:_____

Worksheet

NAME_____ DATE _____

SPECIMEN NO. _____

LESSON 3–4 PLATELET COUNT

	Count #1		Count #2
Platelets counted:			

Platelets counted:

Side 1 _____   Side 1 _____

Side 2 _____   Side 2 _____

Total _____   Total _____

Average (Total ÷ 2) _____   Average (Total ÷ 2) _____

Calculations:

$$\text{platelets/mm}^3 = \frac{\text{average \# platelets counted} \times \text{depth factor (mm)} \times \text{dilution factor}}{\text{area counted (mm}^2)}$$

$$\text{platelets/mm}^3 = \text{average \# platelets counted} \times 1000$$

$$\text{platelets/mm}^3 = \underline{\hspace{3cm}} \qquad \text{platelets/mm}^3 = \underline{\hspace{3cm}}$$

*Normal platelet count = 150,000 – 400,000/mm³

LESSON 3–5
Prothrombin Time

After studying this lesson, you should be able to:
- Discuss the role of prothrombin in blood coagulation.
- Explain the major use of the prothrombin time test.
- Perform a prothrombin time test.
- State the normal value for the prothrombin time test.
- Define the glossary terms.

GLOSSARY

coagulation / formation of a fibrin clot which aids in stopping bleeding

coagulation factors / plasma proteins which interact to form a fibrin clot

coumarin / a class of anticoagulant administered orally to prevent or slow clotting

embolus / a clot that is carried in the bloodstream

enzyme / a complex substance produced in living cells and which is able to cause or accelerate changes in other substances without being changed itself

fibrin / protein filaments formed in the coagulation process, resulting from the action of an enzyme, thrombin, on another plasma protein, fibrinogen

intravascular / inside the blood vessels

prothrombin / one of the plasma coagulation factors

prothrombin time / a test used as a screening test in coagulation; used to monitor oral anticoagulation therapy

thrombus / a clot which forms in a blood vessel or in the heart

INTRODUCTION

Hemostasis takes place because of the interaction of certain plasma proteins called **coagulation factors.** The process of stopping blood flow by formation of a fibrin clot is called **coagulation.** One of these coagulation proteins is prothrombin, also called factor II. **Prothrombin** is one of the coagulation factors which is produced in the liver and is vitamin K dependent. The hemostasis pathway is initiated normally when damage occurs to blood vessels or body tissue. After hemostasis is initiated by an injury, the prothrombin is converted to thrombin, an enzyme. An **enzyme** is a complex substance produced in living cells which is able to cause or accelerate changes in other substances without being changed itself. Thrombin then catalyzes the conversion of fibrinogen to **fibrin,** which forms the bulk of the actual clot. The simplified reactions are:

I. Prothrombin $\xrightarrow{\text{Thrombokinase}}$ Thrombin

II. Fibrinogen $\xrightarrow{\text{Thrombin}}$ Fibrin

Abnormalities in Hemostasis

The system of hemostasis works remarkably well, with a balance between the rate of thrombus formation and destruction. However, abnormal conditions can occur in which there is unnecessary thrombus formation. A **thrombus** is a clot which forms in a blood vessel. These **intravascular** clots can damage the area they are in by cutting off blood circulation. If a thrombus breaks off from where it is attached and travels in the bloodstream, it is called an **embolus.** Emboli travel through the bloodstream and can block small vessels such as those in vital organs. Emboli can cause serious damage to the heart, lungs, brain and kidneys and may result in death to the patient.

In conditions where there is a tendency to form thrombi, such as phlebitis, heart disease, and certain surgical procedures, the physician may prescribe oral anticoagulants for the patient. Drugs in the **coumarin** group are commonly prescribed. These anticoagulants delay clotting time so there is less chance that a thrombus will form. They act by inhibiting synthesis of prothrombin and the clotting factors VII, IX, and X in the liver. The result is that smaller amounts of these factors are available to participate in the hemostasis reaction.

PROTHROMBIN TIME TEST

The **prothrombin time** is a test which is used as a coagulation screening test. However, its major use is to monitor oral anticoagulant therapy since these anticoagulants affect the synthesis of prothrombin and factors VII and X in the liver. The test was developed by Dr. Quick, who named it "prothrombin time" because he thought it measured only prothrombin. Even though it was later discovered that the test actually measures prothrombin plus four additional factors, it is still called the prothrombin time or "pro time."

Normal Values for Prothrombin Time

The normal values for prothrombin time vary slightly from one laboratory to another because of different techniques being used. When the manual tilt method, described here, or the Fibrometer® method is used, the expected value on citrated samples from healthy individuals is commonly accepted to be 11–13 seconds. When other techniques are used, the laboratory must determine its own expected values.

Use of the Prothrombin Time

When a patient is receiving anticoagulants, a prothrombin time is performed at regular intervals, sometimes weekly. The physician can use the results to regulate the patient's dose of the anticoagulant. The usual goal is to keep the patient's prothrombin time about two or two-and-one-half (2–2½) times the normal. This prolongation is usually sufficient to prevent unwanted clotting, but not so long that the patient suffers abnormal bleeding.

Collection of the Specimen

The specimen for prothrombin time must be drawn with minimal trauma to the vein and surrounding tissue to prevent the release of interfering components into the sample. The blood must be drawn into a tube or syringe containing an anticoagulant compatible with the commercial reagent system being used. Most systems for prothrombin time are compatible with a 3.8% solution of sodium citrate, but the instructions for each method must be consulted. Vacuum tubes are available which contain the proper concentration of citrate (Table 3–1). The blood is centrifuged as soon as possible and the plasma removed to be used in the assay. The plasma should be assayed within two hours of

blood collection and should not stand at 37°C for more than five minutes.

Performing the Assay

The prothrombin time has been automated for several years; however, some laboratories prefer to perform the test manually. Most commercial reagents can be used for either method, but the instructions for each must be checked carefully. Many analyzers for coagulation are on the market, but the Fibrometer® from Becton, Dickinson and Company is a popular choice if the prothrombin time is the only coagulation assay desired. Several diagnostic companies manufacture reagents used in both manual and automated determination of prothrombin.

Manual Method. To perform a manual prothrombin time, the patient plasma and the thromboplastin reagents are pipetted into separate labeled test tubes which are placed in a 37°C waterbath for a

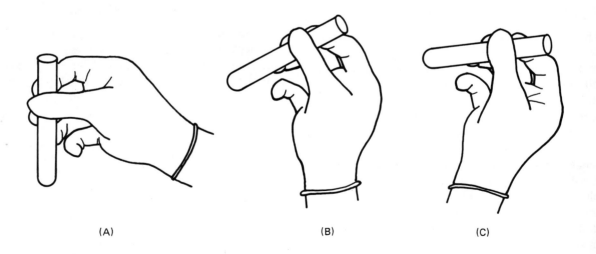

(A)   (B)   (C)

Figure 3–19. Illustrating manual tilt-tube method of determining prothrombin time. (A) Lifting tube out of waterbath, (B) tilting the tube horizontally, and (C) observing formation of fibrin clot.

prescribed amount of time to warm. When the warming time has elapsed, 0.1 ml of the patient plasma is forcibly added to 0.2 ml of reagent. A stopwatch is started at the same time. The tube is allowed to remain in the waterbath about 10 seconds before being lifted up and the outside is wiped to remove water droplets. The tube is held horizontally at just below eye level in front of a good light source. Immediately, the tube is tilted back and forth until a thickening appears (Figure 3–19). This is the fibrin clot. At the first appearance of the clot, the stopwatch is stopped. The time is recorded in seconds. It is generally recommended that manual determinations be performed in triplicate. Timing of the first one will be approximate and the other two should check.

Automated Method. The use of an instrument for prothrombin time determination eliminates the necessity of having a waterbath. Most of the instruments such as the Fibrometer® (Figure 3–20) have built-in heat blocks to warm the samples and reagents. The samples and reagents are pipetted into special cups which fit into the heat wells of the instrument. After the specified warming time has elapsed, the cup containing the reagent is placed in the center well of the instrument. The automatic pipetter on the instrument is used to draw up and then expel the patient sample into the reagent. The timer automatically starts when the sample is expelled. Two wire probes detect the formation of the clot and stop the timer. The time is read directly off the instrument. Automated determinations should be performed in duplicate and the results averaged.

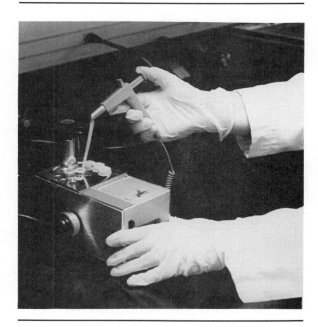

Figure 3–20. Using the Fibrometer® to perform a prothrombin time test. *(Photo courtesy of John Estridge)*

■ The test sample and reagents must be warmed for the times specified in the package inserts and manufacturer's instructions.
■ A quality control program must be established using both normal and abnormal plasmas.

Precautions

There are several precautions that must be observed whether manual or automated methods are used.

■ The temperature of the waterbath or heat block must be kept at 37°C.

The prothrombin time is a useful test for the physician to monitor oral anticoagulant therapy. It is one of the most frequently performed laboratory tests. Patients may have the test performed either at the physician's office or at an outpatient laboratory at the hospital, usually once a week. The results of these regularly performed tests guide the physician in regulating the patient's medication.

LESSON REVIEW

1. What is the role of prothrombin in blood coagulation?
2. How does the physician use the results from the prothrombin time?
3. Explain how a manual prothrombin time is performed. Explain how to perform a prothrombin time using the Fibrometer®.
4. What is the normal value for the prothrombin time test?

5. Define coagulation, coagulation factors, coumarin, embolus, enzyme, fibrin, intravascular, and thrombus.

STUDENT ACTIVITIES

1. Re-read the information on prothrombin time.
2. Review the glossary terms.
3. Practice performing the prothrombin time as outlined on the Student Performance Guide.

Student Performance Guide

NAME _____

DATE _____

LESSON 3–5
PROTHROMBIN TIME

Instructions

1. Practice performing a prothrombin time.
2. Demonstrate the prothrombin time procedure satisfactorily for the instructor. All steps must be completed as listed on the instructor's Performance Check Sheet.
3. Complete a written examination successfully.

Materials and Equipment

- gloves
- centrifuge
- source of thrombokinase (Thromboplastin CaCl$_2$)
- fresh citrated human plasma
- normal controls
- abnormal controls
- distilled water for reconstituting controls
- biohazard container
- surface disinfectant
- laboratory tissue
- hand disinfectant
- test tube rack

For Manual Method

- test tubes (13 x 75)
- waterbath at 37°C
- pipets to transfer 0.1 and 0.2 ml
- stopwatch

For Automated Method

- coagulation instrument, such as Fibrometer®
- supplies for instrument

Procedure

S = Satisfactory
U = Unsatisfactory

You must:	S	U	Comments
1. Wash hands with disinfectant and put on gloves			
2. Obtain blood sample (if not provided)			

You must:	S	U	Comments
3. Centrifuge the specimen as specified in reagent package insert			
4. Remove the plasma to clean test tube. Label with patient identification			
5. *For manual method:* a. Check that waterbath temperature is 37°C			
b. Pipet 0.2 ml of Thromboplastin-CaCl$_2$ reagent into seven labeled tubes (three for the patient, two for each normal and abnormal control)			
c. Place tubes into rack in waterbath			
d. Pipet sufficient patient plasma and control plasmas (0.4–0.5 ml each) to perform the test in triplicate (plus excess) in another set of appropriately labeled tubes			
e. Place tubes into rack in waterbath			
f. Allow patient sample, controls, and reagent to warm the prescribed amount of time			
g. Draw up 0.1 ml patient plasma and forcibly expel into tube containing reagent, starting stopwatch simultaneously			
h. Allow tube to remain in waterbath about ten seconds before picking up and wiping water from outside of tube			
i. *Work Quickly*—pick up the tube, wipe the outside with tissue, start tilting tube slowly back and forth, in front of good light source			
j. Stop the watch at the first sign of thickening (clot) in the moving liquid			
k. Repeat steps g–j. Remember that the first time is approximate, and the second and third should check			
l. Perform steps g–j in duplicate for each control sample			
m. Report results: Report average of patient's second and third times; report the time for the normal control			

6. *For automated method:*
      (Perform steps 1–4 before proceeding)
    a. Turn on instrument. If using automated pipetter, be certain it is turned "OFF"			

b. Label desired number of sample cups and place into heat block. (Patient samples should be run in duplicate.)			

You must:	S	U	Comments
c. Pipet 0.2 ml of reagent into cups, following manufacturer's instructions if using instrument's automatic pipetter			
d. Pipet sufficient patient plasma and controls (0.4–0.5 ml) into separate cups to allow for duplicate testing of patient and controls			
e. Allow all components to warm the prescribed amount of time. Place one sample cup with measured reagent into center well of Fibrometer®			
f. Draw up 0.1 ml of patient plasma			
g. Turn pipetter "ON"			
h. Expel plasma into center cup containing 0.2 ml reagent. The timer will start automatically when the plunger is depressed, if using instrument's pipet			
i. Wait for timer to stop, signaling the formation of a clot			
j. Record the time in seconds			
k. Gently wipe probe wires with laboratory tissue between determinations			
l. Repeat steps e–k using patient plasma			
m. Average the two times and report the results			
n. Repeat steps e–k for each control			
o. Report the time for the normal control			
7. Return all equipment to proper storage			
8. Dispose of all contaminated articles in biohazard container			
9. Wipe counter with surface disinfectant			
10. Remove gloves and discard appropriately			
11. Wash hands with hand disinfectant			

Comments:

Student/Instructor:

Date:_____   Instructor:_____

LESSON 3–6
Erythrocyte Indices

LESSON OBJECTIVES

After studying this lesson, you should be able to:
- State the procedure for determining the erythrocyte indices.
- Write the formulas for each of the three indices.
- Perform the calculations necessary to determine the erythrocyte indices.
- Explain the uses of the erythrocyte indices values.
- List the normal values for the erythrocyte indices.
- Define the glossary terms.

GLOSSARY

indices / plural of index; indexes; erythrocyte indices are values which compare a blood sample to standard values

mean corpuscular hemoglobin / MCH; average red cell hemoglobin concentration; an estimate of the hemoglobin in a red cell in a blood specimen; measured in picograms (pg)

mean corpuscular hemoglobin concentration / MCHC; compares the weight of hemoglobin in a red cell to the size of the cell; reported in percentage or g/dl

mean corpuscular volume / MCV; average red cell volume; an estimate of the volume of a red cell in a blood specimen; measured in femtoliters (fl) or cubic microns (μ^3)

micron / a unit of measurement, 1×10^{-6} meter or one micrometer

picogram / micromicrogram; 1×10^{-12} gram; pg

INTRODUCTION

The erythrocyte **indices** are calculations which yield information concerning the size and the hemoglobin content of the red cells. They are also called the mean corpuscular values. The three indices are: the **mean corpuscular volume (MCV)** the **mean corpuscular hemoglobin (MCH),** and

236

the **mean corpuscular hemoglobin concentration (MCHC).** These indices aid in classifying the anemias.

CALCULATING THE ERYTHROCYTE INDICES

The indices are calculated by formulas using the red cell count, the hemoglobin, and the hematocrit. The validity of the indices results depends on the accuracy of those three values.

Mean Corpuscular Volume

The mean corpuscular volume (MCV) is calculated by using the hematocrit percentage and the red blood cell count (Figure 3–21). The result is reported in femtoliters (fl), formerly cubic **microns,** and gives the average volume of a red cell in an individual blood sample. The formula for the MCV is:

$$MCV = \frac{Hematocrit}{RBC} \times 10$$

Mean Corpuscular Hemoglobin

The mean corpuscular hemoglobin (MCH) is calculated from the hemoglobin and red cell count values. This result estimates the weight of hemo-

$$MCV = \frac{hematocrit\ (in\ percent)}{RBC\ (in\ millions)} \times 10$$

Using a hematocrit of 36% and an RBC of 4.0 million/mm³:

$$MCV = \frac{36}{4.0} \times 10$$

$$MCV = 90\ fl\ (or\ \mu^3)$$

Figure 3–21. Calculation of mean corpuscular volume (MCV)

$$MCH = \frac{hemoglobin\ (in\ grams)}{RBC\ (in\ millions)} \times 10$$

Using a hemoglobin value of 15 g/dl and an RBC of 5.2 million/mm³:

$$MCH = \frac{15.0}{5.2} \times 10$$

$$MCH = 28.8\ pg$$

Figure 3–22. Calculation of mean corpuscular hemoglobin (MCH)

$$MCHC = \frac{hemoglobin\ (in\ grams)}{hematocrit} \times 100$$

Using a hemoglobin value of 15 g/dl and a hematocrit of 44%:

$$MCHC = \frac{15}{44} \times 100$$

$$MCHC = 34\%\ or\ 34\ g/dl$$

Figure 3–23. Calculation of mean corpuscular hemoglobin concentration (MCHC)

globin in a red cell in an individual blood sample. It is expressed in **picograms** (pg). One picogram is equivalent to 10^{-12} gram. The formula for the MCH is:

$$MCH = \frac{Hemoglobin}{RBC} \times 10$$

A sample calculation is shown in Figure 3–22.

Mean Corpuscular Hemoglobin Concentration

The mean corpuscular hemoglobin concentration (MCHC) is calculated from the hemoglobin and hematocrit results. The MCHC expresses the concentration of hemoglobin in the red cells relative to cell size. It is reported in percentage or g/dl since it actually is a comparison of hemoglobin to the hematocrit. The formula is:

$$MCHC = \frac{Hematocrit}{Hct} \times 100$$

A sample calculation is shown in Figure 3–23, page 237.

NORMAL VALUES

The normal range for the MCV is 80–100 femtoliters (fl). A cell with an MCV below 80 fl is said to be *microcytic. Macrocytic* cells are those having an MCV greater than 100 fl.

The normal range for the MCH is 27–32 picograms (pg). A value below 27 pg indicates a low weight of hemoglobin in the red cells and could be found in microcytes or normocytes. A value greater than 32 pg could be found in macrocytes.

The normal range for the MCHC is 33–38% (or g/dl). This relationship compares the concentration of hemoglobin to the packed volume of red cells. It gives the concentration (percentage) of hemoglobin in the red cells. The normal range is 32–37%. Values less than 32% indicate less hemoglobin than is normal for that red cell population. This is referred to as *hypochromia*. A value greater than normal is not possible since it would indicate that the cell is supersaturated or contains more hemoglobin than it can actually hold. The normal values for the erythrocyte indices are shown in Table 3–4.

FACTORS WHICH AFFECT THE INDICES

The indices results can be used to classify the anemias. In iron deficiency anemia, which is characterized by hypochromia and microcytes, all three indices values will be decreased. In the macrocytic anemias, such as pernicious anemia or B_{12} deficiency anemia, the MCV and the MCH are increased.

Sources of Error

There is much chance for error in the calculation of the erythrocyte indices. All of the calculations rely

Table 3-4. Normal values for erythrocyte indices

	Normal Values
MCV	80–100 fl
MCH	27–32 pg
MCHC	33–38%

on the results obtained from the red blood cell counts, the hematocrits, and the hemoglobins. Any error in those results will in turn cause error in the indices results.

AUTOMATION

Almost all medical laboratories now have instrumentation to perform the complete blood count (CBC). These instruments use the values from the hemoglobin, red blood cell count, and hematocrit to calculate the erythrocyte indices. In a physician's office, such automation is not usually available. In such cases, the indices are calculated manually or by using an indices calculator, and are performed infrequently.

Precautions

■ The Hgb, Hct, and RBC values inserted in the formulas must be accurate.
■ The correct values must be inserted in the formulas.
■ The calculations must be performed correctly.

LESSON REVIEW

1. Results from which three hematology procedures are used to calculate the indices?

2. State one use of the indices.
3. What is the normal value for the MCV? Give the formula for calculation.
4. In what units are the MCH and the MCHC reported?
5. What does an MCV greater than 100 femtoliters indicate?
6. Give the normal values for the MCH and MCHC. Give the formulas for their calculation.
7. Define indices, MCV, MCH, MCHC, micron, and picogram.

STUDENT ACTIVITIES

1. Re-read the information on erythrocyte indices.
2. Review the glossary terms.
3. Practice calculating erythrocyte indices as outlined on the Student Performance Guide, using the worksheet.

Student Performance Guide

NAME _____

DATE _____

LESSON 3–6
ERYTHROCYTE INDICES

Instructions

1. Practice the procedure for calculating the erythrocyte indices.
2. Demonstrate the procedure for performing Hgb, Hct, and RBC on a sample and calculating the erythrocyte indices satisfactorily for the instructor. All steps must be completed as listed on the instructor's Performance Check Sheet.
3. Complete a written examination successfully.

Materials and Equipment

- gloves
- hand disinfectant
- tube of venous blood, anticoagulated (or use capillary blood)
- materials for capillary puncture (optional)
- worksheet
- puncture-proof container for sharp objects
- surface disinfectant
- biohazard container

Materials for RBC count:
- RBC blood diluting pipets ⎫ or Unopette®
- pipet filler ⎬ for red cell
- RBC diluting fluid ⎭ count
- hemacytometer and coverglass
- lens paper
- alcohol
- microscope

Materials for hemoglobin determination:
- spectrophotometer
- Drabkin's reagent ⎫ or Unopette®
- Sahli pipet ⎬ for
- cuvettes ⎭ hemoglobin
- test tubes

Materials for hematocrit:
- capillary tubes
- sealing clay
- microhematocrit centrifuge
- microhematocrit reader

Procedure			S = Satisfactory U = Unsatisfactory
You must:	**S**	**U**	**Comments**
1. Wash hands with disinfectant and put on gloves			
2. Assemble appropriate equipment and materials for Hgb, Hct, and RBC procedures			
3. Perform Hgb, Hct, and RBC from either capillary puncture or well-mixed tube of previously-drawn blood, and record results			
4. Calculate the MCV on the worksheet and record the result			
5. Calculate the MCH on the worksheet and record the result			
6. Calculate the MCHC on the worksheet and record the result			
7. Disinfect glassware by immersing in chlorine bleach			
8. Dispose of sharp objects in a puncture-proof container			
9. Discard contaminated materials into biohazard container			
10. Clean equipment and return to proper storage			
11. Clean work area with surface disinfectant			
12. Remove and discard gloves appropriately			
13. Wash hands with hand disinfectant			

Comments:

Student/Instructor:

Date:_____ Instructor:_____

Worksheet

NAME_____ DATE _____

SPECIMEN NO. _____

LESSON 3–6 ERYTHROCYTE INDICES

RBC/mm^3 = _____
Hb (g/dl) = _____
Hct (%) = _____

1. Calculate the MCV:

2. Calculate the MCH:

3. Calculate the MCHC:

LESSON 3–7
Bleeding Time

LESSON OBJECTIVES

After studying this lesson, you should be able to:
- State the purpose of the bleeding time test.
- Name three components that interact to cause hemostasis.
- Name and describe two methods used to determine the bleeding time and list the normal values of each.
- List three conditions in which the bleeding time will be prolonged.
- Perform the Duke bleeding time test.
- Name the incision sites used in the Ivy and Duke bleeding time tests.
- Report the results of a bleeding time.
- List the precautions to be observed in performing a bleeding time.
- Define the glossary terms.

GLOSSARY

coagulation factors / plasma proteins which interact to form the fibrin clot
dysfunction / impaired or abnormal function
hemorrhage / excessive or uncontrolled bleeding
vasoconstriction / a contracting or narrowing of a vessel

INTRODUCTION

The bleeding time test is a screening procedure used to evaluate some aspects of the body's ability to stop bleeding. The bleeding time test is performed by making a small standardized incision of the capillaries. The length of time required for the bleeding to stop is then measured.

HEMOSTASIS

Hemostasis, the cessation of bleeding, involves a series of complex interactions. The components which must interact are (1) the blood vessels, (2) the blood platelets, and (3) the plasma proteins called **coagulation factors.** The blood vessels must have the ability to constrict and slow blood flow

243

after an injury. This property is known as **vasocon-striction.** The platelets react within seconds after an injury to form a plug and to release certain chemical activators. The coagulation factors, proteins in the plasma, are activated by the platelets and the injured tissue.

When all the hemostasis components interact and function properly, a clot is formed and bleeding stops. The failure of the clotting mechanism can be due to the absence, deficiency, or improper function of any of the components. Failure of the hemostatic or clotting mechanism may result in **hemorrhage.**

Several laboratory tests can be performed which will detect deficiencies of the hemostatic system. The bleeding time is one of these tests. It is influenced by the number and function of platelets and the condition of the vessels. The bleeding time may be prolonged in thrombocytopenia, platelet **dysfunction,** and after ingestion of aspirin. The bleeding time is usually normal when there is a deficiency of only one of the coagulation factors.

METHODS OF MEASURING BLEEDING TIME

Two methods for measuring the bleeding time are the Ivy method and the Duke method. The Ivy method, although more difficult to perform correctly, is the preferred method because it can be somewhat standardized. Both of these tests and other coagulation tests must be performed carefully and accurately by well-trained technicians. With both methods it is difficult to obtain reproducible results because of the difficulty of standardizing procedure.

Ivy Bleeding Time

The Ivy bleeding time is performed by incising the forearm and measuring the time required for bleeding to stop. A blood pressure cuff is placed around the patient's arm above the elbow, and the pressure is increased to 40 mm of mercury to standardize the pressure in the capillaries. This

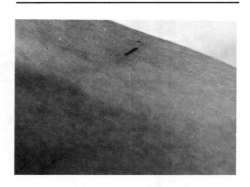

Figure 3–24. Puncture site in Ivy bleeding time *(Photo courtesy of General Diagnostics Division of Warner Lambert)*

pressure is held constant for the entire procedure. The forearm is cleansed with 70% alcohol. A 3 mm deep incision is made in an area that is free of large superficial blood vessels (Figure 3–24). A stopwatch is started when the first drop of blood appears. At thirty second intervals, the blood is blotted with filter paper without touching the puncture site. When the bleeding ceases, the time is noted and the pressure cuff is removed. The time between the first appearance of blood and

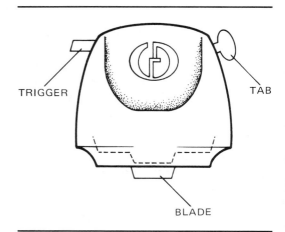

TRIGGER

TAB

BLADE

Figure 3–25. Simplate® device used in performing bleeding time test

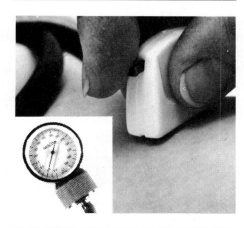

Figure 3–26. Performing a bleeding time test using a Simplate® *(Photo courtesy of General Diagnostics Division of Warner Lambert)*

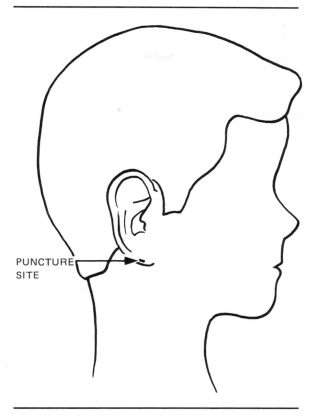

Figure 3–27. Puncture site for Duke bleeding time

he stopping of blood flow is the bleeding time. The normal bleeding time by the Ivy method is one to seven minutes. This method may also be performed using a device called a Simplate® which makes a more standardized incision than a lancet or blade (Figures 3–25 and 3–26). Ivy bleeding times may cause scar formation at incision site. The patient should be informed of this before test is begun.

Duke Bleeding Time

The Duke bleeding time is performed by incising the earlobe and measuring the time required for bleeding to cease. The earlobe is cleansed with alcohol and allowed to dry. A 2–3 mm deep puncture is made with a sterile lancet (Figure 3–27) and timing is begun when the first drop of blood appears. The blood is blotted every thirty seconds with filter paper and without touching the puncture site. The watch is stopped when bleeding ceases. The time elapsed is reported as the bleeding time. The normal bleeding time by the Duke method is one to three minutes.

Precautions

■ Do not perform the bleeding time test if the patient has taken aspirin within seven days of the test.
■ The incision site should be warm to ensure that circulation is good.
■ The incision site should be in an area free of superficial veins, so that only capillaries are punctured.
■ The incision site must be dry before the incision is made.
■ The first drop of blood that appears after the puncture is not wiped away.
■ If bleeding continues more than ten minutes (Duke) or fifteen minutes (Ivy), stop the test and apply pressure to the wound.

■ When blotting the blood with filter paper, the paper should not touch the puncture site, to insure that clot formation is not disturbed.

LESSON REVIEW

1. What does the bleeding time measure?
2. What three components interact to cause hemostasis?
3. Name three conditions in which the bleeding time will be prolonged.
4. Explain the procedure for the Ivy bleeding time.
5. Explain the procedure for the Duke bleeding time.
6. State the normal ranges for bleeding times by the Ivy method and the Duke method.
7. List precautions which should be observed when performing a bleeding time test.
8. What incision site is used for the Ivy bleeding time—for the Duke bleeding time?
9. Define coagulation factors, dysfunction, hemorrhage, and vasoconstriction.

STUDENT ACTIVITIES

1. Re-read the information on bleeding time.
2. Review the glossary terms.
3. Practice explaining the bleeding time procedure to a patient.
4. Practice performing a bleeding time by the Duke method, as outlined on the Student Performance Guide.

Student Performance Guide

NAME _____

DATE _____

LESSON 3–7
BLEEDING TIME

Instructions

1. Practice performing a bleeding time test (Duke method).
2. Demonstrate the procedure for the bleeding time test satisfactorily for the instructor. All steps must be completed as listed on the instructor's Performance Check Sheet.
3. Complete a written examination successfully.

Materials and Equipment

- gloves
- hand disinfectant
- sterile cotton balls or gauze
- 70% alcohol or alcohol swabs
- blood lancets
- filter paper
- stopwatch
- clean microscope slide
- surface disinfectant
- biohazard container
- puncture-proof container for sharp objects

Procedure			S = Satisfactory U = Unsatisfactory
You must:	S	U	Comments
1. Wash hands with disinfectant and put on gloves			
2. Assemble equipment and materials			
3. Explain the procedure to the patient			
4. Cleanse the earlobe with 70% alcohol and allow to dry (or wipe dry with dry sterile gauze)			

You must:	S	U	Comments
5. Puncture the earlobe with a sterile lancet and start the stopwatch			
6. *Do not* wipe away the first drop of blood			
7. Blot the blood with filter paper every thirty seconds by lightly touching the edge of the drop. Do not touch puncture site with filter paper			
8. Stop the watch when blood is no longer absorbed onto the filter paper			
9. Report the bleeding time to the nearest thirty seconds			
10. Treat the puncture site by cleansing gently without disturbing the clot			
11. Clean equipment and return to proper storage			
12. Clean work area with surface disinfectant			
13. Dispose of sharp objects in puncture-proof container			
14. Dispose of contaminated materials in biohazard container			
15. Remove and discard gloves. Wash hands with hand disinfectant			

Comments:

Student/Instructor:

Date:_____ Instructor:_____

LESSON 3–8
Capillary Coagulation

LESSON OBJECTIVES

After studying this lesson, you should be able to:

- List the component of the hemostatic mechanism which is tested by the capillary coagulation procedure.
- List a situation in which the capillary coagulation procedure would be performed.
- Perform a capillary coagulation procedure.
- List the normal capillary coagulation time.
- Name three conditions that may cause a prolonged capillary coagulation time.
- List the precautions to observe when performing the capillary coagulation procedure.
- Define the glossary terms.

GLOSSARY

coagulation / formation of a fibrin clot which aids in stopping bleeding
fibrin / protein filaments formed in the coagulation process, resulting from the action of the enzyme, thrombin, on the plasma protein, fibrinogen

INTRODUCTION

The capillary coagulation test is a simple procedure. It is used to screen for problems in the blood clotting or **coagulation** mechanism. It measures the amount of time needed for the blood to form a **fibrin** clot. This procedure tests the function of the coagulation factors rather than of the platelets or blood vessels. Delayed clotting or lack of clotting can be due to a deficiency in any one or more of the coagulation factors.

The capillary coagulation test is not a specific test. Thus, it has been largely replaced by other tests which are newer and more specific. However, the capillary coagulation test may still be used to screen pediatric patients before surgical procedures such as tonsillectomy or adenoidectomy.

249

PERFORMING THE PROCEDURE

The capillary coagulation test is performed by making a capillary puncture of the fingertip with as little trauma to the tissue as possible. The first drop of blood is wiped away using a sterile cotton or gauze. A stopwatch is started when the second drop of blood appears. At least three special capillary coagulation tubes are filled three-fourths full and laid horizontally on the counter top. The tubes are left undisturbed until two minutes have passed from the starting of the watch. Meanwhile, a gauze is placed over the puncture site and pressure is applied. When two minutes have passed, the first tube filled is picked up and one-half inch of the tube is carefully broken off at one end (Figure 3–28). The two broken ends are gently pulled apart (about one-quarter to one-half inch) to look for the fibrin thread. If a fibrin thread is not seen, breaks are made in the same tube every thirty seconds until a fibrin thread has formed and is observed. If the thread is not observed in the first tube, the second and third tubes are broken in the same manner. The stopwatch is stopped when the fibrin thread is first seen (Figure 3–29). The capillary coagulation time is the time on the stopwatch (or the time elapsed between the appearance of the second drop of blood and the formation of fibrin).

NORMAL VALUES

The normal time for a fibrin thread to appear in the capillary coagulation time test is two to six minutes. There are various factors which can affect the coagulation time. Many of the coagulation factors are produced in the liver and are affected by any disease of or damage to the liver. Production of some of the factors is dependent on vitamin K and a deficiency of that vitamin can

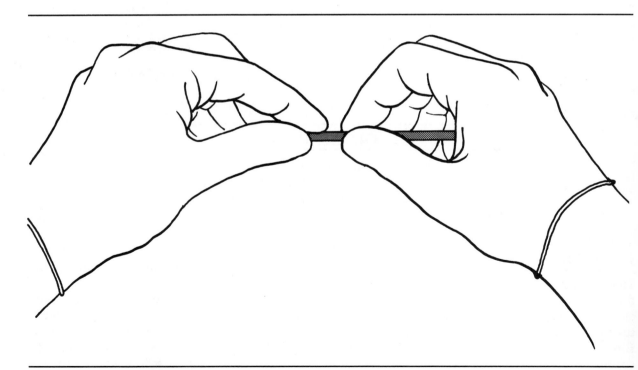

Figure 3–28. Capillary coagulation: breaking the capillary tube

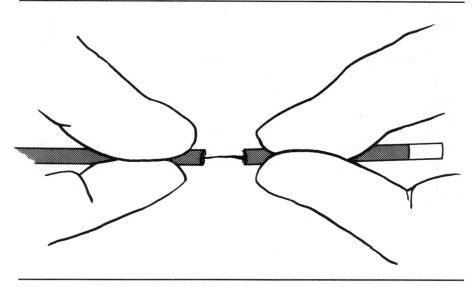

Figure 3–29. Capillary coagulation: appearance of the fibrin thread

prolong the coagulation time. Abnormal capillary coagulation times may also occur when a patient is taking anticoagulant medication, or if an individual has a deficiency of one or more factors.

Precautions

■ Use only tubes made specially for coagulation tests; they have a smaller diameter than regular capillary tubes and contain no anticoagulant.
■ Fill at least two or three tubes since the fibrin may not form before the first tube is used up.
■ Excessive pressure should not be applied near the puncture site.
■ Break the tubes carefully to avoid cutting the fingers or destroying the fibrin thread before it is observed.
■ Break the tubes in the order of filling.
■ Start the stopwatch when the second drop of blood appears.
■ Stop the watch when the fibrin thread is first observed.

LESSON REVIEW

1. What is the capillary coagulation time?
2. The capillary coagulation time is most frequently performed on what age patient?
3. How many capillary tubes should be filled?
4. When are the capillary tubes broken?
5. What is the normal capillary coagulation time?
6. What signals the end of the test?
7. What type of capillary tubes are used and why?
8. What three conditions could cause a prolonged capillary coagulation time?
9. What component of hemostasis is tested in the capillary coagulation time?
10. Define coagulation and fibrin.

STUDENT ACTIVITIES

1. Re-read the information on capillary coagulation.
2. Review the glossary terms.
3. Practice performing a capillary coagulation time as outlined on the Student Performance Guide.

Student Performance Guide

NAME _____

DATE _____

LESSON 3–8
CAPILLARY COAGULATION

Instructions

1. Practice the procedure for capillary coagulation.
2. Demonstrate the procedure for performing the capillary coagulation time satisfactorily for the instructor. All steps must be completed as listed on the instructor's Performance Check Sheet.
3. Complete a written examination successfully.

Materials and Equipment

- gloves
- hand disinfectant
- capillary puncture materials
- stopwatch
- capillary coagulation tubes
- surface disinfectant
- biohazard container
- puncture-proof container for sharp objects

Procedure			S = Satisfactory U = Unsatisfactory
You must:	**S**	**U**	**Comments**
1. Wash hands with disinfectant and put on gloves			
2. Assemble equipment and materials			
3. Perform capillary puncture using proper procedure			
4. Wipe away the first drop of blood with sterile gauze			
5. Start the stopwatch when the second drop of blood appears and fill one capillary coagulation tube three-fourths full			

You must:	S	U	Comments
6. Place the filled capillary tube on the counter top			
7. Fill two additional tubes and place them on the counter top in the order in which they were filled			
8. Place gauze over puncture site and have patient apply pressure			
9. Observe the stopwatch until two minutes have passed (from start)			
10. Pick up the first tube filled (at the two-minute time) and gently break approximately one-half inch from end			
11. Look carefully for a fibrin thread. If a thread is not observed, continue breaking a segment every thirty seconds			
12. Break one-half inch segments from the second tube every thirty seconds if a thread is not seen in the first tube			
13. Continue breaking the segments every thirty seconds until a fibrin thread is observed			
14. Stop the stopwatch when the fibrin thread is observed			
15. Record the total time elapsed as the capillary coagulation time			
16. Dispose of lancets and capillary tubes in a puncture-proof container for sharp objects			
17. Discard contaminated materials into biohazard container			
18. Clean equipment and return to proper storage			
19. Clean work area with surface disinfectant			
20. Remove and discard gloves appropriately			
21. Wash hands with hand disinfectant			

Comments:

Student/Instructor:

Date:_____   Instructor:_____

UNIT 4

Introduction to Serology

UNIT OBJECTIVES

After studying this unit, you should be able to:
- Perform ABO slide typing.
- Perform ABO tube typing.
- Perform Rh slide typing.
- Perform a slide test for pregnancy.
- Perform a slide test for infectious mononucleosis.
- Perform a slide test for rheumatoid factors.

OVERVIEW

Immunology is the study of the body's responses which protect us from disease or provide immunity. Most people think of immunity as the production of antibodies in response to foreign substances which are called antigens. Serology, a branch of immunology, is a term used for laboratory procedures which utilize the antigen-antibody reaction in the tests. Serology was named because early laboratories used serum for testing. Today, serological procedures may use serum, whole blood, or urine for testing.

Modern serology laboratories detect, identify, and measure antibodies to aid in the diagnosis of diseases such as infectious mononucleosis and rheumatoid arthritis. Other serological procedures may use antibodies to identify substances such as hormones, as in the pregnancy test.

Immunohematology, or blood banking, is a specialized branch of immunology which uses serological procedures to study and identify the blood groups. Procedures in blood banking may be simple, such as routine ABO and Rh blood typing. Or, blood banking may involve more complex procedures such as identifying tissue antigens for organ transplantation.

The exercises in Unit 4 are an introduction to techniques, such as agglutination and agglutination inhibition, which are commonly used in serology laboratories and require minimum equipment and time.

LESSON 4–1
ABO Slide Typing

GLOSSARY

agglutination / clumping of cells or particles; in serology due to reaction of the particle with antibody

antibody / serum protein produced in response to a foreign substance (antigen); abbreviated Ab

antigen / a substance which causes the formation of antibodies; abbreviated Ag

antiserum / serum containing antibodies

blood group antibody / a serum protein that reacts specifically with a blood group antigen

blood group antigen / a substance or structure on the red cell membrane which causes antibody formation and reacts with that antibody

immunoglobulins / serum proteins produced in response to antigens; antibodies; abbreviated Ig

serology / laboratory study of serum and the reactions between antigens and antibodies

INTRODUCTION

Immunohematology, or blood banking, is the study of human blood groups. In clinical laboratories, the department which tests blood for transfusion is usually called the blood bank or transfusion services department.

The ABO system is the major human blood group system. A patient's ABO group (or type) must be determined before a blood transfusion can be given. Blood groups must also be considered in organ transplantation, questions of paternity, forensic investigations, and genetic studies.

ABO typing may be performed using a slide test described in this lesson or a tube test (Lesson 4–2). The slide method is quick, easy, and requires no special equipment. However, the tube test is the preferred method and is used most commonly in medical laboratories.

ABO SYSTEM

The ABO blood group system was discovered around 1900. All humans can be placed into one of four major groups: A, B, AB, or O. In the United States, approximately 45% of the population is type O and 41% is type A. Only 10% of the population is B and 4% is AB.

Antigens

The ABO grouping is based on the presence or absence of two **blood group antigens,** which are substances found on the surface of the red blood cells. These blood group antigens are products of inherited genes and are named A and B. Individuals are grouped according to the antigens present on their cells: a person who is type A has A antigen; a person who is type B has B antigen; a person who is type AB has A and B antigens; and a person who is type O has neither A nor B antigen (Table 4–1). The slide test is a procedure which detects A and/or B antigen on the red blood cells, a procedure called *forward* or *direct typing*.

Antibodies

The discovery of the A and B antigens was accompanied by the discovery of the corresponding **blood group antibodies** in human blood. An **antibody** is a serum protein molecule that reacts with an antigen. Antibodies are also called **immunoglobulins** (Ig). There are five classes of immunoglobulins in humans: IgG, IgM, IgA, IgD, and IgE. The antibodies of the ABO system are of the IgM class. If the antigen is on a particle such as a cell, the antibody can cause **agglutination** or clumping of the cells. This reaction can be easily seen. Antibodies are named according to the antigen they react with: an antibody that reacts with A antigen (A red cells) is called anti-A; an antibody that reacts with B antigen (B red cells) is called anti-B. O cells are named because they have no A or B antigen; therefore, there is no anti-O antibody.

Blood group antibodies of the ABO system occur naturally in serum. If an antigen is missing from an individual's cells, the antibody specific for the missing antigen will be present. For example, an individual who is type A will have anti-B antibody in their serum. An individual who is type O will have anti-A and anti-B antibodies

Table 4–1. Table of ABO antigens and antibodies

ABO group	Antigen on Red Blood Cells	Antibody in Serum
A	A	anti-B
B	B	anti-A
AB	A and B	neither anti-A nor anti-B
O	neither A nor B	both anti-A and anti-B

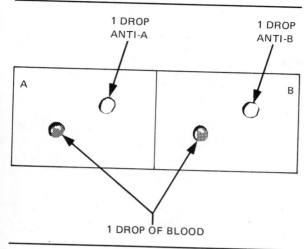

Figure 4–1. ABO slide typing: microscope slide with antisera and blood added

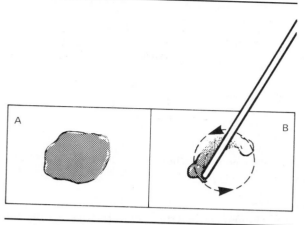

Figure 4–2. ABO slide typing: mixing antisera and blood

since O cells have neither A nor B antigen (Table 4–1). Testing serum for the presence of the blood group antibodies is called *reverse* or *indirect typing*.

Importance of ABO Typing

ABO typing is performed so that blood may be matched if a transfusion is necessary. An individual should be transfused with blood of the same ABO group. The rule to follow in transfusing blood is to avoid giving the patient an antigen he does not already have. In an emergency, O blood may be used because it contains neither A nor B antigen. For this reason, people of blood group O have been called universal donors.

PRINCIPLE OF ABO SLIDE TYPING

The slide test detects the A or B antigens on red cells by using the principle of agglutination. This procedure may be called direct or forward typing and is accomplished by combining cells of unknown type with a known **antiserum** and observing for agglutination. If the antigen present on the cells corresponds to the antibody in the antiserum, agglutination will occur. If the antigen

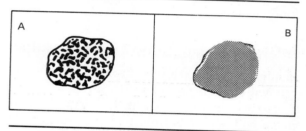

Figure 4–3. Agglutination of blood cells by anti-A in ABO typing. Reaction shown indicates type A blood.

is not present on the cells, no agglutination will be observed.

Performing ABO Slide Typing

Slide typing is performed using a clean microscope slide which has been marked into two halves using a wax pencil. One drop of anti-A is added to the left side and one drop of anti-B to the right side. A small drop of well-mixed blood, capillary or venous, is placed on each side of the slide (Figure 4–1). The anti-A is mixed with one drop of the blood using a wooden applicator stick. The procedure is repeated using a clean applicator stick for anti-B and the other drop of blood (Figure 4–2).

Table 4–2. Reactions of ABO groups with anti-A and anti-B

Blood Group	Reactions of Cells with:	
	anti-A	anti-B
A	+	0
B	0	+
AB	+	+
O	0	0

+ = agglutination
0 = no agglutination

The slide is then rocked gently for two minutes and observed under good light for agglutination. Agglutination will appear as a clumping together of the red cells (Figure 4–3, page 259). The results should be recorded as positive (+) or negative (0) for each antibody

Interpretation of Slide Typing Results

If only the A antigen is present on the red cells, the cells will agglutinate with anti-A but not with anti-B. If only B antigen is present, the cells will agglutinate with anti-B but not with anti-A. Type O blood will show no agglutination with either anti-A or anti-B. Type AB blood will show agglutination with both anti-A and anti-B (Table 4–2).

Precautions

■ All reagents must be in date and equipment must be clean.
■ Manufacturer's instructions for the use of antisera should be followed.
■ Care should be taken to prevent contamination of antisera.

■ If capillary blood is used, the slide typing must be completed before clotting occurs.
■ Timing should be observed carefully; drying around the edges of the cell mixture should not be confused with agglutination.
■ Reactions should be observed under good lighting conditions.
■ Results should be recorded as soon as they are observed to avoid error.
■ Forward typing should be confirmed by reverse typing.
■ Slides must be discarded into biohazard container.

LESSON REVIEW

1. What antigens present on red blood cells determine the ABO groups?
2. Name the four groups in the ABO system and give the frequency of each.
3. What antibody is present in the serum of a person who is type B—type O?
4. What agglutination results would be observed when testing type A blood with anti-A and anti-B—when testing type AB blood?
5. What is being tested in forward typing?
6. Define agglutination, antibody, antigen, antiserum, blood group antibody, blood group antigen, immunoglobulin, and serology.

STUDENT ACTIVITIES

1. Re-read the information on ABO typing.
2. Review the glossary terms.
3. Practice performing ABO slide typing as outlined on the Student Performance Guide, using the worksheet.

Student Performance Guide

NAME _____

DATE _____

LESSON 4–1
ABO SLIDE TYPING

Instructions

1. Practice performing ABO slide typing.
2. Demonstrate the procedure for ABO slide typing satisfactorily for the instructor. All steps must be completed as listed on the instructor's Performance Check Sheet.
3. Complete a written examination successfully.

Materials and Equipment

- gloves
- hand disinfectant
- blood samples, anticoagulated venous
- commercial anti-A serum
- commercial anti-B serum
- Pasteur pipets and bulb or disposable plastic pipets
- clean microscope slides (or typing slides)
- wax pencil
- wooden applicator sticks
- light source
- blood typing worksheet
- stopwatch
- surface disinfectant
- biohazard container
- puncture-proof container for sharp objects

Note: Package insert should be consulted for specific instructions before test is performed.

Procedure			S = Satisfactory U = Unsatisfactory
You must:	**S**	**U**	**Comments**
1. Wash hands with disinfectant and put on gloves			
2. Assemble equipment and materials			
3. Place a clean microscope slide on the work area			

You must:	S	U	Comments
4. Mark the slide into two halves using a wax pencil			
5. Label the left side "A" and the right side "B"			
6. Place one drop of anti-A on the "A" side (do not allow dropper to touch slide)			
7. Place one drop of anti-B on the "B" side (do not allow dropper to touch slide)			
8. Add one drop of well-mixed blood to each side of the slide using the Pasteur pipet (the drop of blood should be no larger than the drop of antibody)			
9. Mix the blood and antiserum on side A into a smooth round circle about the size of a quarter using a clean wooden applicator stick			
10. Repeat the same procedure on side B using a clean applicator stick			
11. Rock the slide gently for two minutes and look for agglutination using strong light			
12. Record agglutination results on worksheet: + = agglutination, 0 = no agglutination			
13. Determine the blood group and record			
14. Repeat steps 3–13 on additional blood samples			
15. Discard specimens and slides appropriately			
16. Clean equipment and return to proper storage			
17. Clean work area with surface disinfectant			
18. Remove gloves and discard appropriately			
19. Wash hands with hand disinfectant			

Comments:

Student/Instructor:

Date:_____   Instructor:_____

Worksheet

NAME_____   DATE _____

LESSON 4–1 ABO SLIDE TYPING

| | Agglutination Results* | | Interpretation |
Sample #	anti-A	anti-B	ABO group
_____	_____	_____	_____
_____	_____	_____	_____
_____	_____	_____	_____
_____	_____	_____	_____
_____	_____	_____	_____

*Record results as:
0 = no agglutination
+ = agglutination

LESSON 4–2
ABO Tube Typing

LESSON OBJECTIVES

After studying this lesson, you should be able to:
- Explain reverse or indirect typing.
- Perform ABO forward and reverse typing by the tube method.
- Interpret the results of tube typing tests.
- List the precautions to be observed in performing ABO tube typing.
- Define the glossary terms.

GLOSSARY

blood bank / place where blood is typed, tested, and stored until it is needed for transfusion

serofuge / a centrifuge which spins small tubes or serological tubes

INTRODUCTION

Tube typing is a more sensitive and reliable method of determining a patient's blood type than slide typing. Tube typing is widely used in **blood banks** and in clinical laboratories. Tube typing consists of (1) direct or forward typing, which identifies the antigens on the cells, and (2) confirmatory or reverse typing, which identifies the blood group antibodies in the serum. A centrifuge or serofuge may be used to speed up the reaction. A **serofuge** is a specialized centrifuge which spins small test tubes at a high—usually fixed—speed.

TUBE TYPING

Tube typing refers to typing carried out in a test tube rather than on a slide. With tube typing, the cells that are used must be a 2–5% saline sus-

pension of red blood cells, instead of the whole blood used in slide typing.

Direct or Forward Typing

Forward or direct typing identifies the antigen present on a patient's red blood cells by reacting suspension of the patient's cells with anti-A and anti-B and observing agglutination after centrifugation. If a centrifuge is not available the reaction may be observed after allowing the tubes to sit at room temperature for fifteen to thirty minutes.

A 2–5% cell suspension is made by adding eighteen to nineteen drops of saline to one drop of the patient's blood. Two tubes labeled "A" and "B" are set up: one drop of anti-A is placed in the "A" tube and one drop of anti-B is placed in the "B" tube. One drop of the patient's 2–5% cell

Table 4–3. Forward and reverse typing results for ABO blood groups

ABO Group	Forward Typing Reactions of Cells with:		Reverse Typing Reactions of Serum with:		
	anti-A	anti-B	A cells	B cells	O cells
O	0	0	+	+	0
A	+	0	0	+	0
B	0	+^{i}	+	0	0
AB	+	+	0	0	0

0 = no agglutination
+ = agglutination

suspension is added to each tube and the contents are mixed. The tubes are centrifuged for thirty seconds to enhance the reaction. The tubes are then removed from the centrifuge. They are shaken gently to remove the cells from the bottom of the tube and are observed for agglutination. A clumping of the cells indicates the antigen present on the cells corresponds to the antibody placed in the test tube (Table 4–3).

Reverse or Indirect Typing

Reverse (or indirect or confirmatory) typing identifies the antibodies present in a patient's serum or plasma by reacting the patient's serum with a 2–5% suspension of group A cells and a 2–5% suspension of group B cells and observing agglutination. Two drops of the patient's serum are added to each of three tubes marked "a," "b," and "control." One drop of the group A cell suspension is added to tube "a," one drop of group B cell suspension is added to tube "b," and one drop of a 2–5% suspension of patient cells to "control" tube. The contents of the tubes are mixed and the tubes are centrifuged for thirty seconds. The tubes are then shaken gently and observed for agglutination. A positive test, agglutination, indicates that antibody is present in the serum which corresponds to the antigen on cells added to the tube. The control tube should always be negative for agglutination since it contains only the patient's serum and cells. The results of forward and reverse typing should be compared to insure that

they agree (Table 4–3). (Reverse typing should confirm the results of forward typing.)

Precautions

■ Follow manufacturer's directions regarding the use of all reagents.
■ Cells used for tube typing must be a 2–5% cell suspension.
■ Avoid shaking tubes too vigorously, which might disperse agglutination.

LESSON REVIEW

1. What is reverse typing?
2. What antibodies would be present in the serum of a person who is type A—type AB?
3. How is a 2–5% cell suspension made?
4. How are the results of tube typing tests interpreted?
5. Define blood bank and serofuge.

STUDENT ACTIVITIES

1. Re-read the information on ABO tube typing.
2. Review the glossary terms.
3. Practice performing ABO tube typings as outlined on the Student Performance Guide, using the worksheet.

Student Performance Guide

NAME _____

DATE _____

LESSON 4–2
ABO TUBE TYPING

Instructions

1. Practice performing ABO tube typing.
2. Demonstrate ABO tube typing satisfactorily for the instructor. All steps must be completed as listed on the instructor's Performance Check Sheet.
3. Complete a written examination successfully.

Materials and Equipment

- gloves
- hand disinfectant
- specimens for typing: EDTA anticoagulated specimen (or tube of clotted blood) for each individual typed
- physiological saline (0.85% or .15M NaCl)
- Pasteur pipets and rubber bulb or disposable plastic pipets
- anti-A serum
- anti-B serum
- A cells (2–5% saline suspension)
- B cells (2–5% saline suspension)
- serofuge or centrifuge capable of spinning 13 × 75 mm tubes at 2000–2500 rpm (optional)
- test tubes, 13 × 75 mm
- test tube racks
- blood typing worksheet
- surface disinfectant
- biohazard container
- puncture-proof container for sharp objects
- chlorine bleach

Note: Package insert should be consulted for specific instructions before test is performed.

Procedure			S = Satisfactory U = Unsatisfactory
You must:	**S**	**U**	**Comments**
1. Wash hands with disinfectant and put on gloves			
2. Assemble equipment and materials			
3. Obtain a blood sample and perform ABO forward tube typing following steps 4–13			
4. Place one drop of well-mixed blood into a test tube; add eighteen to nineteen drops of saline, and label the tube "patient cells" (2–5%):			
5. Label two test tubes "A" and "B"			
6. Place one drop of anti-A in tube "A"			
7. Place one drop of anti-B in tube "B"			
8. Place one drop of the 2–5% patient cell suspension in each tube and mix			
9. Place tubes in serofuge and spin thirty seconds. *Note:* Balance the serofuge by placing tubes opposite each other. (If no serofuge is available, allow tubes to stand at room temperature for 15–30 minutes and go to step 11)			
10. Allow the serofuge to come to a complete stop and remove tubes			
11. Shake each tube gently to remove cells from bottom of tube and observe for agglutination using good light			
12. Record results from each tube on worksheet: 0 = no agglutination, + = agglutination			
13. Determine the blood group of the sample and record			
14. Obtain a blood sample and perform ABO reverse typing following steps 15–25			
15. Centrifuge the blood sample, remove plasma or serum from sample, and place in a clean test tube			
16. Label three test tubes "a," "b," and "control"			
17. Place two drops of serum (or plasma) into each tube			

You must:	S	U	Comments
18. Place one drop of a 2–5% suspension of A cells into tube "a" and mix			
19. Place one drop of a 2–5% suspension of B cells into tube "b" and mix			
20. Place one drop of patient's 2–5% cell suspension into "control" tube and mix			
21. Place tubes in serofuge, balance, and spin thirty seconds			
22. Remove the tubes from the serofuge after it stops completely			
23. Shake each tube gently and observe for agglutination			
24. Record the results from each tube on worksheet: 0 = no agglutination, + = agglutination			
25. Determine the blood group of the sample and record			
26. Compare results of forward typing of the sample with results of reverse typing of the same sample. Reverse typing should confirm results of forward typing			
27. Discard specimens appropriately			
28. Disinfect reusable glassware with chlorine bleach			
29. Clean equipment and return to proper storage			
30. Clean work area with surface disinfectant			
31. Remove gloves and discard appropriately			
32. Wash hands with hand disinfectant			

Comments:

Student/Instructor:

Date:_____   Instructor:_____

Worksheet

NAME _____ DATE _____

LESSON 4–2 ABO TUBE TYPING

Specimen No.	Direct (Forward) Typing*		Inter-pretation	Indirect (Reverse) Typing			Inter-pretation
	anti-A	anti-B	ABO Group	A cells	B cells	Control	ABO Group
____	____	____	____	____	____	____	____
____	____	____	____	____	____	____	____
____	____	____	____	____	____	____	____
____	____	____	____	____	____	____	____
____	____	____	____	____	____	____	____

*Record results as:
 0 = no agglutination
 + = agglutination

LESSON 4–3
Rh Slide Typing

LESSON OBJECTIVES

After studying this lesson, you should be able to:
- Explain the importance of the Rh blood group system.
- Name the most important antigen in the Rh system.
- Name two ways in which immunization to the Rh D antigen may occur.
- Name two problems which may occur as a result of immunization to the D antigen.
- Explain why Rh (D) immune globulin is used.
- Perform Rh slide typing.
- Interpret the results of Rh slide typing.
- Explain the significance of the D^u antigen.
- List the precautions which should be observed while performing the Rh slide typing procedure.
- Define the glossary terms.

GLOSSARY

hemolytic disease of the newborn (HDN) / a disease in which antibody from the mother destroys the red cells of the fetus

immunization / process by which an antibody is produced in response to an antigen

Rh (D) immune globulin / a concentrated, purified solution of human anti-D used for injection; RhIG

INTRODUCTION

Testing for antigens of the Rh system is a routine procedure in blood banks and clinical laboratories. These antigens may be detected by the slide method or the tube method. The slide method is discussed in this lesson.

THE Rh BLOOD GROUP SYSTEM

The Rh blood group, discovered in the 1940s, is the second most important human blood group system. The system is named Rh because the rhesus monkey was being used in the experiments when the system was discovered.

270

The antigens of the Rh system are products of inherited genes and are present on the surface of red blood cells. The major antigen in the Rh system is the D antigen. Red blood cells that possess the D antigen are called Rh positive. Cells that lack the D antigen are called Rh negative. Eighty-five percent of the U.S. population is Rh positive (Rh+) and the other fifteen percent of the population is Rh negative (Rh–). There are now several other known antigens which are part of the Rh system. However, the D antigen is the strongest of the antigens and is the only one that is tested for routinely.

Unlike the ABO system, the Rh system does *not* have antibodies which occur naturally. However, an antibody to D antigen (anti-D) may be produced by an Rh negative person who is immunized or sensitized with the D antigen.

Immunization to the D antigen and subsequent production of anti-D may occur if an Rh negative person is transfused with Rh positive blood. If the Rh negative person is transfused a second time with Rh positive blood, a severe transfusion reaction may occur when the anti-D reacts with the D positive transfused cells.

Hemolytic Disease of the Newborn

When an Rh negative mother gives birth to an Rh positive baby, immunization sometimes occurs, followed by production of anti-D by the mother. The effect may be seen in subsequent Rh positive pregnancies when the mother's antibodies may enter the fetus' bloodstream and attack the unborn baby's red blood cells, a condition called **hemolytic disease of the newborn,** or **HDN.** The effects on the fetus may be mild or severe and may range from mild jaundice to anemia or brain damage. In severe cases, stillbirth or miscarriage may occur.

It is now possible to prevent most cases of Rh hemolytic disease of the newborn by administering **Rh (D) immune globulin** (RhIG) to the mother. RhIG is a concentrated solution of human anti-D antibody which, when injected into the mother, will prevent her from making the anti-D antibody.

This injection must be given within seventy-two hours after delivery of an Rh D positive baby or after termination of pregnancy. Expectant mothers should be typed during the first trimester of pregnancy. This helps to identify mothers who are at risk of having a baby with HDN so that the fetus may be monitored for signs of stress.

Nomenclature

The two commonly used methods of naming the antigens in the Rh system are the Fisher-Race method and the Wiener method. The names of the antigen and antibody in both systems are given in Table 4–4. Manufacturers of blood bank reagents may use one or both systems in labeling reagents.

Weak D Antigen: D^u

Some individuals have a form of the D antigen which is weak. This weak antigen is called the D^u antigen. Blood cells containing the D^u antigen may give a negative reaction in routine slide or tube typing. All blood samples that are negative by routine slide or tube typing should be tested for the D^u antigen before assuming that the sample is Rh negative. The D^u test will not be covered in this lesson for two reasons: (1) most laboratories will not allow non-certified workers to perform the test, and (2) the test involves techniques and principles not covered in this text.

Importance of Rh Typing

It is important to test for the D antigen in all patients who are to receive transfusions so that the proper type of blood will be given. Rh negative patients should always be transfused with Rh

Table 4–4. Fisher-Race and Wiener nomenclature for Rh system

Nomenclature	Antigen	Antibody
Fisher-Race	D	anti-D
Wiener	Rh_0	anti-Rh_0

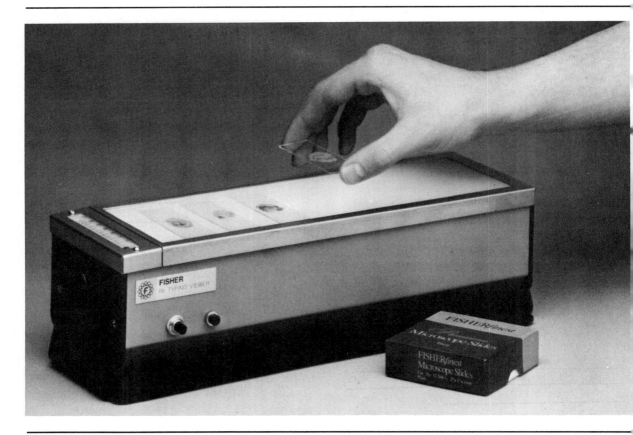

Figure 4–4. Rh slide typing using viewbox *(Photo courtesy of Fisher Scientific Co.)*

negative blood. Testing for the D antigen is also a way of identifying females who might be at risk of giving birth to an infant with HDN. Since the blood group antigens are inherited, identification of these antigens may aid in establishing parentage in legal or civil cases.

Rh SLIDE TYPING PROCEDURE

The D antigen may be identified using a slide typing technique. A control should always be run as part of the test, since the patient's serum contains no natural antibody for reverse or confirmatory typing. Slide typing is performed by (1) mixing one drop of anti-D with one drop of blood on

a microscope slide and (2) mixing one drop of control serum, usually 22% or 30% bovine albumin, with one drop of blood on another slide. The slides are placed on a heated, lighted viewbox to heat them to 37°C, and are rocked gently (Figure 4–4). The slides are observed for two minutes for agglutination and the results are recorded and interpreted. It is important to follow the manufacturer's directions in the use of anti-D.

INTERPRETATION OF RESULTS

If the cells are Rh positive, agglutination should be observed on the anti-D slide only. If the cells are Rh negative, no agglutination should be seen

Table 4–5. Interpretation of results of Rh slide typing

Reactions of cells with:		
anti-D	control serum	Interpretation
+	0	Rh (D) positive
0	0	Rh (D) negative (confirm with D^u test)
+	+	unable to interpret; repeat test using another method

+ = agglutination
0 = no agglutination

in either slide (Table 4–5). The control slide should always be negative for agglutination. If positive results are observed in the control, the test is invalid and should be repeated by the tube method. Positive control results may be due to contaminated control serum or abnormalities in the patient blood sample. Rh negative results should be confirmed by a tube test and a D^u test.

Precautions

■ Always follow manufacturer's instructions for use of reagents.
■ Do not observe heated slides for more than two minutes before interpreting results.

■ Rh slide typing should be performed at 37°C, using a lighted viewbox.
■ Negative slide typing results should be confirmed with a tube test and a D^u test.

LESSON REVIEW

1. What is the major antigen in the Rh system?
2. What circumstances must exist before anti-D is produced by an individual?
3. What is the weak D antigen?
4. Explain how hemolytic disease of the newborn occurs.
5. Why is Rh D typing performed?
6. What two problems may occur after immunization to the D antigen?
7. Define hemolytic disease of the newborn, immunization, and Rh (D) immune globulin.

STUDENT ACTIVITIES

1. Re-read the information on Rh slide typing.
2. Review the glossary terms.
3. Practice performing Rh slide typing on several blood samples as outlined on the Student Performance Guide, using the worksheet.

Student Performance Guide

NAME _____

DATE _____

LESSON 4–3
Rh SLIDE TYPING

Instructions

1. Practice performing Rh slide typing.
2. Demonstrate the procedure for Rh slide typing satisfactorily for the instructor. All steps must be completed as listed on the instructor's Performance Check Sheet.
3. Complete a written examination successfully.

Materials and Equipment

- gloves
- hand disinfectant
- clean microscope slides
- wooden applicator sticks
- anti-D serum (anti-Rh_o)
- Rh control serum (22% or 30% bovine albumin)
- blood specimen
- lighted viewbox
- blood typing worksheet
- wax pencil
- stopwatch
- surface disinfectant
- biohazard container

Note: Package insert should be consulted for specific instructions before test is performed.

Procedure			S = Satisfactory U = Unsatisfactory
You must:	**S**	**U**	**Comments**
1. Wash hands with disinfectant and put on gloves			
2. Assemble equipment and materials			
3. Turn on viewbox			
4. Label two clean microscope slides "D" and "C" (control)			
5. Place one drop of anti-D serum on the "D" slide			

You must:	S	U	Comments
6. Place one drop of Rh control serum (albumin) on the "C" slide			
7. Place one large drop of well-mixed whole blood on each slide			
8. Mix blood and anti-D well with an applicator stick, spreading the mixture over two-thirds of the slide			
9. Repeat procedure for the control slide using a clean applicator stick			
10. Place slides on the lighted viewbox			
11. Tilt the viewbox slowly back and forth for two minutes to mix the contents on the slides			
12. Observe for agglutination at the end of two minutes			
13. Record results on worksheet: + = agglutination, 0 = no agglutination			
14. Determine the Rh type and record on worksheet			
15. Repeat steps 4–14 on at least two other blood samples			
16. Discard specimens and slides appropriately			
17. Clean equipment and return to proper storage			
18. Clean work area with surface disinfectant			
19. Remove gloves and discard appropriately			
20. Wash hands with hand disinfectant			

Comments:

Student/Instructor:

Date:_____   Instructor:_____

Worksheet

NAME_____ DATE _____

LESSON 4–3 Rh SLIDE TYPING

| Sample # | Agglutination Results* | | Interpretation† |
	anti-D	Control (albumin)	Rh type
_____	_____	_____	_____
_____	_____	_____	_____
_____	_____	_____	_____
_____	_____	_____	_____
_____	_____	_____	_____

*Record results as:
  0 = no agglutination
  + = agglutination
†Record interpretation as:
  Rh positive or
  Rh negative

LESSON 4-4
Urine Pregnancy Test

LESSON OBJECTIVES

After studying this lesson, you should be able to:
- Name the hormone present in pregnant females.
- Explain the principle of pregnancy tests.
- Explain the principle of agglutination inhibition.
- Perform a slide test for pregnancy.
- Interpret the results of a pregnancy test.
- Name a cause of a false positive pregnancy test.
- List precautions to observe when performing a slide test for pregnancy.
- Define the glossary terms.

GLOSSARY

agglutination inhibition / interference of agglutination
EIA / enzyme immunoassay
HCG / human chorionic gonadotropin, a hormone found in pregnant women; sometimes called uterine chorionic gonadotropin (UCG)

INTRODUCTION

Most pregnancy tests are designed to detect human chorionic gonadotropin, or **HCG,** a hormone normally found in the serum and urine of pregnant women. It is sometimes called uterine chorionic gonadotropin, or UCG. The urine or serum may be used for testing. Pregnancy tests may be performed as either tube tests or slide tests. Tube test results are usually available after two hours. Slide tests are carried out on a glass or cardboard slide and results are usually available within a few minutes. The slide test is rapid, sensitive, and easy to perform.

PRINCIPLE OF PREGNANCY TESTS

Most pregnancy tests employ serological methods to detect the HCG hormone. Some of these tests are based on the principle of **agglutination inhibition.** In an agglutination inhibition test, the substance being tested, when present, will inhibit agglutination. Absence of agglutination is a posi-

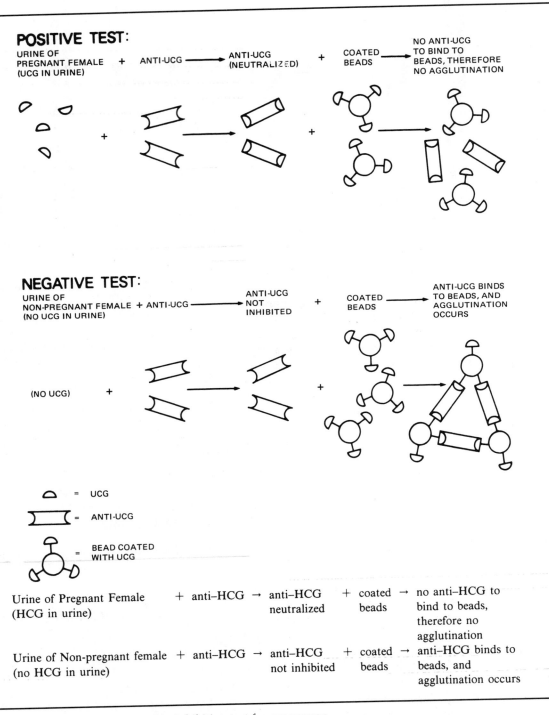

Figure 4–5. Principle of agglutination inhibition test for pregnancy

tive test result. If the substance being tested is not present, agglutination will occur and will be interpreted as a negative test.

Another type of recently introduced pregnancy test is the **EIA,** or enzyme immunoassay. These tests also use antigen–antibody reaction, but give a colored reaction which must be interpreted.

SPECIMEN

The urine sample tested should be the first urine voided in the morning since the hormone will be more concentrated then. The hormone HCG appears in the urine and serum about one week after the missed onset of menstruation. The level of HCG rises during early pregnancy, begins to decline about the third month of pregnancy, and disappears a few days after delivery.

COMPONENTS OF HCG TESTS

Urine test kits are available from a variety of manufacturers. The majority of the kits rely on the following test components:

1. *HCG hormone.* Present in the urine of pregnant females.
2. *Anti-HCG.* This is an antibody which will react with HCG. It is produced by inoculating HCG into an animal so that the animal will produce antibodies against the HCG. The serum is then harvested from the animal, purified, packaged and sold as the source of anti-HCG for a variety of pregnancy tests.
3. *Indicator particles.* Suspensions of latex beads or cells (usually red cells) which are coated with HCG hormone.

GENERAL PROCEDURE FOR AGGLUTINATION INHIBITION TEST FOR PREGNANCY

A portion of a urine sample is mixed with anti-HCG. If HCG is present in the urine (if the patient is pregnant), the HCG will bind to the antibody (anti-HCG) and "neutralize" or inhibit the activity of the antibody. This reaction is not visible. If the urine sample is from a non-pregnant female, no reaction will occur with the antibody, since the urine will have no HCG.

After the urine and the anti-HCG antibody are mixed together, HCG-coated particles are added to the mixture to make the reaction visible. If the patient is pregnant, the antibody will have been inhibited by the patient's HCG, will be unable to bind to the HCG-coated beads, and no agglutination will be seen. If the patient is not pregnant, the antibody will combine with the HCG-coated particles and cause agglutination or clumping of the particles (Figure 4–5).

Precautions

■ Control samples (positive and negative urines) should always be tested at the same time as the patient sample to be certain that reagents are reacting properly.

■ Many early pregnancies (the first one to two weeks) have undetectable levels of HCG. Therefore, negative tests should be repeated in one to two weeks.

■ Specimens should be tested within 24 hours and kept refrigerated until tested.

■ Serological tests for HCG may give false positive results due to elevated levels of pituitary hormones, and rare conditions such as choriocarcinoma and hydatiform mole.

LESSON REVIEW

1. Explain the principle of pregnancy tests.
2. What hormone is tested?
3. List two methods of performing pregnancy tests.
4. What is a cause of a false positive test—a false negative test?

5. What two types of specimens can be used in a pregnancy test?
6. Describe the principle of agglutination inhibition.
7. When does the HCG hormone first appear in pregnancy? When does it disappear?
8. What precautions should be observed in performing the slide test for pregnancy?

9. Define agglutination inhibition, EIA, and HCG.

STUDENT ACTIVITIES

1. Re-read the information on the pregnancy test.
2. Review the glossary terms.
3. Practice performing a slide test for pregnancy as outlined on the Student Performance Guide.

Student Performance Guide

NAME _____

DATE _____

LESSON 4–4
URINE PREGNANCY TEST

Instructions

1. Practice performing a slide test for pregnancy.
2. Demonstrate the slide test procedure for pregnancy satisfactorily for the instructor. All steps must be completed as listed on the instructor's Performance Check Sheet.
3. Complete a written examination successfully.

Materials and Equipment

- gloves
- hand disinfectant
- urine specimen
- stopwatch
- positive and negative urine controls
- slide test kit for pregnancy (kit should include slide, dispensers, stirrers, reagents)
- surface disinfectant
- biohazard container

Note: The procedure should be modified to conform to the manufacturer's instructions for the kit being used.

Procedure			S = Satisfactory U = Unsatisfactory
You must:	**S**	**U**	**Comments**
1. Wash hands with disinfectant and put on gloves			
2. Assemble equipment and materials			
3. Place one drop of antiserum in the center of the slide			
4. Obtain urine sample. Insert tip of dispenser into urine sample, squeeze, and release pressure to draw up specimen			
5. Hold dispenser perpendicular over slide and squeeze to release one drop of urine beside the drop of antiserum			
6. Mix urine and antiserum with stirrer provided			
7. Rock slide to mix for appropriate time interval			
8. Apply one drop of indicator particles to mixture on slide			
9. Mix indicator particles with antiserum and spread mixture over entire circled area of slide using stirrer			
10. Rock slide slowly in a figure-eight motion for appropriate time interval			
11. Observe slide for agglutination at the end of the time interval and record results			
12. Repeat steps 3–11 using a positive urine control and a negative urine control			
13. Wash reusable equipment and discard disposable supplies in biohazard container			
14. Dispose of specimen as instructed			
15. Clean work area with surface disinfectant			
16. Remove gloves and discard appropriately			
17. Wash hands with hand disinfectant			

Comments:

Student/Instructor:

Date:_____   Instructor:_____

LESSON 4–5
Slide Test for Infectious Mononucleosis

LESSON OBJECTIVES

After studying this lesson, you should be able to:
- Name the cause of infectious mononucleosis.
- List five clinical symptoms of infectious mononucleosis.
- Name two types of tests which are performed to diagnose infectious mononucleosis.
- Perform a slide test for infectious mononucleosis.
- Interpret the results of a slide test for infectious mononucleosis.
- Define the glossary terms.

GLOSSARY

heterophile antibody / antibody which is increased in infectious mononucleosis

lymphocytosis / an increase above normal in the number of lymphocytes in the blood

INTRODUCTION

Infectious mononucleosis (IM) is a contagious disease which may have vague clinical symptoms and may mimic other diseases. Serological tests are often the basis for an early diagnosis of the disease, and may also be used to follow the course of the disease. The most common serological test used is a rapid slide test which tests serum for the presence of antibodies called **heterophile antibodies.** The slide test gives quick, reliable results and is simple to perform. Tests are also available which test for antibodies to Epstein-Barr virus, the cause of IM.

INFECTIOUS MONONUCLEOSIS

Infectious mononucleosis (IM) is commonly called "mono" or "kissing disease." IM is a viral disease which affects mostly the fifteen- to twenty-five-year-old age group. The disease is a result of infection of the lymphocytes by the Epstein-Barr virus (EBV). Clinically, the symptoms are nonspecific and may include fatigue, fever, sore throat, weakness, headache, and swollen lymph nodes. In order to properly diagnose IM, hematological and serological test results must be considered along with the clinical symptoms.

Hematological Test for IM

The hematological test for IM includes a white cell count and evaluation of the patient's lymphocytes. In IM, a **lymphocytosis,** or increase in lymphocytes, usually occurs and the lymphocytes have an unusual or "atypical" appearance.

Serological Test for IM

Persons with IM produce an antibody called **heterophile antibody** by the sixth to tenth day of the illness. Detection of this heterophile antibody combined with the hematological and clinical findings can provide the basis for the diagnosis of IM. The serological test is usually positive after the first week of illness. However, if a negative test results, the test may be repeated in another week if clinical symptoms are still present.

SLIDE TEST FOR INFECTIOUS MONONUCLEOSIS

The procedure for detecting the heterophile antibody of IM discussed in this lesson is the one developed by Ortho Diagnostics and marketed under the name Monospot®. Several other tests are available which follow the same general principles as this one. Manufacturer's instructions for each kit should be strictly followed.

Serological kits for infectious mononucleosis usually provide all necessary reagents, materials, and controls. The laboratory must provide the specimen to be tested, which is usually a small sample of the patient's plasma or serum.

The slide test is a rapid method of detecting heterophile antibody in serum. The procedure is based on agglutination of horse erythrocytes by the heterophile antibody present in IM. There are other antibodies which will also react with horse erythrocytes. Therefore, the serum is reacted with absorbents to remove these other antibodies before it is reacted with the horse cells.

The test is performed using a glass slide which has two squares (I and II) etched on the slide. The reagents are mixed thoroughly and a drop of indicator cells (horse erythrocytes) is added to a corner of each square using the capillary pipet provided. One drop of Reagent I is then placed in the center of square I and one drop of Reagent II is placed in the center of square II. One drop of serum is placed in the center of each square using the plastic pipet provided in the kit (Figure 4–6).

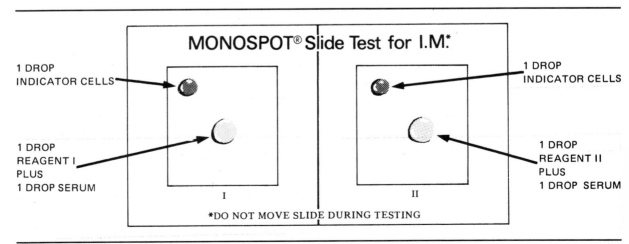

Figure 4–6. Monospot® slide with reagents added

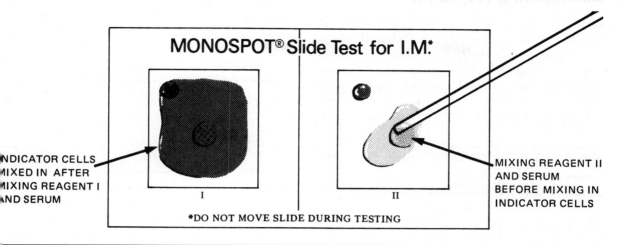

Figure 4–7. Mixing reagents on Monospot® slide using wooden applicator

The serum and reagent I are mixed using at least ten stirring motions with a clean wooden applicator stick. The cells are blended in so that the entire surface of the square is covered. The contents of square II are mixed in the same manner as square I (Figure 4–7). A timer is started as soon as mixing is completed and the slide is observed for one minute for agglutination of the horse cells. During this time the slide should not be moved or picked up. At the end of one minute the results are recorded and interpreted. Positive and negative serum controls provided with the kit should be tested in the same manner to insure that all reagents are reacting properly.

INTERPRETATION OF RESULTS

The presence or absence of heterophile antibody of infectious mononucleosis will be indicated by the presence or absence of agglutination, as indicated in Table 4–6.

Table 4–6. Interpretation of results of Monospot® test

Positive test:	Negative test:
Agglutination pattern is stronger on the left side of the slide (square I) than on the right side of the slide (square II)	A. Agglutination pattern is stronger on the right side of the slide (square II) than in square I
	or
	B. No agglutination appears in either square
	or
	C. Agglutination is equal in both squares of the slide

Precautions

■ Slide should not be moved during the one-minute incubation period.

■ Agglutination appearing after one minute or when the slide is picked up should not be interpreted as a positive result.

■ Manufacturer's instructions for kits must be adhered to.

LESSON REVIEW

1. What causes infectious mononucleosis?
2. What are the clinical symptoms of IM?
3. What information can be gained from the hematological test?
4. What does the serological test detect?
5. What precautions should be followed in performing and interpreting a slide test for IM?
6. How soon after the disease begins will the serological test be positive?
7. Define heterophile antibody and lymphocytosis.

STUDENT ACTIVITIES

1. Re-read the information on the slide test for infectious mononucleosis.
2. Review the glossary terms.
3. Practice performing the slide test for infectious mononucleosis as outlined on the Student Performance Guide.

Student Performance Guide

NAME _____

DATE _____

LESSON 4–5
SLIDE TEST FOR INFECTIOUS MONONUCLEOSIS

Instructions

1. Practice performing the slide test for infectious mononucleosis.
2. Demonstrate the procedure for the slide test for infectious mononucleosis satisfactorily for the instructor. All steps must be completed as listed on the instructor's Performance Check Sheet.
3. Complete a written examination successfully.

Materials and Equipment
- gloves
- hand disinfectant
- serum
- stopwatch
- surface disinfectant
- test kit for infectious mononucleosis (kit should include instructions, slide, serum dispensers, stirrers, reagents)
- biohazard container
- chlorine bleach

Note: Procedure given is for Monospot® test by Ortho Diagnostics. Package insert should be consulted before test is performed. If another kit is used, the manufacturer's instructions should be followed.

Procedure			S = Satisfactory U = Unsatisfactory
You must:	**S**	**U**	**Comments**
1. Wash hands with disinfectant and put on gloves			
2. Assemble equipment and materials			
3. Place the Monospot® slide on the work surface			

You must:	S	U	Comments
4. Mix the reagent vials several times by inversion			

5. Fill the capillary pipet to the top mark:
   a. Place the rubber bulb on the end of the capillary pipet with the heavy black line
   b. Insert the pipet into the vial of indicator cells
   c. Allow the pipet to fill by capillary action to the top mark			

6. Place the index finger over the hole in the bulb and squeeze gently to dispense one-half the cells onto a corner of square I of the slide (the level of the cells should now be at the lower mark on the pipet)			
7. Deliver the remaining cells to a corner of square II			
8. Place one drop of thoroughly-mixed Reagent I in the center of square I			
9. Place one drop of thoroughly-mixed Reagent II in the center of square II			
10. Add one drop of serum to the center of each square using the disposable plastic pipet provided			
11. Mix Reagent I with the serum using *at least ten* stirring motions with a clean wooden applicator stick			
12. Blend in the indicator cells in square I with the applicator stick using *no more than ten* stirring motions, and spreading the mixture over the entire surface of the square			
13. Repeat steps 11–12 using Reagent II in square II, using a clean applicator stick			
14. Start the stopwatch upon completion of the mixing of both squares			
15. Observe for agglutination at the end of one minute (no longer) without moving the slide or picking it up			
16. Record the agglutination in each square and interpret the results: If the agglutination pattern is stronger in square I than in square II, the test is positive for the heterophile antibody of infectious mononucleosis. Any other combination of reactions is negative			
17. Record test results as positive or negative			

You must:	S	U	Comments
18. Repeat test procedure (steps 3–17) using positive and negative control sera			
19. Discard contaminated materials into biohazard container			
20. Dispose of specimen appropriately and disinfect reusable materials			
21. Clean work area with surface disinfectant			
22. Remove gloves and discard appropriately			
23. Wash hands with hand disinfectant			

Comments:

Student/Instructor:

Date:_____ Instructor:_____

LESSON 4–6
Slide Test for Rheumatoid Factors

LESSON OBJECTIVES

After studying this lesson, you should be able to:
- Explain the significance of rheumatoid factors.
- Explain the principle of latex agglutination tests.
- Perform a qualitative latex agglutination test for rheumatoid factors.
- Perform a quantitative latex agglutination test for rheumatoid factors.
- Interpret the results of a latex agglutination test for rheumatoid factors.
- Define the glossary terms.

GLOSSARY

autoantibody / an antibody which is directed against self (reacts with a self-antigen)

reciprocal / inverse; one of a pair of numbers (as 2/3, 3/2) which has a product of one

rheumatoid arthritis / an inflammatory disease characterized by inflammation of the joints

rheumatoid factors / autoantibodies against human IgG which are often present in the serum of patients with rheumatoid arthritis

titer / reciprocal of the highest dilution which gives the desired reaction

INTRODUCTION

Arthritis, an inflammation of the joints, can occur in several diseases. Among these are gout, rheumatic fever, osteoarthritis and **rheumatoid arthritis.** Several types of serological tests are available which aid in distinguishing rheumatoid arthritis from arthritis of other causes. Most of these tests are based on the detection of rheumatoid factors in the patient's serum. This lesson describes a rapid slide test for the detection of rheumatoid factors.

RHEUMATOID FACTORS

Seventy-five to 85 percent of persons with rheumatoid arthritis have elevated levels of **rheumatoid factors** (RF) in their serum. Rheumatoid factors are **autoantibodies,** usually of the IgM

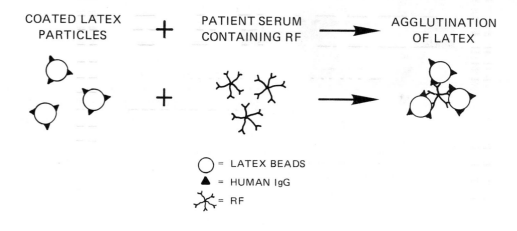

Figure 4–8. Principle of agglutination test for rheumatoid factors. Rheumatoid factors in serum react with IgG-coated particles to cause agglutination.

class, directed against human IgG. Rheumatoid factors are not usually elevated in other forms of arthritis. Because of this, the test for rheumatoid factors is useful in the diagnosis of rheumatoid arthritis.

PRINCIPLE OF SLIDE AGGLUTINATION TEST FOR RF

Most RF slide agglutination tests use latex particles to visualize the reaction. In the RF test, these particles are coated with a specially treated human immunoglobulin (IgG). If rheumatoid factors are present in a patient's serum, the RF, which are autoantibodies, will bind to the IgG coating the particles and cause agglutination (see Figure 4–8). Many commercial kits are available which test for RF. These kits provide the coated latex particles, positive and negative control sera, buffer, and other materials necessary to perform the test.

QUALITATIVE LATEX AGGLUTINATION TEST FOR RF

The usual specimen for a slide agglutination test is serum. The serum is diluted 1:20 using the glycine

buffer included in the test kit. This dilution is necessary because most normal individuals have low levels of RF. The dilution assures that only significant levels of RF will be detected.

To perform the test, one drop each of positive control serum, negative control serum, and diluted patient serum are placed in separate rings on a black glass slide. One drop of well-mixed latex reagent is dispensed into each ring. The latex reagent is then mixed with each serum using a clean stirrer or spreader for each. The mixture is spread over the entire surface of the ring. The slide is then rocked or rotated for the appropriate time (usually two to three minutes) and observed for agglutination under a bright light.

INTERPRETATION OF RESULTS

Agglutination appears as small white clumps against the black background of the slide. A negative test (absence of agglutination) appears as a milky white solution in the ring of the slide (see Figure 4–9). The positive control serum should be positive (show agglutination). The negative control serum should be negative (show no ag-

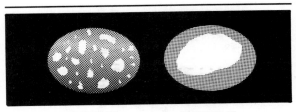

POSITIVE = AGGLUTINATION (WHITE CLUMPS)
NEGATIVE = NO AGGLUTINATION
(MILKY WHITE SOLUTION)

Figure 4–9. Example of latex agglutination. Reaction of coated latex particles used in RF test with negative serum and positive serum.

glutination). Lack of agglutination with the patient serum indicates the level of rheumatoid factors is within normal range. Agglutination with the patient serum indicates an elevation of rheumatoid factors in the serum. A quantitative test should then be performed to determine the level of rheumatoid factors.

Significance of Results

The amount of RF present can be useful in monitoring disease since levels tend to parallel the patient's condition. Persons with active rheumatoid arthritis usually have higher levels of rheumatoid factors than those with inactive disease. Diagnosis of rheumatoid arthritis should not be based on the RF test alone since some other diseases, particularly inflammatory diseases, may also cause a positive RF test. Since only 75–85% of those with rheumatoid arthritis have increased levels of RF, a negative test does not rule out the diagnosis of rheumatoid arthritis.

QUANTITATIVE LATEX AGGLUTINATION TEST FOR RF

A quantitative test for RF is performed by testing a series of dilutions of the patient's serum to determine the RF titer. The highest serum dilution

showing agglutination (positive reaction) is recorded. The **titer,** which is the **reciprocal,** or inverse, of the highest dilution giving a positive result, is reported. For example: dilutions of 1:40, 1:80, and 1:160 were made from a serum which was positive in the qualitative test. When the dilutions were tested for RF, the 1:40 and 1:80 dilutions showed agglutination, and the 1:160 dilution was negative. The RF titer of this serum would be reported as a titer of 80 (the reciprocal of the 1:80 or 1/80 serum dilution).

LESSON REVIEW

1. What are rheumatoid factors?
2. An elevated level of RF is often associated with what disease?
3. Explain the principle of latex agglutination tests.
4. Describe the appearance of a positive test and a negative test.
5. What is the difference in a qualitative and quantitative agglutination test?
6. What is the significance of a positive slide agglutination test for rheumatoid factors—of a negative slide agglutination test for rheumatoid factors?
7. Define autoantibody, reciprocal, rheumatoid arthritis, rheumatoid factors, and titer.

STUDENT ACTIVITIES

1. Re-read the information on slide test for rheumatoid factors.
2. Review the glossary terms.
3. Practice performing qualitative and quantitative slide agglutination tests for rheumatoid factors as outlined on the Student Performance Guide.

Student Performance Guide

NAME _____

DATE _____

LESSON 4–6
SLIDE TEST FOR RHEUMATOID FACTORS

Instructions

1. Practice performing a slide test for rheumatoid factors.
2. Demonstrate the slide test for rheumatoid factors satisfactorily for the instructor. All steps must be completed as listed on the instructor's Performance Check Sheet.
3. Complete a written examination successfully.

Materials and Equipment

hand disinfectant
gloves
timer
test tubes (13 × 75 mm)

- test tube rack
- serum sample for testing
- pipets for delivering .05 ml (50µl), 0.5 ml, 0.95 ml
- rheumatoid factor slide test kit which includes:
    RF latex reagent
    RF positive control serum
    RF negative control serum
    glycine diluent
    ringed black glass slide
    dispenser-spreaders
- surface disinfectant
- biohazard container
- applicator sticks (if spreaders are not in kit)
- chlorine bleach

Note: Instructions given are general. The procedure should be modified to conform to the manufacturer's instructions for the kit being used.

Procedure			S = Satisfactory U = Unsatisfactory
You must:	**S**	**U**	**Comments**
1. Wash hands with disinfectant and put on gloves			
2. Assemble materials and equipment			
3. Allow all reagents to reach room temperature before performing test			

4. Prepare a 1:20 dilution of the test serum:
    a.   Pipet 0.05 ml (50μl) of serum into a 13 × 75 tube
    b. Pipet 0.95 ml of glycine diluent into the tube and mix well			

5. Dispense one drop of positive control serum into ring on slide			
6. Dispense one drop of negative control serum into ring on slide			
7. Dispense one drop of diluted patient serum into ring on slide using dispenser-spreader included in kit (save dispenser for mixing specimen)			
8. Mix the RF latex reagent well by inversion			
9. Dispense one drop of well-mixed RF latex reagent into each ring containing a control or test serum			
10. Use the spreader end of the dispenser (used to dispense serum) to thoroughly mix serum with reagent, spreading the mixture over the entire surface of the ring. *Note:* Be sure to use a separate spreader-mixer for each serum or control sample. A wooden applicator stick may be used if no spreaders are available.			
11. Rock the slide in a figure-eight motion for the appropriate time (usually 2–3 minutes) to continue mixing			
12. Observe the rings for agglutination immediately at the end of the appropriate time period			
13. Record the results of the controls and patient serum (+ = agglutination, 0 = no agglutination)			
14. Perform the quantitative test (steps 15–18) if the patient sample is positive for agglutination; if it is negative, go to step 19			

You must:	S	U	Comments

15. Prepare a two-fold serial dilution of patient serum:
   a.   Label 5 test tubes: 1 (1:40), 2 (1:80), 3 (1:160), 4 (1:320), and 5 (1:640)
   b.   Pipet 0.5 ml of glycine diluent into each tube
   c.   Pipet 0.5 ml of 1:20 dilution of patient serum (from qualitative test) into tube 1 (1:40) and mix contents of tube well
   d.   Transfer 0.5 ml from tube 1 to tube 2 and mix well
   e.   Transfer 0.5 ml from tube 2 to tube 3 and mix well
   f.   Transfer 0.5 ml from tube 3 to tube 4 and mix well
   g. Transfer 0.5 ml from tube 4 to tube 5 and mix well			

16. Use each dilution (tubes 1–5) as a separate test specimen and perform the agglutination test as in steps 5–13			
17. Record the results for each tube			
18. Record the serum RF titer (the reciprocal of the highest dilution which shows agglutination)			
19. Disinfect glass slide with chlorine bleach and return to storage			
20. Return all reagents and materials to proper storage			
21. Discard specimens and contaminated items appropriately			
22. Clean and disinfect work area			
23. Remove gloves and discard appropriately			
24. Wash hands with hand disinfectant			

Comments:

Student/Instructor:

Date:_____   Instructor:_____

UNIT 5
Urinalysis

UNIT OBJECTIVES

After studying this unit, you should be able to:
- Describe proper urine collection and preservation methods.
- Perform a physical examination of urine.
- Perform a chemical examination of urine.
- Identify components of urine sediment.
- Perform a microscopic examination of urine sediment.

OVERVIEW

The urinary system is an excretory system consisting of the kidney, ureters, bladder, and urethra. The kidney is the organ in which urine is formed. Three processes are involved in urine formation: (1) filtration of waste products, salts, and excess fluid from the blood, (2) reabsorption of water and solutes from the filtrate, and (3) secretion of ions and certain drugs into the urine.

The filtering unit is called the *glomerulus.* The part which secretes substances, reabsorbs substances and concentrates the filtrate is called the *tubule.* Together, these two parts form the *nephron.* There are approximately one million nephrons in each kidney. Each minute more than 1000 ml of blood flows through the kidney to be cleansed. In the glomerulus, certain substances are filtered out of the blood. The remaining filtrate then passes into the tubule where various changes occur. Some tubular cells reabsorb certain constituents such as glucose. Other tubular cells have the ability to secrete certain substances such as potassium and hydrogen ions. In another part of the tubule most of the water in the filtrate is reabsorbed. The portion which is not reabsorbed forms the *urine.* This urine passes out of the kidney into the bladder through a tube called the

297

ureter. The *bladder* is used for temporary storage of the urine until it is excreted by the body through a tube called the *urethra*.

An examination of the urine, a urinalysis, may be performed for two purposes: (1) to check for certain metabolic end products which indicate particular diseases; or (2) to observe physical, chemical, and microscopic characteristics which indicate disease or damage to the urinary tract itself. This unit demonstrates that urinalysis test results can and do make a difference in the diagnosis and treatment of the patient.

LESSON 5-1
Collection and Preservation of Urine

LESSON OBJECTIVES

After studying this lesson, you should be able to:
- Instruct a male and female patient to correctly collect a clean-catch urine.
- Instruct a male and female patient to correctly collect a mid-stream urine.
- List causes of contamination in urine specimens.
- Explain the reason for adding preservatives to some urine specimens.
- State the normal 24-hour urine volume for adults.
- Name three factors that influence urine volume.
- Define the glossary terms.

GLOSSARY

anuria / absence of urine production

clean-catch urine / a mid-stream urine sample collected after the urethral opening and surrounding tissues have been cleansed

mid-stream urine / a urine sample collected in the middle of voiding

nocturia / excessive urination at night

oliguria / decreased production of urine

polyuria / excessive production of urine

INTRODUCTION

Examination of a urine specimen can yield many results which are helpful in the diagnosis and treatment of patients. However, proper collection of the sample is essential in order for the test results to be valid.

TYPE OF SPECIMEN

The preferred specimen for most examinations is the first urine voided in the morning. This specimen will be the most concentrated; the volume and concentration usually varies during the day. The patient may be instructed to collect a clean-catch urine sample or a mid-stream urine sample.

Mid-Stream Urine Specimen

If the urine specimen is to be used for a routine urinalysis, a mid-stream sample may be used. A **mid-stream urine** sample is one in which the patient collects the urine only in the middle of voiding.

Clean-Catch Urine Specimen

A **clean-catch urine** sample must be collected for bacteriological examinations. To collect a clean-catch sample the patient first cleanses the urethral opening and the surrounding tissues. After the area has been cleansed the patient then collects a mid-stream sample. Occasionally, it may be necessary to obtain the urine by catheterization, a procedure performed only by specially trained personnel.

PROCEDURE FOR COLLECTING A CLEAN-CATCH URINE SAMPLE

A clean-catch urine specimen is necessary if it is to be tested for the presence of bacteria. Most hospitals and doctors' offices use a kit containing towelettes and a sterile disposable urine container. Male and female patients should be instructed to carefully collect the desired urine specimen.

Instructions to the Male

The male patient should retract the foreskin on the penis (if not circumcised) using a towelette. A second towelette should be used to cleanse the urethral opening with a single stroke directed from the tip of the penis toward the ring of the glans. The towelette should then be discarded and the cleansing procedure repeated using two more towelettes. The patient should begin to void into the toilet. The urine stream should be interrupted to collect the urine into the supplied container. Only the middle portion of the urine flow should be included in the sample. After the specimen has

been collected, the container should be closed. The patient should avoid touching the inside of both the container and the lid. The information on the label should then be completed and attached to the specimen container.

Instructions to the Female

The female patient should position herself comfortably on the toilet seat and should swing one knee to the side as far as possible. She should spread the outer vulval folds (labia majora) using a towelette and the inner side of one inner fold (labium minora) should be wiped with a towelette using a single stroke from front to back. The towelette should then be discarded and a second towelette used to repeat the procedure on the opposite side. A third towelette is used to cleanse the urethral opening with a single front-to-back stroke. The patient should then begin to void into the toilet. The urine stream should be interrupted to collect the urine in a container. Only the middle portion of the urine flow should be included in the sample. Touching only the outside of the container and lid, the container should then be closed. The information on the label should be completed and attached to the container.

PROCEDURE FOR COLLECTING A MID-STREAM URINE SAMPLE

For a routine chemical and microscopic analysis of urine, it is not necessary to have a clean-catch specimen. The sample preferred is the first morning sample of urine. However, a urine sample taken randomly during the day may be used. The cleansing procedures above are not necessary, but the urine should be collected mid-stream.

SOURCES OF CONTAMINATION

Urine collection procedures must be followed correctly. If they are not, the urine specimen may become contaminated with epithelial cells, blood cells, microorganisms, or excessive mucus. Pre-cleaned or sterile disposable containers, made of either plastic or plastic-coated paper, are widely used to collect urine samples. If reusable contain-ers are used, they must be thoroughly washed and dried first. If a bacterial culture is to be per-formed on the urine, a sterile container must be used.

HANDLING AND PRESERVING SPECIMENS

The way a urine specimen is handled after col-lection can affect the results of many of the tests. A urine specimen should be examined within one hour of voiding. If this is not possible, the urine may be refrigerated at 4–6° Celsius for up to eight hours. A urine specimen which cannot be refriger-ated or which has to be transported over a long distance can have a preservative added to it. The laboratory may give the patient a container with preservative added for the patient to take home and collect a specimen (i.e., 24-hour urine).

When a urine sample is allowed to sit at room temperature, any bacteria present will multiply rapidly. When this occurs, the specimen will have an unpleasant, ammonia-like odor. A delay before testing can also increase the decomposition of *casts* and the cellular components of the sample. The addition of a preservative will retard the growth of bacteria and slow the destruction of other urine components. The preservative must be carefully chosen to prevent interference with the tests which have been ordered. Some commonly used pre-servatives are toluene, formalin, and thymol. No preservative of any kind should be added to a urine which is to be used for bacteriological studies.

URINE VOLUME

When a routine urinalysis is performed, the vol-ume of the specimen is usually not recorded. However, there are certain quantitative tests which

Table 5–1. Normal 24-hour urine volumes

Age	Volume (ml/24 hours)
Newborn	20–350
One year	300–600
Ten years	750–1500
Adult	750–2000

are performed on urine collected in a 24-hour period. The volume of these samples should be carefully measured using a graduated cylinder and then recorded.

The urinary volume depends on various fac-tors: the fluid intake, the fluid lost in exhalation and perspiration, and the status of renal and car-diac functions of the person. Excessive production of urine is called **polyuria.** The term **nocturia** refers to excessive urination at night. **Oliguria** is insufficient production of urine. The absence of urine production is **anuria.**

The normal volume of urine produced every 24 hours varies according to the age of the individ-ual (Table 5–1). Infants and children produce smaller volumes than adults. The normal 24-hour urine volume for newborns is between 20 and 350 ml. At the age of one year 300–600 ml is normal for twenty-four hours. For ten-year-olds the volume may range from 750–1500 ml in twenty-four hours. The normal adult volume is 750–2000 ml in twenty-four hours, with 1500 ml being average.

LESSON REVIEW

1. How is a clean-catch urine sample collected?
2. When is a clean-catch urine sample required?
3. What is a mid-stream urine specimen?
4. What are the sources of contamination of a urine specimen?
5. When is a urine preservative necessary?
6. Name three commonly used urine preserva-tives.

7. What is the major disadvantage of using preservatives in urine?
8. Is the urine volume recorded for routine specimens?
9. What is the normal 24-hour urine volume for each age group?
10. Name three factors that influence urine volume.
11. How does improper collection affect urinalysis test results?
12. Why is the first morning specimen preferred for urinalysis?
13. Define anuria, clean-catch urine, mid-stream urine, nocturia, oliguria, and polyuria.

STUDENT ACTIVITIES

1. Re-read the information on collection and preservation of urine.
2. Review the glossary terms.
3. Explain collection and preservation of urine specimens to the instructor.
4. Design patient instruction cards for the collection of clean-catch urine specimens (male and female).
5. Practice giving instructions for obtaining clean-catch urine samples (male and female) as outlined on the Student Performance Guides.

Student Performance Guide

NAME _____

DATE _____

LESSON 5–1
COLLECTION AND PRESERVATION
OF URINE: MALE PATIENT

Instructions

1. Practice instructing male patients in the proper method of urine collection.
2. Explain the procedures for collecting and preserving urine samples satisfactorily for the instructor. All steps must be completed as listed on the instructor's Performance Check Sheet.
3. Complete a written examination successfully.

Materials and Equipment

- gloves
- hand disinfectant
- clean, graduated urine containers and lids (disposable)
- towelettes
- labels
- marking pen
- biohazard container

Procedure			S = Satisfactory U = Unsatisfactory
You must:	**S**	**U**	**Comments**
1. Wash hands with disinfectant and put on gloves			
2. Assemble equipment and materials			

3. Explain to male patient the procedure for collecting a clean-catch urine:
  a. Collect the first urine passed in the morning
  b. Retract foreskin (if not circumcised) with towelette
  c. Use one of the towelettes to clean the urethral opening using a single stroke directed from the tip of the penis toward the ring of the glans
  d. Discard towelette
  e. Repeat the cleansing procedure with two more towelettes
  f. Void into the toilet and continue to void but interrupt the stream to collect the urine into the specimen container. Only the middle portion of the urine flow should be included in the sample. Do not touch the inside of the container or the inside of the lid
  g. Close the container and wash hands			

4. Obtain specimen from patient, complete the information on the label (patient number, name, date, time of collection), and attach it to the specimen container			
5. Store specimen as instructed until testing can be performed			
6. Remove and discard gloves appropriately			
7. Wash hands with hand disinfectant			

Comments:

Student/Instructor:

Date:_____   Instructor:_____

Student Performance Guide

NAME _____

DATE _____

LESSON 5–1
COLLECTION AND PRESERVATION OF URINE: FEMALE PATIENT

Instructions

1. Practice instructing female patients in the proper method of urine collection.
2. Explain the procedures for collecting and preserving urine samples satisfactorily for the instructor. All steps must be completed as listed on the instructor's Performance Check Sheet.
3. Complete a written examination successfully.

Materials and Equipment

- gloves
- hand disinfectant
- clean, graduated urine containers and lids (disposable)
- towelettes
- labels
- marking pen
- biohazard container

Procedure			S = Satisfactory U = Unsatisfactory
You must:	**S**	**U**	**Comments**
1. Wash hands with disinfectant and put on gloves			
2. Assemble equipment and materials			

3. Explain to female patient the procedure for collecting a clean-catch urine:
   a. Collect the first urine passed in the morning
   b. Sit comfortably on the toilet seat and swing one knee to the side as far as possible
   c. Spread the outer folds around the urethral opening using a towelette. Wipe the inner side of the inner fold with a single stroke from front to back using another towelette, and then discard the towelette
   d. Use a second towelette and repeat step c on the opposite side of the urethral opening
   e. Use a third towelette and cleanse the urethral opening with a single front-to-back stroke
   f. Void into the toilet and continue to void, but interrupt the stream to collect the urine in the container. Only the middle portion of the urine flow should be included in the sample. Do not touch the inside of the container or the inside of the lid
   g. Close the container and wash hands			

4. Obtain specimen from patient, complete the information on the label (patient number, name, date, time of collection), and attach it to the specimen container			
5. Store specimen as instructed until specimen can be tested			
6. Remove and discard gloves appropriately			
7. Wash hands with hand disinfectant			

Comments:

Student/Instructor:

Date:_____   Instructor:_____

LESSON 5–2
Physical Examination of Urine

LESSON OBJECTIVES

After studying this lesson, you should be able to:
- List three causes of abnormal odor of urine.
- Explain why normal urine has a yellow color.
- List three abnormal colors of urine and give a cause for each.
- List two conditions that may affect transparency of urine.
- Explain what determines the specific gravity of urine.
- Demonstrate the proper use of the urinometer and refractometer.
- Perform a physical examination of urine.
- Define glossary terms.

GLOSSARY

hematuria / presence of red blood cells in urine

ketones / substances produced during increased metabolism of fat; sometimes called ketone bodies

melanin / a dark pigment

myoglobin / protein found in muscle tissue

porphyrins / a group of pigments which are intermediates in the production of hemoglobin

refractometer / an instrument for measuring refraction

specific gravity / ratio of weight of a given volume of a solution to the weight of the same volume of water; a measurement of density

turbid / having a cloudy appearance

urinometer / a float with a calibrated stem used for measuring specific gravity

urochrome / yellow pigment which gives color to urine

INTRODUCTION

A routine urinalysis consists of physical, chemical, and microscopic examinations of urine. The physical examination of urine can provide useful information to the physician and should be the first part of the urinalysis performed.

The physical examination of urine includes observing the odor, color, transparency, and specific gravity. The physical examination is the easiest and quickest part of a routine urinalysis and can be performed at the time the urine is being prepared for other procedures.

Changes in physical characteristics of urine can provide significant clues to renal or metabolic disease. However, variations in odor, color, and transparency do not always reflect pathologic changes. Sometimes, these variations are caused by the handling of the specimen (i.e., temperature of storage). For accurate evaluation of physical characteristics of urine, the sample should be examined immediately after voiding.

ODOR OF URINE

Normal, freshly voided urine has a characteristic aromatic and not unpleasant odor. Changes in odor of urine may be due to diet, disease, or the presence of microorganisms.

The odor of the urine of a patient with uncontrolled diabetes is described as fruity. This is because of the presence of **ketones,** products of fat metabolism.

If urine is allowed to stand, bacteria may break down urea to form ammonia; the resulting odor is similar to ammonia. A freshly voided sample of urine which has a foul, pungent odor suggests urinary tract infection.

Foods such as garlic and asparagus can also produce an abnormal odor. Although odor may be striking in certain diseases, it is not a reliable enough characteristic to use alone in detecting disease.

Table 5–2. Table of urine colors and their causes

Color	Cause
Pale yellow to amber	Normal
Red, red-brown	Red cells, hemoglobin, myoglobin
Wine-red	Porphyrins
Brown-black	Melanin, hemoglobin in acidic urine
Yellow-brown, green-brown	Bilirubin, bile pigments

COLOR OF URINE

The normal color of urine is yellow; however, variations in color may be caused by diet, medication, and disease (Table 5–2). The urine color can sometimes provide a clue for the diagnosis of certain diseases.

Yellow urine. The pigment that produces the normal yellow to amber color of urine is **urochrome.** As the urine concentration varies, so will the intensity of the color. Dilute urine samples are pale while the more concentrated urine samples are darker.

Red urine. The abnormal color seen most frequently is red or red-brown urine. This may be due to **hematuria**—the presence of red blood cells—or to the presence of hemoglobin or **myoglobin. Porphyrins** may cause the urine to be red or wine-red.

Brown/black urine. Hemoglobin will become brown in acidic urine that has been standing. **Melanin** will also cause urine to become dark or black on standing.

Yellow-brown or green-brown urine. Bilirubin or bile pigments may cause urine to be yellow-brown or green-brown. These urines may have a yellow-green foam when shaken. Urine specimens containing bilirubin should be handled with caution to avoid possible exposure of laboratory personnel to the hepatitis organism.

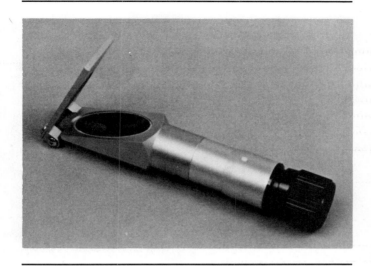

Figure 5–1. Refractometer *(Photo by John Estridge)*

TRANSPARENCY OF URINE

Fresh urine is normally clear immediately after voiding. As the urine reaches room temperature, or after refrigeration, it may become **turbid,** or cloudy. Depending on the pH of the urine, this cloudiness may be due to urates or phosphates. Mucus or white blood cells in the urine also can cause a cloudy appearance; red blood cells in urine give it a cloudy-red appearance. Fat causes urine to appear opalescent. Bacteria cause turbidity in urine when present in high numbers.

It is essential that the sample be well mixed while observing the urine for transparency. The cause of cloudiness will usually become evident during the microscopic examination.

SPECIFIC GRAVITY

The **specific gravity** of a solution is the ratio of the weight of a given volume of the solution (urine) to the weight of an equal volume of water. The specific gravity of urine indicates the concentration of solids such as urea, phosphates, chlorides, proteins, and sugars which are dissolved in the urine.

The ability of the kidneys to concentrate is reflected by the specific gravity of the urine produced. Urine samples of small volume usually are more concentrated than those of large volume. Dehydration may cause urine to become highly concentrated.

The normal specific gravity of urine ranges from 1.005–1.030, with most samples falling between 1.010 and 1.025. Specific gravity is measured with a refractometer (Figure 5–1) or a urinometer (Figure 5–2).

To use the **refractometer,** one drop of well-mixed urine is put into the instrument and the value is read directly off a scale viewed through the ocular. The refractometer must be calibrated daily with distilled water (which has a specific gravity of 1.000).

The urinometer method requires a larger volume of urine (about 40–50 ml). The **urinometer,** which is a float with a calibrated stem, is placed into the sample with a slight spinning motion. The value is read at the meniscus of the urine. The float will rise higher in a concentrated

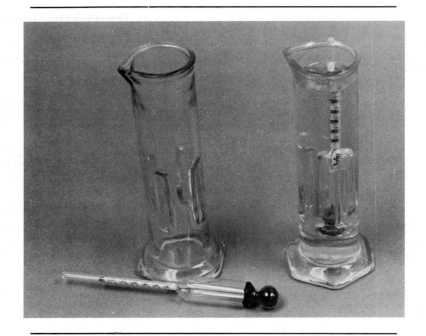

Figure 5–2. Urinometer *(Photo by John Estridge)*

urine and will sink lower in a dilute sample. The urinometer should also be calibrated daily with distilled water.

PERFORMING A PHYSICAL EXAMINATION OF URINE

To perform a physical examination of urine, a fresh urine specimen must be obtained. The urine should be observed for odor, color, and transparency after it is well mixed (by gentle swirling). The specific gravity of the urine should then be measured using a refractometer or urinometer. These observations and measurements should be recorded and the urine should be retained for chemical and microscopic examinations. The normal values for the physical characteristics of urine are shown in Table 5–3.

Table 5–3. Physical characteristics of normal urine

Characteristic	Normal
Transparency	Clear
Color	Straw to amber
Specific gravity	1.005–1.030

Precautions

■ The urine should be gently, but thoroughly, mixed before making physical observations.
■ Wipe up any urine spills with disinfectant.
■ Test urinometer and refractometer daily with distilled water to check reliability.

LESSON REVIEW

1. What observations are included in the physical examination of urine?
2. What are some of the causes of abnormal odors of urine?
3. What gives urine its normal color?
4. What is the significance of variations in urine color and what are causes of variations?
5. What is the normal transparency of urine?
6. What are some causes of cloudy urine?
7. What is the normal specific gravity of urine?
8. What kidney function is reflected by the specific gravity of urine?
9. Define hematuria, ketones, melanin, myoglobin, porphyrins, refractometer, specific gravity, turbid, urinometer, and urochrome.

STUDENT ACTIVITIES

1. Re-read the information on physical examination of urine.
2. Review the glossary terms.
3. Compare the specific gravities of lighter-colored urines with those of darker-colored urines.
4. Divide a urine sample. Put one part in the refrigerator; place the other part on the counter at room temperature. Observe each for transparency changes and odor changes at the end of one hour, two hours, or more.
5. Practice performing physical examinations of several urine samples as outlined on the Student Performance Guide, using the worksheet.

Student Performance Guide

NAME _____

DATE _____

LESSON 5–2
PHYSICAL EXAMINATION OF URINE

Instructions

1. Practice the procedure for performing a physical examination of urine.
2. Demonstrate the procedure for a physical examination of urine satisfactorily for the instructor. All steps must be completed as listed on the instructor's Performance Check Sheet.
3. Complete a written examination successfully.

Materials and Equipment

- gloves
- hand disinfectant
- conical centrifuge tube, glass or clear plastic
- test tube rack
- fresh urine sample
- dropping pipet
- refractometer
- urinometer
- distilled water
- urinalysis report form
- soft tissue or soft paper towels
- surface disinfectant
- biohazard container
- chlorine bleach

Note: Consult manufacturer's directions before performing the test.

Procedure			S = Satisfactory U = Unsatisfactory
You must:	**S**	**U**	**Comments**
1. Wash hands with disinfectant and put on gloves			
2. Assemble equipment and materials			
3. Obtain a fresh urine specimen			
4. Mix the urine gently by swirling and pour approximately 5 ml into a conical centrifuge tube			

You must:	S	U	Comments
5. Observe and record the color of the urine (straw, yellow, red, etc.)			
6. Notice the odor of the urine			
7. Observe and record the transparency of the urine (clear, slightly cloudy, turbid)			
8. Measure the specific gravity by using both the refractometer and urinometer: A. Refractometer (1) Place one drop of distilled water on the glass plate of the refractometer and close gently			
(2) Look through ocular and read the specific gravity from the scale. For water the specific gravity should read 1.000. (If it does not, calibrate with the screwdriver provided with the refractometer)			
(3) Wipe the water from the glass plate, place one drop of urine on the plate and close gently			
(4) Look through the ocular, read the specific gravity from the scale and record			
(5) Clean the glass plate with disinfectant and dry with a soft tissue			
B. Urinometer (1) Pour 40–50 ml of urine into the glass cylinder (approximately three-fourths full)			
(2) Insert urinometer with spinning motion, gently			
(3) Read the specific gravity from the scale on the stem of the urinometer as it stops spinning and record			
(4) Rinse equipment and repeat B1–B3 with distilled water (specific gravity of water should be 1.000)			
9. Discard urine sample properly			
10. Disinfect and clean equipment and return to proper storage			
11. Clean work area with disinfectant			
12. Remove and discard gloves appropriately			
13. Wash hands with hand disinfectant			

Comments:

Student/Instructor:

Date:_____   Instructor:_____

Worksheet

NAME_____ DATE _____

SPECIMEN NO. _____

LESSON 5–2 PHYSICAL EXAMINATION OF URINE

Physical Examination	Normal Values

1. Volume (ml): _____   750–2000 ml (adult)
   (only report for 24-hour urines)

2. Transparency: _____ clear   clear

                      _____ hazy (slightly cloudy)

                      _____ cloudy (turbid)

3. Color: _____   straw to amber

4. Specific gravity: _____   1.005–1.030

LESSON 5-3
Chemical Examination of Urine

LESSON OBJECTIVES

After studying this lesson, you should be able to:
- Name chemical tests routinely performed on urine and explain the principle of each.
- Use and interpret a reagent strip.
- List a condition that may cause an abnormal result in each of the chemical tests routinely performed on urine.
- Perform four confirmatory chemical tests on urine.
- Discuss the precautions that must be observed in chemical testing of urine.
- Define the glossary terms.

GLOSSARY

bilirubin / product formed in the liver from the breakdown of hemoglobin

glomerular / pertaining to the glomerulus, the filtering unit of the kidney

glycosuria / glucose in the urine; glucosuria

ketonuria / ketones in the urine

pH / an expression of the degree of acidity or alkalinity of a solution

proteinuria / protein in the urine, usually albumin

urobilinogen / a derivative of bilirubin formed by the action of intestinal bacteria

INTRODUCTION

Tests can be performed on urine samples to detect the presence of certain compounds or chemicals. These tests are usually considered to be a part of a routine urinalysis. When performed correctly, these tests can provide valuable information to the physician. In some situations, the urine chemical test results can be critical to the diagnosis.

315

METHODS OF CHEMICAL ANALYSIS

Reagent strips are the most widely used technique of detecting chemicals in urine and are available in a variety of types (Figure 5–3). A reagent strip is a firm plastic strip to which pads containing chemical reactants are attached. Most reagent strips contain reagent areas that test pH, protein, glucose, ketone, bilirubin, and blood. Some strips may also test for urobilinogen, specific gravity, leukocytes, and bacteria. The presence (or absence) of these chemicals in the urine provides information on the patient's carbohydrate metabolism, kidney and liver function, and acid-base balance.

Reagent strips are designed to be used only once and discarded. Exact directions for the use of the strips are included in each package. These instructions must be followed precisely for accurate results. A color comparison chart is also included, usually on the label of the reagent strip container. Positive results may be checked by confirmatory tests. The performance of the strips should be checked by testing strips with urine controls (positive and negative) which may be purchased or made. (See Preparation of Reagents, Appendix N, page 505.)

PERFORMING THE CHEMICAL TESTS BY REAGENT STRIP

Chemical testing should be performed within one hour of urine collection. If tests cannot be performed within this time, the specimen may be refrigerated for up to eight hours. Refrigerated specimens should be allowed to return to room temperature prior to testing.

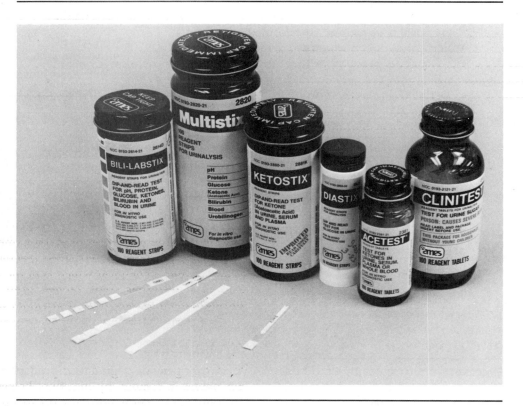

Figure 5–3. Various types of reagent strips used for urine testing (*Photo by John Estridge*)

Chemical testing is performed by dipping a reagent strip into a fresh urine. The color changes on the reagent pads should be visually compared to the color chart after the appropriate time period (Color Plate No. 17). Although in most labs reagent strips are visually interpreted by the technician, there are instruments which can detect the color changes electronically. When such instruments are used, the moistened reagent strip is inserted into the instrument and the results are displayed on a lighted panel. Using such an instrument eliminates technician error due to differences in timing or interpretation of colors.

PRINCIPLES OF CHEMICAL TESTS

pH

The **pH** is a measure of the degree of acidity or alkalinity of the urine. A pH below seven indicates an acid urine; a pH above seven indicates alkaline urine. Normal, freshly voided urine may have a pH range of 5.5–8.0. The pH of urine may change with diet, medications, kidney disease, and metabolic diseases such as diabetes mellitus. Chemical indicators in the pH reagent pad change colors in a range from yellow-orange for acid urine to green-blue in alkaline urine.

Protein

The condition in which protein is present in the urine is called **proteinuria.** This is an important indicator of renal disease, but can also be caused by other conditions such as urinary tract infection. At a constant pH, the development of any green color on the protein reagent pad is due to the presence of protein. Colors range from yellow for negative to yellow-green or green for positive.

Glucose

The presence of glucose in urine is called **glycosuria.** This condition indicates that the blood glucose level has exceeded the renal threshold. This condition may occur in diabetes mellitus. The reagent strip is specific for glucose and uses the enzymes glucose oxidase and peroxidase, which react with glucose to form colors ranging from green (low concentration) to brown (high concentration).

Ketone

When the body metabolizes fats incompletely, ketones are excreted in the urine, a condition called **ketonuria.** The ketone test is based on the development of colors ranging from light pink to maroon when ketones react with nitroprusside. Ketonuria may be present in diabetes and starvation or fasting. Since ketones will evaporate at room temperature, urine should be tightly covered and refrigerated if not tested promptly.

Bilirubin

Bilirubin is a breakdown product of hemoglobin. When it is present in urine, it may be an indication of liver disease, bile duct obstruction, or hepatitis. Therefore, samples suspected of containing bilirubin should be handled cautiously because of the possibility of hepatitis. These samples should also be protected from light until testing is completed, since direct light will cause decomposition of bilirubin. The test for bilirubin is based on the coupling of bilirubin with a dye to form a color.

Blood

Presence of blood in the urine may indicate infection or trauma of the urinary tract or bleeding in the kidneys. Hemoglobin and red cells may be detected by the formation of a color due to the enzyme peroxidase (in red cells) reacting with orthotolidine, a chemical which is in the reagent pad. The resulting color ranges from orange through green to dark blue. Myoglobin will also cause a positive reaction on the reagent strip.

Urobilinogen

Urobilinogen is a degradation product of bilirubin which is formed by intestinal bacteria. The urobilinogen level is normally 0.1 to 1.0 Ehrlich units (E.U.) per deciliter of urine. It may be increased in hepatic disease or hemolytic disease. The reagent strip will detect urobilinogen in concentrations as low as 0.1 E.U. The reagent pad contains a chemical which reacts with urobilinogen to form a pink-red color.

Nitrite

Gram negative bacteria can convert urinary nitrate to nitrite. The nitrite produced reacts with chemicals in the nitrite reagent pad to form a pink color. A positive nitrite test is an indication of possible bacterial urinary tract infection.

Leukocytes

The presence of leukocytes in urine may also indicate infection. The esterase enzyme in granular leukocytes reacts with chemicals in the leukocyte reagent pad to form a purple color.

Specific Gravity

Some reagent strips also test for specific gravity. The specific gravity of the urine reflects the kidneys' ability to concentrate the urine. The reagent strip pad contains an indicator which turns various colors depending on the ion concentration of the urine. Specific gravities between 1.000 and 1.030 can be measured.

Normal Values

Normal urine, when tested with a reagent strip, is negative for glucose, ketone, bilirubin, bacteria, leukocyte esterase, and blood. Normal urine may be negative or contain a trace of protein. Normal, freshly voided urine usually has a pH of 5.5–8 (Table 5–4). Positive or abnormal results should be confirmed according to laboratory policy. Some laboratories retest with a reagent strip; others use confirmatory tests. Positive nitrite or leukocyte esterase tests should be confirmed microscopically.

CONFIRMATORY TESTS

Sometimes it may be necessary to measure chemicals in urine other than by the reagent strip method. The other methods are called confirmatory tests because the most common use is to confirm a positive (or negative) result obtained using the reagent strip. Confirmatory tests are more time consuming and require more reagents and equipment than the reagent strip method. Four most commonly used confirmatory tests are those for protein, reducing sugars, ketone, and bilirubin.

Protein. Most simple tests for urine protein involve treating the urine with an acid to cause the protein to precipitate and therefore become visible. The amount of precipitate formed is roughly proportional to the concentration of protein present. Acids that are commonly used are acetic, nitric, and sulfosalicylic acids.

Reducing sugars. A copper reduction test such as Clinitest® is the most common test performed to detect reducing sugars such as lactose and galactose in urine. The test is based on the reduction of copper ions in the Clinitest® tablet by substances such as glucose, galactose, or lactose. Therefore, the test is not specific for glucose. If a reducing sugar is present in the urine, the color changes from blue to green and then orange depending on

Table 5–4. Normal values for urine chemical tests

Substance Tested	Normal Value
pH	5.5-8
protein	negative to trace
glucose	negative
ketone	negative
bilirubin	negative
blood	negative
urobilinogen	0.1-1.0 E.U./dl
bacteria (nitrite)	negative
leukocyte esterase	negative

the amount of sugar present. Since the Clinitest® is not specific for glucose, and a number of substances such as penicillin, salicylates, and reducing sugars may cause positive results, Clinitest® results should not be used as the sole basis for adjusting insulin dosage.

Ketone. The Acetest® is a test for ketones and is available in tablet form. The test is based on the same principle as that found in the reagent strip. If ketones are present in urine, a drop of urine added to the tablet will produce a purple color. A strip such as Ketostix® or Ketodiastix® may also be used to confirm presence of ketones.

Bilirubin. The Ictotest® is a specific test for bilirubin and is four times as sensitive as the reagent strip method. The test is composed of a tablet and absorbent mat. A few drops of urine are placed on the mat, the tablet is placed over the moist area, and water is dropped on the tablet. If bilirubin is present, a purple color will develop on the mat within thirty seconds.

Precautions

■ Reagent strips should be tested with positive controls on each day of use to be sure that strips are working properly.

■ Failure to observe color changes at the appropriate time intervals may cause inaccurate results.

■ Reagents and reagent strips must be stored properly to retain reactivity.

■ Observe color changes and color charts under good lighting.

■ Proper collection and storage of urine is necessary to insure preservation of components such as bilirubin and ketones.

■ Use care in performing the Clinitest® procedure because of the heat that is generated and the caustic nature of the reagents.

■ Do not allow the pads of the reagent strips to touch the fingers or other surfaces.

■ Wipe up any spills promptly with surface disinfectant.

LESSON REVIEW

1. What chemical tests are routinely performed on urine using reagent strips?
2. Explain briefly how a reagent strip is used.
3. What type of urine specimen is preferred for chemical testing?
4. Name four confirmatory tests performed on urine.
5. Name a condition that may cause an increase of the following chemicals in urine: protein, ketones, glucose, bilirubin, and nitrite.
6. Name a method of measuring urine protein other than by the reagent strip method.
7. Name a test that may be performed to detect a reducing sugar other than glucose.
8. List precautions that must be observed to insure accurate results in chemical testing of urine.
9. Define bilirubin, glomerular, glycosuria, ketonuria, pH, proteinuria, and urobilinogen.

STUDENT ACTIVITIES

1. Re-read the information on chemical examination of urine.
2. Review the glossary terms.
3. Practice performing chemical examinations on several urine samples as outlined on the Student Performance Guide, using the worksheet.
4. Compare the results of the physical examination of a sample with the chemical examination results. Are they as expected? If protein is present in a sample, is specific gravity high? If blood is positive on a reagent strip, was it detected in the physical examination?

Student Performance Guide

NAME _____

DATE _____

LESSON 5–3
CHEMICAL EXAMINATION
OF URINE

Instructions

1. Practice the procedure for performing a chemical examination of urine.
2. Demonstrate the procedure for a chemical examination of urine satisfactorily for the instructor. All steps must be completed as listed on the instructor's Performance Check Sheet.
3. Complete a written examination successfully.

Materials and Equipment

- gloves
- hand disinfectant
- fresh urine samples
- urine control solutions (positive and negative)
- reagent strips with comparative chart
- stopwatch or timer
- conical graduated centrifuge tubes
- forceps
- centrifuge
- test tubes, 13 × 100 mm and 16 × 125 mm
- dropping pipets
- distilled water
- 20% sulfosalicylic acid
- Clinitest® tablets
- Acetest® tablets
- Ictotest® tablets and absorbent pads
- test tube racks
- worksheet
- urinalysis report forms
- surface disinfectant
- biohazard container

Note: Consult package inserts for specific instructions before performing tests

320

Procedure	S	U	S = Satisfactory U = Unsatisfactory
You must:	**S**	**U**	**Comments**
1. Wash hands with disinfectant and put on gloves			
2. Assemble equipment and materials			
3. Obtain urine sample (or control)			

4. Perform reagent strip test:
  a. Dip reagent strip into urine sample, moistening all pads
  b. Remove strip from urine immediately and tap to remove excess urine
  c. Observe reagent pads and compare colors to color chart at appropriate time intervals
  d. Record results on urinalysis report form
  e. Discard reagent strip into biohazard container			

5. Perform sulfosalicylic acid test for protein (usually performed only if protein is positive by reagent strip method):
  a. Centrifuge five ml of urine to clear the urine if it is cloudy
  b. Place four ml of clear urine into a 13 × 100 mm test tube
  c. Add three drops of 20% sulfosalicylic acid
  d. Mix thoroughly and estimate the amount of turbidity
  e. Record results on urinalysis form as negative, trace, 1+, 2+, 3+, or 4+			

6. Perform Clinitest® for reducing substances:
  a. Place 16 × 125 mm test tube into a test tube rack
  b. Place five drops of urine into the test tube
  c. Place ten drops of distilled water into the test tube
  d. Drop a Clinitest® reagent tablet into the urine-water mixture (use forceps; the Clinitest® tablet will burn fingers)
  e. Observe color while allowing tablet to effervesce or boil until boiling stops and without touching the test tube with fingers
  f. Wait fifteen seconds, shake test tube gently using forceps and compare color to color chart (tube will be hot and opening should be pointed away from the face)
  g. Record results on urinalysis report form as negative, ¼%, ½%, ¾%, 1%, or 2% or more			

You must:	S	U	Comments
7. Perform Acetest® for ketones			
a. Place an Acetest® tablet on a clean piece of white paper or filter paper			
b. Place one drop of urine on top of the tablet			
c. Compare color of tablet to color chart after thirty seconds			
d. Record results on urinalysis report form as negative or positive			
8. Perform Ictotest® for bilirubin			
a. Place five drops of urine on an Ictotest® mat (if bilirubin is present, it will be absorbed onto the mat surface)			
b. Place an Ictotest® reagent tablet on the moistened area of the mat			
c. Let two drops of water flow onto the tablet *Note:* When elevated amounts of bilirubin are present in the urine specimen, a blue to purple color forms on the mat within thirty seconds. The rapidity of the formation of the color and the intensity of the color are proportional to the amount of bilirubin in the urine (a pink or red color is a negative test)			
d. Record results on urinalysis report form as negative or positive			
9. Dispose of urine specimen properly			
10. Dispose of test tube contents properly			
11. Clean equipment and return to proper storage			
12. Clean work area with surface disinfectant			
13. Remove gloves and discard into biohazard container			
14. Wash hands with hand disinfectant			
Comments: Student/Instructor:			

Date:_____   Instructor:_____

Worksheet

NAME_____ DATE _____

SPECIMEN NO. _____

LESSON 5–3 CHEMICAL EXAMINATION OF URINE

Chemical Examination

A. Multistix	Observed Result	Normal Values
pH	_____	5.5–8.0
protein	_____	negative, trace
glucose	_____	negative
ketone	_____	negative
bilirubin	_____	negative
blood	_____	negative
urobilinogen	_____	0.1–1.0 E.U./dl urine
nitrite	_____	negative
leukocyte esterase	_____	negative

Confirmatory Test Results   (circle result)

B. Protein (sulfosalicylic acid)   negative trace 1+ 2+ 3+ 4+

   Reducing substances (Clinitest®)   negative ¼% ½% ¾% 1% 2% or more

   Ketones (Acetest®)   negative   positive

   Bilirubin (Ictotest®)   negative   positive

LESSON 5-4

Identification of Urine Sediment

LESSON OBJECTIVES

After studying this lesson, you should be able to:

- Write a definition of urine sediment.
- Name four types of cells that may be seen in urine sediment.
- Name three types of casts that may appear in urine sediment.
- Explain how casts are formed.
- Name and draw eight crystals which may be seen in urine sediment.
- Identify components of urine sediment using the microscope.
- Define the glossary terms.

GLOSSARY

amorphous / without definite shape
cast / mold; in urinalysis, a protein matrix formed in the tubules that becomes washed into urine
hyaline / transparent, pale
sediment / solid substances which settle to the bottom of a liquid
supernatant / clear liquid remaining at the top after centrifugation or settling of precipitate

INTRODUCTION

Examining urine sediment is part of a routine urinalysis. It may provide beneficial information in evaluating the course and progress of renal disease as well as detecting the presence of infection. The urine must be freshly voided and examined as soon as possible to prevent deterioration of sediment components. Sediment is obtained by centrifugation of 10–15 ml of urine. The **supernatant** urine is carefully poured off and the sediment remaining in the tube is resuspended, placed on a slide, and examined microscopically.

COMPONENTS OF URINE SEDIMENT

The term urine **sediment** usually refers to cells, casts, crystals, and amorphous deposits. These components of urine sediment may be identified microscopically and are usually observed un-

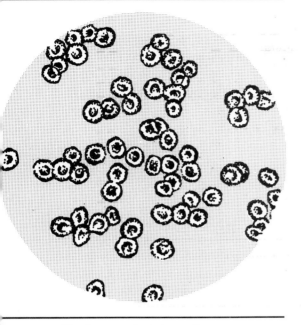

Figure 5–4. Erythrocytes in urine sediment

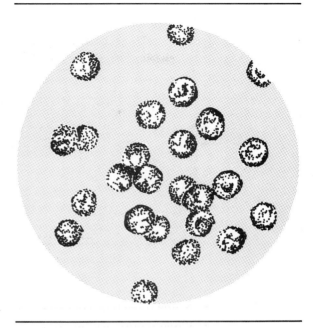

Figure 5–5. Leukocytes in urine sediment

stained. (See Color Plates 17–24 for examples of some components of urine sediment.)

Cells in Urine Sediment

Blood Cells. Normal urine may contain a few blood cells. Blood cells are best identified using the high power (45×) objective.

- Erythrocytes (red blood cells)—Erythrocytes usually look like pale, light-refractive disks when viewed under high power (Figure 5–4 and Color Plates 17, 18, 19, and 21). They have no nuclei. The presence of large numbers of red cells in urine is called *hematuria* and is an abnormal condition indicating disease or trauma.
- Leukocytes (white blood cells)—A few leukocytes may be present in normal urine (Figure 5–5). The type usually present is the segmented neutrophil. Leukocytes in urine may be increased in urinary tract infections. Leukocytes are slightly larger than erythrocytes, may appear granular and have a visible nucleus (Color Plates 17, 18, and 21).

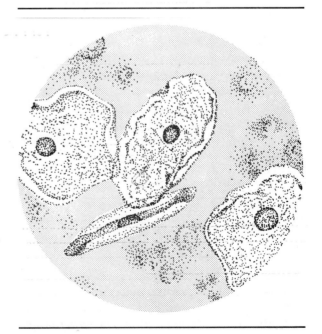

Figure 5–6. Squamous epithelial cells

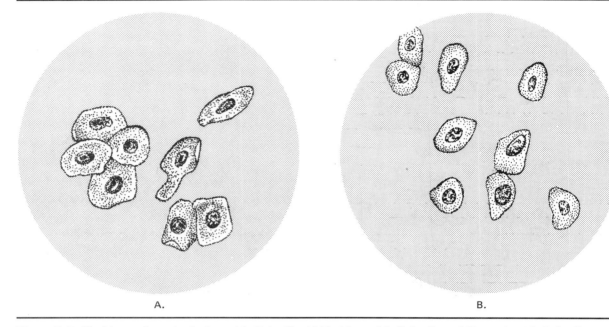

A.

B.

Figure 5–7. Bladder and renal tubular epithelial cells: A) bladder epithelial cells and B) renal epithelial cells

Epithelial Cells. Epithelial cells are constantly being sloughed off from the lining of the urinary tract. The epithelial cells appear large and flat, with a distinct nucleus and much cytoplasm. These cells may be identified using the high power (45×) objective. The most commonly seen cell is the squamous epithelial cell (Figure 5–6, page 325); less commonly seen are the smaller bladder and renal tubular cells (Figure 5–7). The latter may indicate renal disease if they are present in large numbers (Color Plates 17–19).

Microorganisms. Microorganisms should not be present in properly collected, fresh, normal urine. The presence of large numbers of microorganisms indicates infection. Microorganisms are observed using the high power (45×) objective (Figure 5–8).

- Bacteria—Bacteria may appear as tiny round or rod-shaped objects. The rod-shaped bacteria

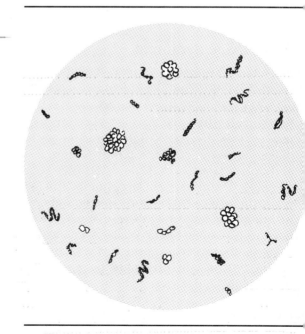

Figure 5–8. Bacteria in urine sediment

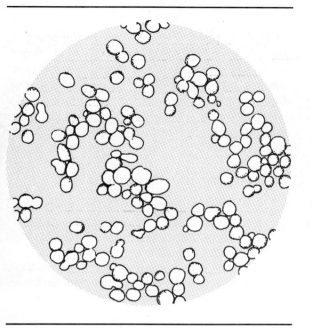

Figure 5–9. Yeasts in urine sediment

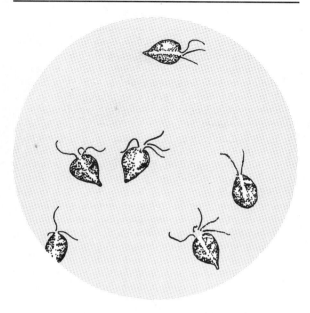

Figure 5–10. Protozoa in urine sediment

are usually more noticeable because the round ones may closely resemble amorphous material.

- Yeast—Yeast cells may be present in urine sediment. They are smaller than erythrocytes but may appear similar to them. Yeasts are ovoid and may be observed budding or in chains (Figure 5–9). To distinguish between yeasts and red cells, add one drop of dilute acetic acid to the urine sediment; red cells will lyse and yeast will not. The most common yeast found is *Candida albicans*.

- Protozoa—*Trichomonas vaginalis* is the most frequently seen parasite in urine. It is a flagellated protozoan that may infect the urinary tract and is usually recognized in urine sediment because of movement of flagella (Figure 5–10).

- Spermatozoa—Spermatozoa may occasionally be observed in urine samples. They are easily recognized and have spherical heads and long thin tails. Spermatozoa should only be reported when they are identified in urine samples of males (Figure 5–11).

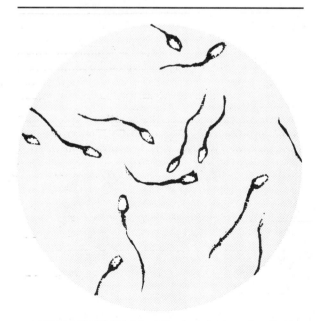

Figure 5–11. Spermatozoa in urine sediment

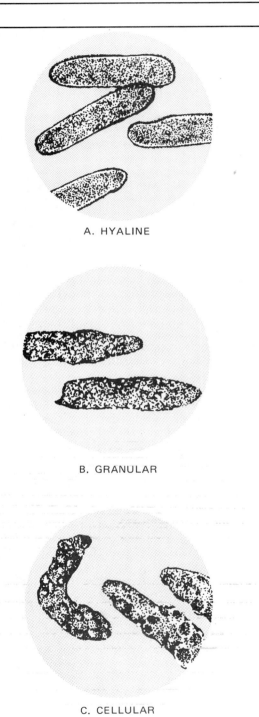

A. HYALINE

B. GRANULAR

C. CELLULAR

Figure 5–12. Casts in urine sediment: A) hyaline, B) granular, and C) cellular

Casts in Urine Sediment

Casts are formed when protein accumulates and precipitates in the kidney tubules and is washed into the urine. The presence of casts in urine, other than an occasional **hyaline** cast, may indicate renal disease. Casts are cylindrical with rounded or flat ends and are classified according to the substances observed in them (Figure 5–12). Some casts may trap cells or debris as they are formed and appear cellular or granular. Casts are viewed using the low power objective (10×) and low light.

- Hyaline—Hyaline casts are occasionally found in normal urine. They are transparent, colorless cylinders and are best seen by reducing the light on the microscope (Color Plate 20).
- Granular—A granular cast contains remnants of disintegrated cells which disappear as fine or coarse granules embedded in the protein.
- Cellular—Cellular casts may contain epithelial cells, red cells, or white cells in the protein.

Crystals and Amorphous Deposits in Urine Sediments

A variety of crystals may be found in normal urine. The formation of crystals is influenced by pH, specific gravity, and temperature of the urine. Although most urine crystals have no clinical significance, there are some rare crystals which appear in urine because of certain metabolic disorders. Therefore, it is important to be able to recognize both normal and abnormal crystals. Crystals, when seen, should be identified and reported.

Normal Crystals in Acid Urine. The normal crystals most commonly seen in acid urine are **amorphous** urates, uric acid, and calcium oxalate.

- Amorphous urates—The amorphous urates may appear in urine as fine granules with no specific shape. Sediment may appear pink in the urine

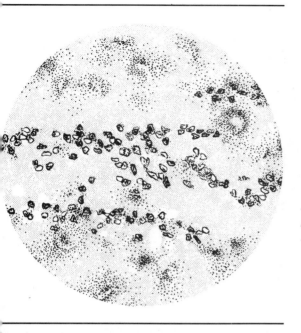

Figure 5–13. Amorphous urates in urine sediment

container but, under the microscope, will appear yellowish (Figure 5–13, Color Plate 24).

- Uric acid—Uric acid may appear as yellow-brown crystals which may have a variety of shapes: irregular, rhombic, clusters, or rosettes (Figure 5–14, Color Plate 22).
- Calcium oxalate—Calcium oxalate forms colorless octahedral crystals which are refractile. They may look like "envelopes," having an X intersecting the crystal, and may vary in size (Figure 5–15).

Normal Crystals in Alkaline Urine. The normal crystals most commonly seen in alkaline urine are amorphous phosphates, triple phosphate, and calcium carbonate.

- Amorphous phosphates—Phosphates may appear as colorless, amorphous, granular masses in urine sediment. Amorphous phosphates are soluble in 10% acetic acid (Figure 5–16, Color Plate 23).

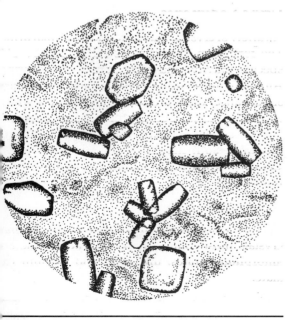

Figure 5–14. Uric acid crystals in urine sediment

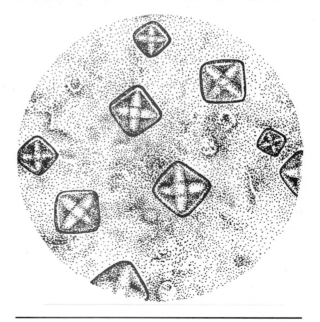

Figure 5–15. Calcium oxalate crystals in urine sediment

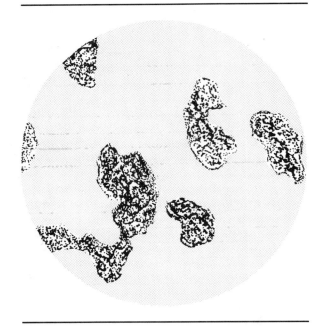

Figure 5–16. Amorphous phosphates in urine sediment

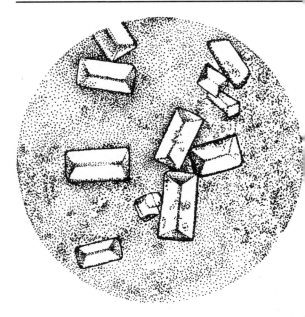

Figure 5–17. Triple phosphate crystals in urine sediment

- Triple phosphate—Ammonium magnesium phosphate (triple phosphate) may form color-less, highly refractile prisms having three to six sides. The crystals are often described as having a coffin-lid appearance (Figure 5–17, Color Plate 23).
- Calcium carbonate—Calcium carbonate forms small, colorless, dumbbell-shaped or leaf-shaped crystals in alkaline urine (Figure 5–18).

Abnormal Crystals in Urine. Abnormal crystals may be seen in the urine of patients with metabolic disease or after administration of drugs such as sulfonamides. Some rare crystals are cystine, tyro-sine, leucine, cholesterol, and sulfonamide.

- Cystine—Cystine may form colorless, refrac-tile, flat, hexagonal crystals, usually having unequal sides. Presence of these crystals in urine indicates disease such as *cystinuria* (Fig-ure 5–19).

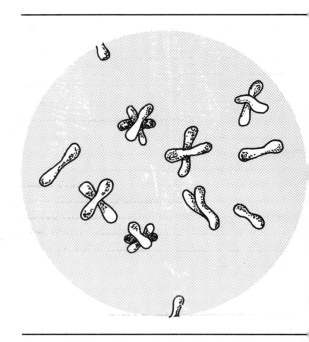

Figure 5–18. Calcium carbonate crystals in urine sediment

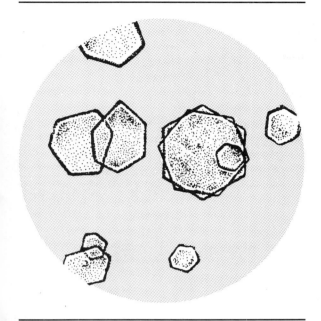

Figure 5–19. Cystine crystals in urine sediment

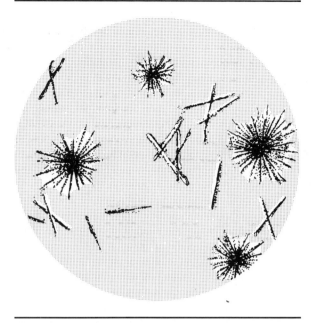

Figure 5–20. Tyrosine crystals in urine sediment

- Tyrosine—Tyrosine forms fine needles arranged in sheaves. Presence of these crystals indicates liver disease or damage (Figure 5–20).
- Leucine—Leucine crystals appear as oily spheres which may be yellow-brown in color and are refractive. Presence of these crystals in urine is an indication of liver disease or damage (Figure 5–21).
- Cholesterol—Cholesterol crystals are colorless, flat plates with notched corners. These crystals are not present in normal urine (Figure 5–22).
- Sulfonamide—Sulfonamide crystals are rarely seen because of the increased solubility of sulfa drugs currently used. Crystals, when seen, appear as bundles of needles with striations (Figure 5–23).

Other Substances in Urine

Mucus threads (from the urinary tract lining) and contaminants such as fibers, hair, talc granules,

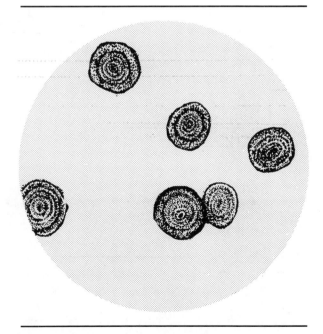

Figure 5–21. Leucine crystals in urine sediment

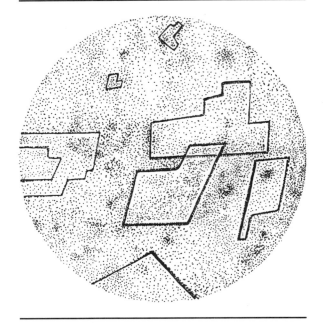

Figure 5–22. Cholesterol crystals in urine sediment

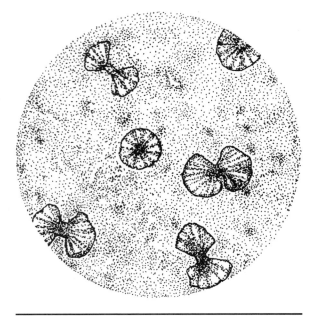

Figure 5–23. Sulfonamide crystals in urine sediment

and oil droplets may sometimes appear in urine sediment. These substances must be recognized and should not be confused with substances in the sediment that are clinically significant. Mucus threads, when seen, are reported (Figure 5–24); contaminants or artifacts are not (Figure 5–25, Color Plate 24).

Precautions

■ Urine samples should be handled with care and spills should be wiped with a surface disinfectant. If urine comes in contact with skin, wash the area with a hand disinfectant.

■ Urine sediment must be observed using reduced light on the microscope.

LESSON REVIEW

1. Define urine sediment.
2. Is identification of urine sediment a part of a routine urinalysis?
3. What is the significance of blood cells in urine sediment?
4. Name four types of cells that may be seen in urine sediment.
5. Should microorganisms be found in fresh, properly collected normal urine?
6. Explain how casts are formed.
7. What are three types of casts that may appear in urine sediment?
8. What are eight crystals which may be seen in urine sediment? Describe the appearance of each.
9. Define amorphous, cast, hyaline, sediment, and supernatant.

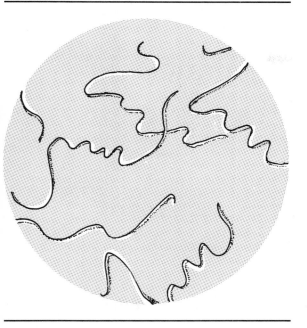

Figure 5–24. Mucus threads in urine sediment

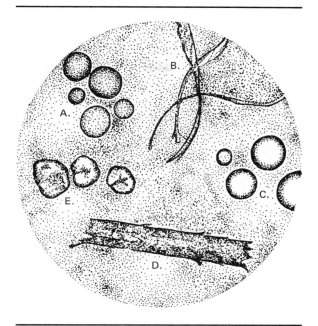

Figure 5–25. Examples of artifacts which may be seen in urine sediment: A) air bubbles, B) fibers, C) oil droplets, D) hair, and E) starch granules

STUDENT ACTIVITIES

1. Re-read the information on identification of urine sediment.
2. Review the glossary terms.

3. Practice microscopic identification of the components of one or more urine sediments as outlined on the Student Performance Guide. Compare your responses with those obtained by the instructor or fellow students.
4. Use unlabeled illustrations provided by the instructor to identify the components of urine sediment.

Student Performance Guide

NAME _____

DATE _____

LESSON 5–4
IDENTIFICATION OF
URINE SEDIMENT

Instructions

1. Practice identification of urine sediment.
2. Identify components of urine sediment microscopically or using visual aids satisfactorily for the instructor. All steps must be completed as listed on the instructor's Performance Check Sheet.
3. Complete a written examination successfully.

Materials and Equipment

- gloves
- hand disinfectant
- urine sediments
- microscope
- glass slides
- coverglasses
- visuals depicting various components of sediment
- surface disinfectant
- biohazard container
- disposable glass or plastic pipet

Procedure			S = Satisfactory U = Unsatisfactory
You must:	**S**	**U**	**Comments**
1. Wash hands with disinfectant and put on gloves			
2. Assemble equipment and materials			
3. Obtain a sample of urine sediment			
4. Place one drop of resuspended urine sediment onto a clean glass slide			
5. Place coverglass over drop of urine			

You must:	S	U	Comments
6. Place slide on microscope stage securely			
7. Focus microscope using low power (10×)			
8. Scan slide using reduced light on microscope			
9. Observe and identify casts if present			
10. Rotate high power (45×) objective into position			
11. Scan slide and identify any blood cells, bacteria, yeasts, or epithelial cells which may be present			
12. Identify any crystals or amorphous deposits present			
13. Discard sediment properly and discard slide in puncture-proof biohazard container			
14. Repeat steps 3–13 using another urine sediment			
15. Clean and return equipment to proper storage			
16. Clean work area with surface disinfectant			
17. Remove and discard gloves appropriately			
18. Wash hands with hand disinfectant			
19. Use unlabeled illustrations provided by instructor to identify components of sediment not seen on slides			

Comments:

Student/Instructor:

Date:_____ Instructor:_____

LESSON 5-5

Microscopic Examination of Urine Sediment

LESSON OBJECTIVES

After studying this lesson, you should be able to:
- Discuss the proper specimen to use for microscopic examination of urine.
- Describe how to prepare urine sediment from a urine specimen.
- List the normal values for erythrocytes, leukocytes, casts, and bacteria in urine.
- Prepare a slide for examining urine sediment.
- Perform a microscopic examination of urine sediment and report the results.
- List the precautions to be observed when microscopically examining urine.

INTRODUCTION

The microscopic examination of urine is the third part of the routine urinalysis. A microscopic examination of urine sediment provides helpful information in evaluating the course and progression of renal disease. The examination also helps to diagnose some infections and metabolic diseases.

Early morning specimens are preferred for routine urinalysis because the specimen is usually more concentrated. If the urine is too dilute, red blood cells, white blood cells, and epithelial cells may lyse and the amount and types of urine sediment seen may be misleading. The urine should be examined as soon as possible after collection to prevent cellular deterioration. The specimen should be a mid-stream or clean-catch specimen to avoid contamination of the specimen with epithelial cells and microorganisms.

OBTAINING THE URINE SEDIMENT

To obtain the sediment, 10 to 15 ml of urine should be poured into a clean, graduated conical centrifuge tube. The tube should be centrifuged at a standard speed (usually 1500 to 2000 rpm) for five minutes. The supernatant urine is then carefully poured off, leaving approximately 0.5 ml in the tube. The sediment remaining in the tube is resuspended by gently shaking the tube.

Table 5–5. Normal values for components of urine sediment

Component	Normal Value
RBC/HPF	rare
WBC/HPF	0–4
epith/HPF	occasional (may be higher in females)
casts/LPF	occasional hyaline
bacteria	negative
mucus	negative to 2+
crystals	types present vary with pH (crystals such as cystine, leucine, tyrosine, and cholesterol are considered abnormal)

PERFORMING THE MICROSCOPIC EXAMINATION

A drop of resuspended sediment is placed directly onto a clean microscope slide and covered with a overslip. The slide is first examined with the low power objective (10×) and reduced light to locate elements that are present in low numbers, such as casts. Ten to fifteen low power fields (LPF) are scanned and the average number of casts per LPF is counted and recorded.

The high power objective (45×) is used to identify erythrocytes, leukocytes, epithelial cells, yeasts, bacteria, and crystals (ten to fifteen high power fields should be scanned). The diaphragm of the microscope should be adjusted during the scanning to obtain the proper amount of light. The average number of erythrocytes, leukocytes, and epithelial cells per high power field (HPF) is recorded. Table 5–5 lists the normal values for urine sediment.

METHOD OF COUNTING CELLS AND MAGNIFICATION

The method of counting cells and the magnification used may differ among laboratories. Therefore, the method used should always be that of the laboratory where the test is being performed.

The counts for RBC, WBC, and epithelial cells represent an average of the number of cells seen in each of the 10 high power fields (HPF) scanned. The results may be reported as 0, rare, occasional or as a range such as 2–4 or 4–6.

The count for casts represents an average of the number of casts seen in each of the 10 low power fields (LPF) scanned. Casts should be categorized as hyaline, granular, or cellular. The method of reporting casts is like that for cells.

Microorganisms such as yeasts (budding) and protozoa such as *Trichomonas* should be reported if seen. Bacteria are usually reported only if large numbers are seen in a fresh urine sample that has been properly collected.

Mucus threads and crystals should be reported if seen, and crystals should be identified. Mucus and bacteria are usually reported as negative, 1+, 2+, 3+, and 4+. Spermatozoa are only reported in males.

Precautions

■ The light level on the microscope should be reduced. The fine adjustment should be used, especially to see casts.
■ Red blood cells and yeasts appear very similar. Yeasts usually cannot be positively identified unless budding is observed.
■ All spills should be wiped up promptly with surface disinfectant.

LESSON REVIEW

1. What kind of urine is the best specimen to use when identifying urine sediment? Why?
2. What power of magnification should be used to initially examine a slide of urine sediment?
3. What are the major components of urine sediment that are usually encountered?
4. How is a urine sediment prepared?
5. What centrifuge speed is commonly used to prepare the urine sample?
6. What volume of sample is centrifuged?
7. List the normal values for RBC, WBC, casts, and bacteria.
8. Explain the procedure for performing a microscopic examination of urine sediment.

STUDENT ACTIVITIES

1. Re-read the information on microscopic examination of urine sediment.
2. Practice performing a microscopic examination of one or more urine sediments as outlined on the Student Performance Guide using the worksheet.
3. Compare the results of the microscopic examination of urine with those obtained by fellow students or the instructor.
4. Draw three components which were observed in urine sediment. Is the presence of each normal or abnormal?

Student Performance Guide

NAME _____

DATE _____

LESSON 5–5
MICROSCOPIC EXAMINATION
OF URINE SEDIMENT

Instructions

1. Practice the procedure for preparing and examining urine sediment.
2. Demonstrate the procedure for preparing and examining urine sediment satisfactorily for the instructor. All steps must be completed as listed on the instructor's Performance Check Sheet.
3. Complete a written examination successfully.

Materials and Equipment

- gloves
- hand disinfectant
- fresh urine sample
- conical graduated centrifuge tubes
- centrifuge
- microscope
- glass slides
- coverglasses
- worksheet (urinalysis report form)
- surface disinfectant
- biohazard container
- disposable glass or plastic pipets
- puncture-proof container for sharp objects
- stopwatch or timer (if centrifuge lacks timer)

Procedure			S = Satisfactory U = Unsatisfactory
You must:	**S**	**U**	**Comments**
1. Wash hands with disinfectant and put on gloves			
2. Assemble equipment and materials			
3. Obtain a urine sample			
4. Pour 10 to 15 ml of well-mixed urine into a clean conical centrifuge tube			
5. Place filled tube in centrifuge, insert balance tube, and close lid (centrifuge must be balanced)			
6. Centrifuge at 1500 to 2000 rpm for five minutes			
7. Remove tube from centrifuge after rotor stops spinning			
8. Pour off supernatant urine, leaving approximately 0.5 ml of urine in tube			
9. Resuspend urine sediment by shaking the tube			
10. Place one drop of resuspended urine onto a clean glass slide			
11. Place coverslip over drop of urine			
12. Place slide on microscope stage and focus using low power (10×) and low light			
13. Scan ten to fifteen low power fields, count the number of casts per field, and record the average			
14. Identify the type(s) of casts present and record			
15. Rotate the high power objective (45×) into position			
16. Scan ten to fifteen fields on high power			
17. Count the number of RBC, WBC, and epithelial cells per high power field and record the average for each			
18. Observe the sample for the presence of microorganisms, crystals, or mucus and record if present. If crystals are present, identify type			
19. Complete the urinalysis report form			
20. Discard specimen appropriately			

You must:	S	U	Comments
21. Discard slide into puncture-proof container			
22. Clean and return equipment to proper storage			
23. Clean work area with surface disinfectant			
24. Remove and discard gloves appropriately			
25. Wash hands with hand disinfectant			
Comments:			
Student/Instructor:			

Date:_____   Instructor:_____

Worksheet

NAME_____ DATE _____

SPECIMEN NO. _____

LESSON 5–5 MICROSCOPIC EXAMINATION OF URINE

Microscopic Examination					Normal Values
WBCs:	_____/HPF				0-4
RBCs:	_____/HPF				rare
Epithelial cells:	_____/HPF				occasional (higher in females)
Casts:	_____/LPF				occasional, hyaline
Type:	_____				
Yeasts:	negative	1+ 2+ 3+ 4+			negative
Bacteria:	negative	1+ 2+ 3+ 4+			negative
Mucus:	negative	1+ 2+ 3+ 4+			negative–2+
Crystals:	_____ none seen_____ present				
Type:	_____				
Other:	_____				

UNIT 6
Introduction to Bacteriology

UNIT OBJECTIVES

After studying this unit, you should be able to:
- Identify three basic bacterial shapes and two Gram stain reactions.
- Prepare a bacterial smear.
- Perform a Gram stain.
- Transfer bacteria from one medium to another.
- Collect throat and urine specimens for bacterial culture.
- Perform a throat culture.
- Perform a rapid test for Group A *Streptococcus*.
- Perform a urine culture.

OVERVIEW

The main objective of bacteriological procedures is to identify the organisms responsible for illness so that the physician can properly treat the patient. These procedures may be performed in physicians' offices or in the microbiology department of the medical laboratory.

Identifying bacteria involves consideration of their morphology, their Gram stain reactions, and the results of certain biochemical reactions. The morphology and the Gram stain reaction of an organism can be disclosed by preparing a bacterial smear and performing a Gram stain. The procedures for performing these are presented in Lessons 6–1, 6–2, and 6–3.

To further identify the bacteria, laboratory personnel must grow the bacteria on appropriate growth media. The procedures for the actual collection of the specimens from the patient, the transfer to proper growth media, and the selection of media are presented in Lessons 6–4, 6–5, and 6–6.

Lesson 6–6 and Lesson 6–7 present information concerning three commonly performed procedures. The procedures for performing both a culture and a rapid test for Group A *Streptococcus* are described in Lesson 6–6. In Lesson 6–7 a method for performing a urine culture and a colony count is included.

Although the strains of organisms utilized in these lessons are not considered highly pathogenic, safety precautions are still of utmost importance. All bacterial specimens should be handled as though capable of causing disease. Principles of aseptic technique must always be observed. A laboratory coat should be worn while performing these procedures to prevent bacterial stains from being splashed on clothing. A laboratory coat also prevents contamination of the worker with the bacteria.

It is equally important that a good surface disinfectant be used to wipe benchtops before and after each laboratory session and anytime an accidental spill of culture material occurs. Washing the hands often with a hand disinfectant and before and after handling any specimens is also essential. A method of dealing with spills of bacterial cultures is included in Lesson 6–2.

LESSON 6-1

Identification of Stained Bacteria

LESSON OBJECTIVES

After studying this lesson, you should be able to:
- Explain the principle of the Gram stain.
- Identify gram-positive bacteria on a smear.
- Identify gram-negative bacteria on a smear.
- Identify the coccus form of bacteria.
- Identify the bacillus form of bacteria.
- Identify the spiral form of bacteria.
- Define the glossary terms.

GLOSSARY

bacillus (pl. bacilli) / a rod-shaped bacterium

bacteria / a group of one-celled microorganisms; germs

bacterial morphology / the form or structure of bacteria; color, shape and size

coccus (pl. cocci) / spherical or oval-shaped bacterium

colony / a circumscribed mass of bacteria growing in or upon a solid or semi-solid medium; assumed to have grown from a single organism

gram negative / refers to bacteria which are decolorized in the Gram stain; pink-red in color after being counterstained

gram positive / refers to bacteria which retain the crystal violet dye in the Gram stain; purple-blue in color

Gram stain / a stain which differentiates bacteria according to the chemical composition of their cell walls

spirochete / a slender, spiral microorganism

INTRODUCTION

Many diseases are caused by microorganisms known as **bacteria.** The three basic forms of bacteria are round (oval), rod-shaped, and spiral. The round or oval form is known as a **coccus** (Figure 6-1). Round bacteria which occur predominantly

345

in pairs are called *diplococci*. The rod-shaped form of bacteria is known as a **bacillus** (Figure 6–2) and the spiral one as a **spirochete** (Figure 6–3).

Most bacteria are very small and must be viewed using the oil immersion (100×) objective of the microscope. The sizes of bacteria are usually in the range of 0.1–2.0 micrometers in width and not more than five micrometers long.

Even bacteria which have color usually do not appear to be colored because they are so small. Only when many bacteria of one type are together in a colony is the color visible. A **colony** is a group of bacteria which grew from a single organism.

Since the small size of bacteria makes it difficult to see them with the microscope, stains are applied to the bacteria to make them more visible. The bacterial stain most often used is the Gram stain.

THE GRAM STAIN

The **Gram stain** is a procedure which stains bacteria differentially according to the composition of their cell walls. The Gram stain is performed on a thin smear of the organisms to be studied. The smear is passed through a Bunsen burner flame two or three times to fix the smear to the glass slide. Crystal violet, Gram's iodine, a decolorizer, and a safranin counterstain are then applied, in sequence, to the smear.

After the stain has dried, the smear is ready for microscopic observation. The slide is placed on the microscope stage and the stained area is found with the low power (10×) objective. A drop of immersion oil is placed on the smear and the oil immersion objective (100×) is used to view the organisms. The bacteria which retain the crystal violet and appear blue-purple are called **gram positive.** The bacteria which stain red-pink with safranin are called **gram negative.**

The Gram stain can be used to give the physician information which is helpful in diagnosing and treating infections. By staining the specimen taken directly from a wound, for example, the presence or absence of bacteria in the wound can be verified. If bacteria are present, the stain will identify them as gram negative or gram positive. This information can then be used to choose the proper nutrients on which to grow the bacteria for further study. The Gram stain also helps in the choice of antibiotic treatment since gram negatives and gram positives are, in general, susceptible to different antibiotics.

APPEARANCE OF STAINED BACTERIA

The round bacteria, the cocci, will appear similar to those shown in Figure 6–1. The most common

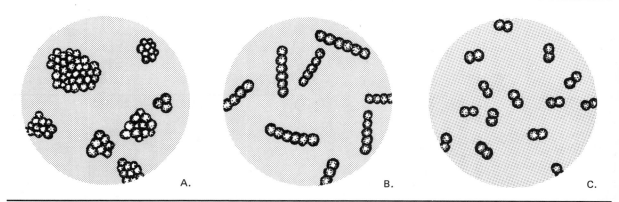

Figure 6–1. Microscopic appearance of round bacteria. A) round bacteria (cocci) in clusters, B) round bacteria (cocci) in chains, and C) diplococci

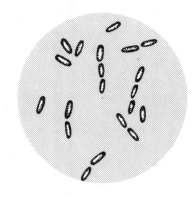

Figure 6–2. Microscopic appearance of rod-shaped bacteria

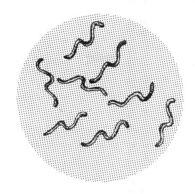

Figure 6–3. Microscopic appearance of spiral bacteria

cocci cultured from humans are *Staphylococcus* and *Streptococcus*. The *Staphylococcus* will appear singly or in grape-like clusters. Since *Staphylococci* are gram positive, they will stain dark blue (see Color Plate 25). *Streptococci* are also gram positive and appear either singly or in a bead-like chain. *Neisseria gonorrhoeae,* the causative agent of gonorrhea, is a diplococcus which is gram negative.

The rod-shaped bacteria may be either gram positive or gram negative. A common gram-negative rod is *Escherichia coli* which is found in the intestinal tract (Figure 6–2 and Color Plate 26).

The spiral forms of bacteria usually stain gram negatively and appear as twisted rods, having from less than one turn to many turns (Figure 6–3). One bacteria with a spiral form is *Campylobacter fetus,* which can cause a variety of serious conditions in humans.

The **bacterial morphology** observed with the microscope is essential information which is used to aid in identifying bacteria. However, other characteristics such as biochemical reactions, antibiotic susceptibility, and growth on certain media must also be utilized to make the final identification of the bacteria.

LESSON REVIEW

1. What is the principle of the Gram stain?
2. How are gram positives identified on a stained smear?
3. How are gram negatives identified on a stained smear?
4. The round bacteria are referred to by what other name?
5. The rod-shaped bacteria are known by what other name?
6. What is another name for the spiral bacteria?
7. Most bacteria are in what size range?
8. Define bacillus, bacteria, bacterial morphology, coccus, colony, gram negative, gram positive, Gram stain, and spirochete.

STUDENT ACTIVITIES

1. Re-read the information on the identification of stained bacteria.
2. Review the glossary terms.
3. Practice identifying the three morphological forms and two Gram stain reactions of bacteria as outlined on the Student Performance Guide.

Student Performance Guide

NAME _____

DATE _____

LESSON 6–1
IDENTIFICATION OF
STAINED BACTERIA

Instructions

1. Practice identifying the three forms of bacteria and their Gram stain reactions.
2. Demonstrate the identification of stained bacteria satisfactorily for the instructor. All steps must be completed as listed on the instructor's Performance Check Sheet.
3. Complete a written examination successfully.

Materials and Equipment

- hand disinfectant
- microscope
- immersion oil
- lens paper
- soft laboratory tissue
- prepared Gram-stained bacterial slides: coccus, bacillus, spirochete
- surface disinfectant

Procedure			S = Satisfactory U = Unsatisfactory
You must:	**S**	**U**	**Comments**
1. Wash hands with hand disinfectant			
2. Assemble equipment and materials			
3. Select one of the prepared slides and secure it on the microscope stage			
4. Locate a stained area of the smear using the low power (10×) objective			
5. Place a drop of immersion oil on the area to be viewed			
6. Rotate the oil immersion lens into place carefully			
7. Identify the type of bacteria (coccus, bacillus, spirochete) by shape			
8. Identify the Gram stain reaction by the color			
9. Repeat steps 3–8 until all three shapes have been identified and both Gram stain reactions have been observed			
10. Wipe the oil off the slides gently with laboratory tissue			
11. Clean equipment and return to proper storage			
12. Clean work area with disinfectant			
13. Wash hands with hand disinfectant			

Comments:

Student/Instructor:

Date:_____   Instructor:_____

LESSON 6–2

Preparation of a Bacteriological Smear

LESSON OBJECTIVES

After studying this lesson, you should be able to:
- Demonstrate aseptic technique.
- Prepare a smear directly from a swab.
- Prepare a smear of *Staphylococcus aureus* from tubed media.
- Prepare a smear of *Escherichia coli* from an agar plate.
- Heat-fix a bacteriological smear.
- List the precautions to be observed in the preparation of a bacteriological smear.
- Define the glossary terms.

GLOSSARY

aseptic techniques / techniques used to maintain sterility or to prevent contamination
culture / to cultivate bacteria in a nutrient medium; a mass of growing bacteria
flame / sterilization of certain materials used in bacteriology by heating or passing through a flame
inoculating loop / a nichrome or platinum wire fashioned into a loop on one end and having a handle on the other end; used to transfer bacterial growth
medium / a nutritive substance, either solid or liquid, in or upon which microorganisms are grown for study

INTRODUCTION

Preparing a bacteriological smear is a relatively simple process which can be performed quickly. The smear can be prepared directly from the specimen such as a throat swab, or from a colony of bacterial growth on a medium. Since the specimen contains live organisms, workers in the bacteriology laboratory must avoid contamination of themselves, the environment, and the specimen by using **aseptic techniques.** These techniques are guidelines to prevent contamination resulting from careless handling of bacteria.

ASEPTIC TECHNIQUES

Many procedures and safety rules fall under the category of aseptic techniques. Such procedures include 1) flaming the loop before and after each use, 2) flaming the mouths of tubes before and after entering the tube (after opening and before closing the tube), and 3) placing all contaminated objects in containers of disinfectant or biohazard containers until disposal. One good way of dealing with bacterial spills is to prepare the work area by placing paper towels on the counter and pouring surface disinfectant on the paper towels until just wet. If a spill occurs, it is easy to simply roll up the towels and discard them into a biohazard container. Safety rules that follow the principles of aseptic techniques include:

* wearing a laboratory coat or apron to protect the clothing from contamination
* keeping the work area clean with a surface disinfectant
* wiping up all spills promptly with disinfectant
* washing hands with hand disinfectant after every procedure
* disposing of all specimens and culture materials by incineration or autoclaving.

THE DIRECT SMEAR

The direct smear is prepared from the swab which was used to obtain the sample. Such a smear could be from a throat culture or wound culture. If the material is also to be transferred to a medium to grow, the slide used must be sterile and free of debris. This is to prevent the transfer of organisms on an unsterile slide onto the swab and consequently onto the medium when it is inoculated. The best procedure is to obtain two swabs.

To prepare the smear, the swab is gently rolled across the surface of the slide (Figure 6–4)

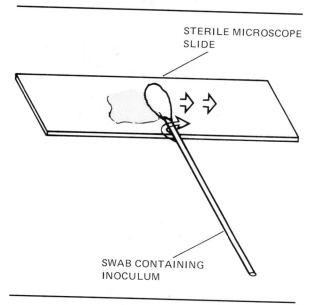

STERILE MICROSCOPE SLIDE

SWAB CONTAINING INOCULUM

Figure 6–4. Preparation of a direct smear from a swab

leaving a thin film of the culture material on the slide. When the film has completely air dried, it is ready to be heat-fixed. This is done by holding the slide by one end with a spring-type clothespin or forceps and passing the smear area through the Bunsen burner flame two or three times (Figure 6–5). When performed correctly, the slide will not be hot enough to burn the fingers. Heat-fixing is necessary to make the organism adhere to the slide throughout the staining process. If the smear is fixed before it is air dried or if it is exposed to extreme heat, the morphology of the organisms will be affected or the slide may break. After the slide has been heat-fixed, it is ready to be stained.

A SMEAR FROM BACTERIA GROWING ON MEDIA

It is also relatively simple to prepare a smear using organisms which are already growing on **media**. A medium (**media**) is a nutritive substance upon which bacteria are placed for growth. The organisms which grow can be referred to as a

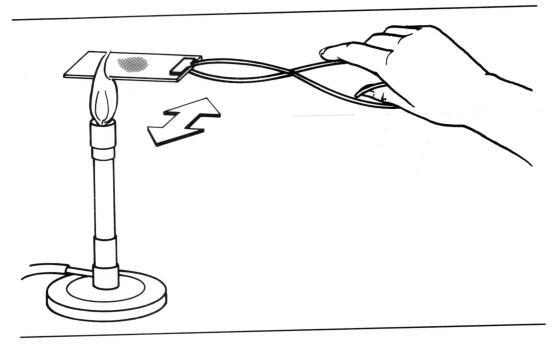

Figure 6–5. Heat-fixing a bacteriological smear

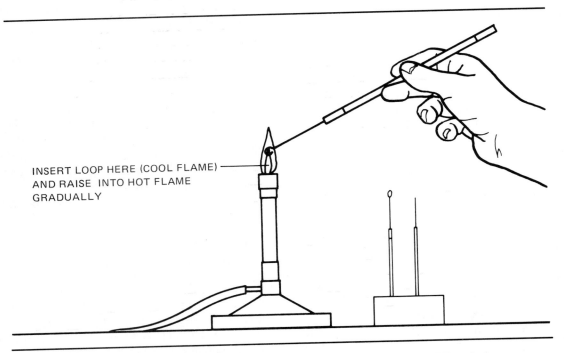

INSERT LOOP HERE (COOL FLAME)
AND RAISE INTO HOT FLAME
GRADUALLY

Figure 6–6. Sterilizing the inoculating loop

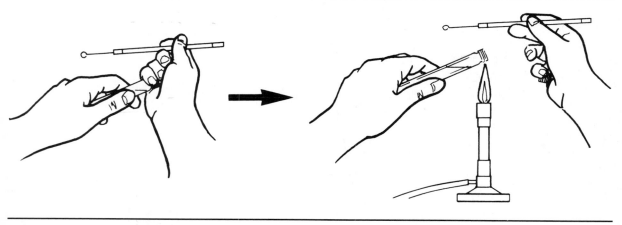

Figure 6–7. Flaming a culture tube

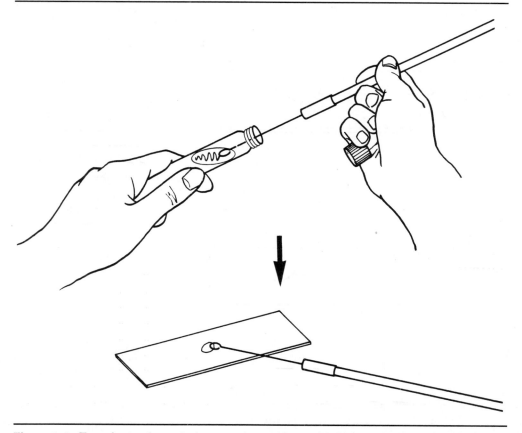

Figure 6–8. Transferring bacteria from a culture tube to a slide

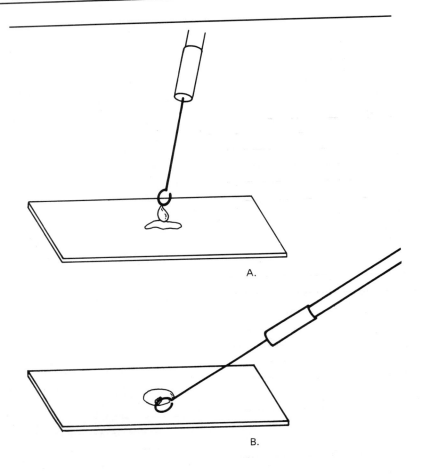

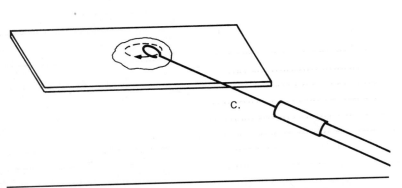

Figure 6–9. Making a bacterial smear using the inoculating loop

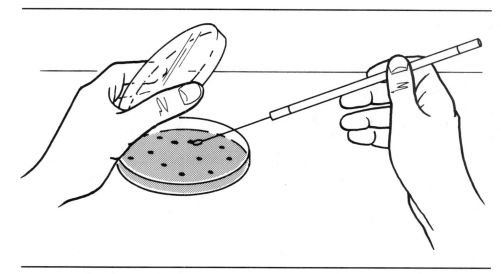

Figure 6–10. Removing bacteria from an agar plate using the inoculating loop

culture of bacteria. If the bacterial culture is contained on tube media, the principles of aseptic technique must be followed. Using aseptic techniques helps to avoid introducing contaminants into the tube or allowing the organisms to escape from the tube into the environment.

In order to remove a portion of the bacterial growth, the tube should be held in the left hand and the **inoculating loop** in the right hand. The loop is sterilized by heating in the Bunsen burner flame until red hot (Figure 6–6, page 352). Spattering of the culture material can be avoided by gradually placing the loop into the cool part of the flame and then into the hot part. The loop is allowed to cool briefly and the cap is removed from the tube using the fourth and fifth fingers of the right hand. Immediately the mouth of the tube is **flamed** by passing it briefly through the burner flame (Figure 6–7, page 353). The cooled loop is then used to remove a pin-point sized portion of the growth and place it onto a glass slide which has already had one loopful of water placed on the surface (Figure 6–8, page 353). The water and the bacteria are mixed together and spread out to an area approximately the size of a nickel (Figure 6–9). The mouth of the tube is again flamed briefly, the cap is replaced on the tube, and the tube is placed into a test tube rack. The inoculating loop is flamed again and replaced in its special holder. The slide is allowed to dry and then is heat-fixed. A smear which is of proper thickness will be almost invisible when completely dried.

The procedure used to make a smear from organisms growing on a medium in a petri dish is similar. However, the petri dish is not flamed; the lid is lifted just enough to allow the entrance of the cooled sterilized loop (Figure 6–10). The smear is then prepared as explained above.

Precautions

■ The Bunsen burner must be situated so that laboratory supplies, hair, or articles of clothing will not catch fire.
■ The prepared smear must be very thin; if it is too thick it will not stain or decolorize properly.
■ After sterilization, the inoculating loop must be cooled in the air briefly before it is touched to the organisms.
■ The inoculating loop should be held only by the handle, and must be replaced in its special holder when not in use.

■ The inoculating loop must always be sterilized after transfer of bacteria and before it is stored in its holder.

■ For the greatest margin of safety, all organisms must be handled as if they are capable of causing disease.

■ To avoid morphological changes in the organisms or breakage of the slide, the smear must be completely dry before heat-fixing.

■ Wash hands with hand disinfectant before and after handling any specimen.

LESSON REVIEW

1. Discuss aseptic technique.
2. Explain why the glass slide used for a bacterial smear must be sterile if a culture and a smear are to be prepared from one swab.

3. Explain the differences in the procedures for transferring organisms from a tube and from a petri dish.
4. Why must the smear be completely dry before it is heat-fixed?
5. List precautions which should be observed when preparing a bacterial smear.
6. Why is it necessary to wear a laboratory apron or coat when working with bacterial cultures?
7. Define aseptic techniques, culture, flame, inoculating loop and medium.

STUDENT ACTIVITIES

1. Re-read the information on the preparation of a bacterial smear.
2. Review the glossary terms.
3. Practice the procedure for preparing bacteriological smears as outlined on the Student Performance Guide.

Student Performance Guide

NAME _____

DATE _____

LESSON 6–2
PREPARATION OF A
BACTERIOLOGICAL SMEAR

Instructions

1. Practice preparing bacteriological smears using organisms on swabs and organisms growing on tube media and in petri dishes.
2. Demonstrate the procedure for preparing bacteriological smears from the three sources satisfactorily for the instructor. All steps must be completed as listed on the instructor's Performance Check Sheet.
3. Complete a written examination successfully.

Materials and Equipment

- hand disinfectant
- educational strain (less pathogenic strain used specifically for teaching, available through catalogs) of *Escherichia coli* growing in a culture tube or petri dish
- educational strain of *Staphylococcus aureus* growing in a culture tube or petri dish
- microscope slides
- inoculating needle or loop
- diamond or carbide-tip etching pencil
- Bunsen burner or electric loop sterilizer
- holder for inoculating loop
- container of water
- test tube rack
- matches or flint-type lighter
- forceps, or spring-type clothespins
- swabs inoculated with organisms and stored in sterile, capped tubes
- surface disinfectant
- biohazard container
- puncture-proof container for sharp objects
- paper towels

Procedure			S = Satisfactory U = Unsatisfactory
You must:	**S**	**U**	**Comments**
1. Wash hands with hand disinfectant			
2. Assemble equipment and materials			
3. Prepare work area: place paper towels on counter; pour surface disinfectant onto them until just wet			
4. Light a Bunsen burner and place it in a safe, accessible area			

5. Prepare one smear from each source listed below:
  A. From a swab:
    (1) Obtain a microscope slide and a swab which has been inoculated with organisms
    (2) Remove the swab from its container being careful not to touch the tip
    (3) Touch the swab to the surface of the slide and apply a film of culture material to the slide by gently rolling the swab on the surface. The size of the area should be a circle approximately ¾ in.–1 in. diameter
    (4) Return the swab to its container
    (5) Allow the smear to air dry completely
    (6) Hold the end of the slide with a clothespin or forceps and pass the smear quickly through the Bunsen flame two to three times to heat-fix. Do not heat the slide excessively; the slide should not be hot enough to burn the fingers when touched
    (7) Allow the slide to cool
    (8) Label the slide using a diamond or carbide-tip etching pencil
    (9) Keep the slide for staining in Lesson 6–3
  B. From the tubed medium:
    (1) Obtain a microscope slide and culture of *Escherichia coli* growing in a culture tube
    (2) hold the culture tube in the left hand and the inoculating loop in the right hand
    (3) Flame the inoculating needle or loop until red hot and cool briefly in the air
    (4) Use the loop to transfer one drop of water to the center of the slide
    (5) Flame the loop again
    (6) Remove the cap from the tube with the little finger of the right hand and flame the mouth of the tube			

You must:	S	U	Comments
(7) Transfer a portion of the bacterial growth to the slide			
(8) Flame tube briefly, replace the cap on the tube and set the tube in the test tube rack			
(9) Mix the water and bacterial material together using the loop and spread out to an area approximately the size of a nickel			
(10) Sterilize the loop and replace it into the holder. *Note:* Avoid spattering the culture material			
(11) Allow the smear to air dry and then heat-fix as in steps A (6) to A (9) above			
C. From a petri dish:			
(1) Obtain a microscope slide and a petri dish culture of *Staphylococcus aureus*			
(2) Flame the inoculating loop or needle until red hot and allow to air cool briefly			
(3) Transfer one drop of water to the center of a glass slide			
(4) Flame the loop again			
(5) Lift the lid of the petri dish just enough to allow entrance of the inoculating loop or needle			
(6) Touch the sterile loop to a bacterial colony and transfer a portion of the colony to the water on the glass side			
(7) Close the petri dish			
(8) Use the loop to mix the bacteria and water together and spread them into an area about the size of a nickel			
(9) Sterilize the loop and place in holder. *Note:* Avoid spattering the culture material			
(10) Allow the smear to dry and heat-fix the slide as in steps A (6) to A (9)			
6. Turn off the Bunsen burner			
7. Store slides for staining			
8. Return materials to proper storage			
9. Clean and return equipment to proper storage			
10. Roll up paper towels and discard appropriately			
11. Clean work area with surface disinfectant			

You must:	S	U	Comments
12. Wash hands with hand disinfectant			

Comments:

Student/Instructor:

Date:_____ Instructor:_____

LESSON 6–3
The Gram Stain

LESSON OBJECTIVES

After studying this lesson, you should be able to:
- Perform the Gram stain procedure.
- Observe gram-positive cocci on the *Staphylococcus aureus* smear.
- Observe gram-negative rods on the *Escherichia coli* smear.
- List precautions to be observed when performing the Gram stain.
- Define the glossary terms.

GLOSSARY

bibulous paper / a special absorbent paper which is used to dry slides
counterstain / a dye which adds a contrasting color
mordant / a substance which fixes a dye or stain to an object

---

NTRODUCTION

he Gram stain is a procedure which is performed
outinely in bacteriology laboratories. Most bacte-
ial cells are so small and possess so little color that
hey are difficult to observe microscopically unless
 stain is applied. The Gram stain is the most
ommon staining technique used for bacteria. The
ram stain is performed on a bacteriological smear
vhich has been previously heat-fixed and allowed
o cool.

The staining procedure consists of applying a
equence of dye, mordant, decolorizer, and
ounterstain to a bacterial smear. The counter-
tain adds a contrasting color. The dyes are taken
ıp differentially according to the chemical compo-
ition of the cell walls of the organisms present.

PERFORMING THE GRAM STAIN

The heat-fixed bacteriological smear should be
supported over a pan, beaker, or sink during the
staining procedure. The support may be provided
by parallel metal or glass rods (Figure 6–11).
However, there are also various staining racks
manufactured and these should be used if available.

To perform the Gram stain, the smear is placed
on the supporting rods and a dye called crystal
violet is poured onto the slide (Figure 6–11). After
the manufacturer's recommended time has passed
(usually one minute), the slide is rinsed by gently
pouring tap water onto it. Gram's iodine, which is
a mordant, is then added to the slide. A **mordant** is
a substance which causes a dye to adhere to the
object being stained. When the Gram's iodine has

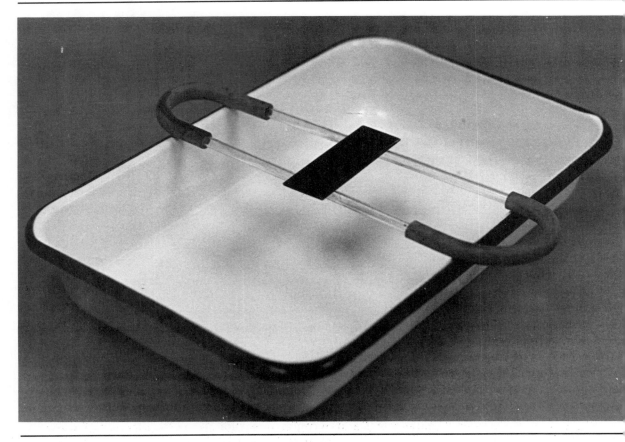

Figure 6–11. Slide staining rack *(Photo by John Estridge)*

been on the slide for the required time (usually one minute), the slide is again rinsed with water. A decolorizer, such as alcohol, is added to the slide briefly (three to five seconds) or until no more purple runs off the smear. The slide is again rinsed with water.

At this point in the staining process the gram-positive organisms will be purple-blue because their cell wall composition allows retention of the dye (Table 6–1). The gram-negative organisms will appear colorless because their cell-wall composition allows removal of the dye along with some of the cell wall constituents (Table 6–1). Prolonged decolorization can remove the dye even from the gram-positive cells. After the decolorizing procedure is finished, the slide is flooded with a

red dye called safranin for approximately one minute. The safranin, which is a counterstain, will have no effect on the gram-positive cells but the now colorless gram-negative cells will be stained red-pink (Table 6–1). The slides are washed by pouring distilled water on them and blotting gently with a special absorbent paper called **bibulous paper**. When the slides are completely dry, they are ready to be observed microscopically.

OBSERVING THE STAINED BACTERIOLOGICAL SMEAR

The stained smear should be observed using the oil immersion (100×) objective after the stained area has been located using the low power (10×

Table 6–1. Steps of Gram stain procedure

	Procedure	Result
STEP 1	Primary stain: Apply crystal violet stain (purple) ↓ Rinse slide	All bacteria stain purple
STEP 2	Mordant: Apply Gram's iodine ↓ Rinse slide	All bacteria remain purple
STEP 3	Decolorize: Apply alcohol ↓ Rinse slide	Purple stain is removed from gram-negative cells
STEP 4	Counterstain: Apply safranin stain (red) ↓ Rinse slide and dry	Gram-negative cells appear pink-red; gram-positive cells appear purple

objective. Gram-negative organisms will appear pink-red and gram-positive organisms will appear blue-purple. *Staphylococcus aureus* is a gram-positive coccus and *Escherichia coli* is a gram-negative bacillus.

■ Decolorization, in particular, should be performed with care to avoid false gram negatives.

Precautions

■ The staining apparatus should be arranged so that the stains will not spill onto countertops.
■ A lab coat or apron should be worn to prevent splashing of stain onto clothing.
■ The manufacturer's directions for the staining procedure must be followed carefully; the times may be different for each lot of reagents.

LESSON REVIEW

1. Explain how to perform a Gram stain.
2. What is the appearance of the gram-positive cocci on the *Staphylococcus aureus* smear?
3. Describe the appearance of the *Escherichia coli* smear.
4. List precautions to be observed when performing the Gram stain.
5. What is the purpose of the Gram's iodine?

6. What is the purpose of the decolorizer?
7. Which bacteria are stained by the safranin?
8. What paper is used to dry the slides more quickly?
9. Define bibulous paper, counterstain, and mordant.

STUDENT ACTIVITIES

1. Re-read the information on the Gram stain.
2. Review the glossary terms.
3. Practice performing the Gram stain as outlined on the Student Performance Guide.

Student Performance Guide

NAME _____

DATE _____

LESSON 6–3
THE GRAM STAIN

Instructions

1. Practice performing the Gram stain procedure using smears of a gram-negative and gram-positive culture (or smears prepared in Lesson 6–2).
2. Demonstrate the procedure for the Gram stain satisfactorily for the instructor. All steps must be completed as listed on the instructor's Performance Check Sheet.
3. Complete a written examination successfully.

Materials and Equipment

- hand disinfectant
- Gram stain kit or individual Gram stain reagents (in plastic squeeze bottles)
- unstained heat-fixed smears of gram-positive cocci (*Staphylococcus aureus*) or smears prepared in Lesson 6–2
- unstained heat-fixed smears of gram-negative rods (*Escherichia coli*) or smears prepared in Lesson 6–2
- staining rack
- forceps or spring-type wooden clothespins
- Pasteur pipet with rubber bulb
- paper towels or soft laboratory tissue
- bibulous paper
- microscope
- immersion oil
- lens paper
- surface disinfectant
- biohazard container

Note: Follow manufacturer's instructions for specific staining times.

Procedure			S = Satisfactory U = Unsatisfactory
You must:	**S**	**U**	**Comments**
1. Wash hands with hand disinfectant			
2. Assemble equipment and materials			
3. Place smear of gram-positive cocci on the staining rack with smear side up			
4. Flood the slide with crystal violet for the manufacturer's recommended time (approximately one minute)			
5. Rinse the stain off the slide by pouring water gently from a beaker, a small diameter laboratory hose, or a plastic squeeze bottle			
6. Tilt the slide to remove excess water			
7. Flood the slide with Gram's iodine			
8. Leave the Gram's iodine on the slide for the recommended time (one minute)			
9. Rinse the slide gently with water			
10. Tilt the slide to remove excess water			
11. Add 95% ethyl alcohol decolorizer by the drop onto the slide using a Pasteur pipet with bulb or plastic squeeze bottle			
12. Tilt the slide immediately; a purple color should run off the slide			
13. Decolorize quickly two to three times (steps 11–12) or until no purple color runs off the slide. *Note:* Do not decolorize longer than three to five seconds or gram positives will appear gram negative			
14. Rinse the slide immediately with a gentle stream of tap water to remove the decolorizer			
15. Counterstain the smear by adding the safranin dye for the recommended time (one minute)			
16. Rinse the slide gently with tap water			
17. Tilt the slide to remove excess water			

You must:	S	U	Comments
18. Wipe the back of the slide with paper towel or soft tissue to remove water and dye			
19. Place the smear between two sheets of bibulous paper and gently blot dry, or allow slide to air dry by standing the slide on end			
20. Place the dry smear on the microscope stage			
21. Use the low power (10×) objective to locate the stained area			
22. Place a drop of immersion oil on the stained area			
23. Rotate the oil immersion objective into place carefully			
24. Observe that the *Staphylococcus* organisms are gram-positive cocci and are arranged in clusters			
25. Rotate low power objective into position			
26. Remove slide			
27. Repeat steps 3–23 using the smear of gram-negative rods			
28. Observe that the *Escherichia coli* are gram-negative rods			
29. Rotate low power objective into place			
30. Remove slide			
31. Clean oil immersion objective and condenser thoroughly			
32. Return equipment to proper storage			
33. Wipe oil off slides gently and store or discard into puncture-proof container			
34. Clean work area with surface disinfectant			
35. Wash hands with hand disinfectant			

Comments:

Student/Instructor:

Date:_____   Instructor:_____

LESSON 6–4
Inoculation of Media

LESSON OBJECTIVES

After studying this lesson, you should be able to:
- Transfer bacteria from one medium to another.
- Streak an agar plate and an agar slant.
- Inoculate broth medium.
- Utilize aseptic technique during the transfer of bacteria.
- List the precautions to be observed in culture transfer.
- Define the glossary terms.

GLOSSARY

aerosol / a suspension of fine solid or liqud particles in the air

agar plate / agar medium dispensed into sterile petri dishes and allowed to solidify

agar slant / agar medium dispensed into tubes and allowed to solidify at an angle

broth / liquid nutrient medium in tubes

incubator / temperature-controlled chamber into which inoculated media is placed so that bacterial growth will occur

inoculation / the introduction of organisms into media

inoculum / the portion of culture organisms which is being introduced into a medium

quadrant / one fourth; one quarter of an agar plate

INTRODUCTION

The transfer of culture material from one medium or source to another medium is **inoculation.** The medium used may be solid or liquid and may be in either a culture tube or a petri dish. Aseptic techniques must be strictly observed to insure safety and to avoid contamination of the culture by unwanted bacteria.

INOCULATION OF A TUBE OF BROTH MEDIUM

At times it may be necessary to inoculate a tube broth medium. The organisms may be transferr from an **agar slant** or other source into the **bro** A broth is a liquid medium; an agar slant conta agar, so it solidifies. If an agar slant is used, t procedure can be performed by holding bo

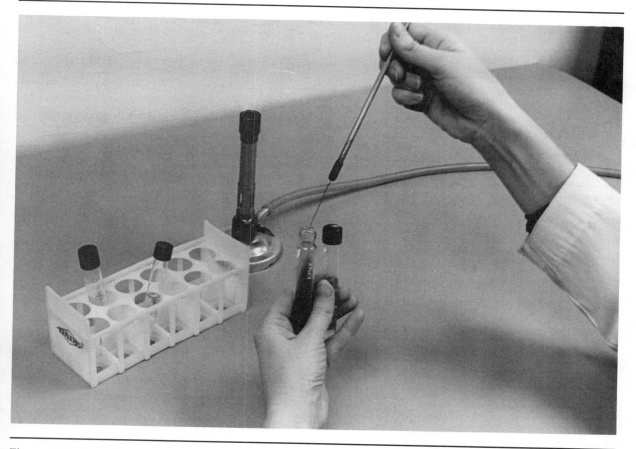

Figure 6–12. Transferring organisms from agar slant to broth *(Photo by John Estridge)*

tubes in the left hand and the inoculating loop in the right (Figure 6–12). The loop should be flamed. The cap can then be removed from the agar tube, using the fourth and fifth fingers of the right hand (which is still holding the loop). The mouth of the tube is briefly flamed and a portion of culture picked up on the flamed and cooled loop. The loop is withdrawn, the mouth of the tube is briefly flamed, and the cap is replaced on the agar tube. The cap is then removed from the second tube (broth), the mouth of the tube is flamed briefly, and the loop is immersed into the broth, agitated several times to disperse the **inoculum,** the portion of culture being transferred (Figure 6–13). The loop is withdrawn, the mouth of the tube is flamed, and the cap is replaced on the broth tube. The loop is

then flamed and replaced into its holder. The broth tube, with cap slightly loosened, is placed in a test tube rack in the **incubator** set at 37°C and left overnight or for 18 to 24 hours.

This method prevents the loop or the caps from being laid on the countertop and thus prevents contamination. If these procedures are performed carelessly, the surroundings and/or personnel may become contaminated. One way contamination may occur is through the formation of aerosols. **Aerosols** are formed when a broth is shaken, a loop spatters in the flame, or something happens which causes the organisms to become airborne.

A broth can also be inoculated by using a swab. The swab which contains the inoculum is

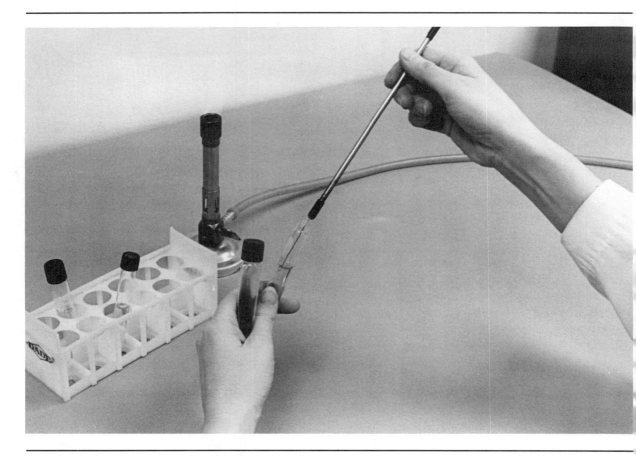

Figure 6–13. Inoculation of broth *(Photo by John Estridge)*

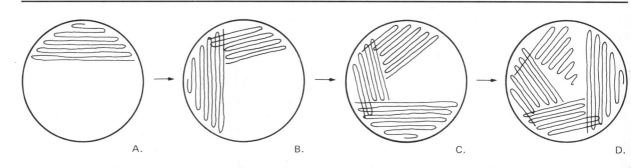

Figure 6–14. Streaking an agar plate in four quadrants

inserted into the broth and agitated to disperse the culture material. The tip is then pressed against the inner surface of the tube to express any remaining material. The swab is then withdrawn from the tube. The tube is then flamed and capped as in the procedure utilizing the loop. The swab should be placed in a biohazard container to be autoclaved or incinerated.

INOCULATION OF AN AGAR PLATE

The transfer of organisms from an agar slant onto an **agar plate** is performed in a similar manner. The tube is held in the left hand, the loop in the right hand, and the cap of the tube is removed with the fingers of the right hand. The loop and the mouth of the tube are then flamed. When the organisms have been removed from the tube with the loop, the mouth of the tube is flamed, and the cap is replaced. The tube is set in the test tube rack. The left hand is then free to lift the lid on the agar plate (petri dish). To avoid contamination or formation of aerosols, the lid is lifted only about two and one-half inches—just enough to allow entrance of the loop. The inoculum is spread with the loop by streaking it across a **quadrant** (one quarter) of the agar surface (Figure 6–14). The loop is then flamed and cooled. The petri dish is turned one quarter turn and the inoculum is spread into the second quadrant with the loop crossing the first quadrant two or three times. The loop is again flamed and cooled, and the inoculum is spread into the third quadrant by entering the second quadrant with the loop two or three times (Figure 6–14). When streaking the organism from the third quadrant into the fourth, the loop should enter the previously streaked third quadrant only two or three times.

Because the loop is flamed between the streaking of each quadrant, the number of organisms introduced into each quadrant is fewer than the number in the one before. When a plate is streaked in this manner, the final quadrant should contain only a few organisms. This technique is called streaking for isolated colonies and is illustrated in Figure 6–14.

After streaking, the plate is labeled on the bottom. It is then placed overnight (18 to 24 hours) in the incubator set at 37°C to allow for growth of the organisms. Agar plates are incubated upside down to prevent condensate (which forms on the lid) from dropping onto the agar surface. If the plate was streaked properly, quadrant four should contain only a few isolated colonies of the organism after the overnight incubation period.

INOCULATION OF AN AGAR SLANT

Organisms may also be transferred onto an agar slant in a culture tube to allow growth. Aseptic techniques are used, including flaming the mouth of the tube and the loop. When the cap has been removed, the inoculum can be introduced into the tube by a swab or loop. A swab can be used in the same manner as a loop with the inoculum being spread in a zig-zag manner from the far end of the slant toward the opening of the tube. Alternately, the swab may be used to introduce the inoculum onto the slant and the loop is then used to spread the inoculum (Figure 6–15). The mouth of the tube is again flamed briefly and the cap is replaced on the tube. The loop is flamed, cooled, and replaced in its holder. The slant tube, with cap slightly loosened, is then placed in a test tube rack in the 37°C incubator overnight.

Each laboratory will have its particular way of performing these basic procedures. However, every method must contain good aseptic techniques. If aseptic measures are not followed, bacteria in the air or even from the skin will be introduced and will grow along with the inoculum. Perfection of the streaking method will result in scattered, isolated, pure colonies of bacteria which can be picked up and transferred for further studies.

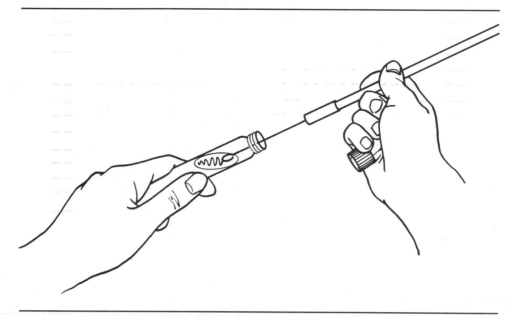

Figure 6–15. Inoculation of an agar slant

Precautions

■ Aseptic techniques must be observed at all times.

■ The loop should be checked periodically to be sure it has a smooth surface. A misshaped loop may tear the agar surface when streaking the inoculum.

■ The loop must be cooled after flaming; a hot loop will kill the organisms, damage agar surfaces, and cause aerosols to form.

■ The loop must be replaced into its special holder between uses.

LESSON REVIEW

1. What is an inoculum?
2. What is an aerosol?
3. How can aerosol formation be avoided?

4. How is an agar plate streaked to produce isolated colonies?
5. Why are isolated colonies needed?
6. How is the number of organisms reduced from quadrant to quadrant?
7. What kind of pattern is used to inoculate an agar slant?
8. Why is aseptic technique important?
9. Explain the procedure for transferring organisms from a culture tube onto a plate.
10. Define aerosol, agar plate, agar slant, broth, incubator, inoculation, inoculum, and quadrant.

STUDENT ACTIVITIES

1. Re-read the information on the inoculation of media.
2. Review the glossary terms.
3. Practice the procedures for transferring organisms to broths, agar slants, and petri dishes as outlined on the Student Performance Guide.

Student Performance Guide

NAME _____

DATE _____

LESSON 6–4
INOCULATION OF MEDIA

Instructions

1. Practice inoculating broth, agar slant, and petri dish media.
2. Demonstrate the procedure for inoculating broth, agar, and petri dish media satisfactorily for the instructor. All steps must be completed as listed on the instructor's Performance Check Sheet.
3. Complete a written examination successfully.

Materials and Equipment

- hand disinfectant
- inoculating loop or needle
- Bunsen burner or electric loop sterilizer
- matches or flint-type lighter
- agar slants (tryptose or comparable agar)
- agar plates (tryptose or comparable agar)
- broth tubes (tryptose or comparable)
- sterile swabs
- educational strains of *Staphylococcus aureus* or *Escherichia coli* growing on tubed media
- test tube racks
- incubator (37°C)
- surface disinfectant
- biohazard container
- paper towels

Procedure			S = Satisfactory U = Unsatisfactory
You must:	**S**	**U**	**Comments**
1. Wash hands with hand disinfectant			
2. Assemble equipment and materials			
3. Prepare work area: place paper towels on counter; pour surface disinfectant onto them until just wet			
4. Light the Bunsen burner			

You must:	S	U	Comments
5. Select the culture to be transferred			
6. Select a tube of broth, an agar slant, and an agar plate to be inoculated			
7. Label each appropriately with the following: name of culture used, your name, and the date. Agar plates are always labeled on the bottom of the petri dish			
8. Inoculate the agar slant: a. Hold the tube containing the bacterial culture and the agar slant tube in the left hand			
b. Hold the inoculating loop in the right hand similar to a pencil			
c. Flame the loop and cool it			
d. Remove the cap from the tube containing the bacterial growth with the fifth finger of the right hand			
e. Flame the mouth of the open tube briefly			
f. Remove a portion of the bacterial growth with the loop (try to get a part of an isolated colony)			
g. Withdraw the loop from the tube, flame the mouth, replace the cap. Limit the movement of the loop through the air to avoid aerosols			
h. Remove the cap from the tube containing the agar slant and flame the mouth			
i. Inoculate the slant, starting at the far end of the slant and continuing in a zigzag motion toward the mouth of the tube			
j. Withdraw the loop, flame it, and replace it in its holder. *Note:* Avoid spattering the culture material			
k. Flame the mouth of the tube and replace the cap on the tube (do not tighten)			
l. Place the slant in a test tube rack			
9. Inoculate the broth: a. Repeat steps 8 a through 8 g, substituting the broth in place of the agar slant. Observe aseptic technique			
b. Remove the cap from the broth tube			
c. Insert the loop containing the bacterial growth beneath the surface of the broth and agitate to disperse the organisms throughout the broth			
d. Withdraw the loop, flame it, and replace it in holder. *Note:* Avoid spattering culture material			

You must:	S	U	Comments
e. Flame the mouth of the tube briefly and replace the cap on the broth tube (do not tighten)			
f. Place broth in a test tube rack			
10. Inoculate the agar plate:			
a. Place the petri dish containing the agar plate on the counter			
b. Hold the tube containing the bacterial growth in the left hand and the inoculating loop in the right hand			
c. Flame the loop and allow to cool			
d. Remove the cap from the tube, briefly flame the mouth of the tube, and use the loop to obtain a portion of a colony of the bacterial culture			
e. Withdraw the loop, flame the mouth of the tube, replace the cap onto the tube, and place tube in test tube rack			
f. Open the petri dish lid with the left hand just enough (two and one-half inches) to allow the entrance of the loop			
g. Streak one quadrant by spreading the organisms, making six to eight streaks			
h. Flame the loop and cool it			
i. Turn the petri dish one quarter turn			
j. Streak the second quadrant making six to eight streaks, entering the previously streaked quadrant two to three times			
k. Repeat steps i–j for the third quadrant			
l. Begin the streaks in the fourth quadrant as in the other quadrants; continue making the streaks, decreasing the width and increasing the distance between the streaks to form a "tornado-like" pattern			
11. Turn off the Bunsen burner. *Note:* Never leave lighted burner unattended			
12. Place the broth and slant tubes into a test tube rack in a 37°C incubator (leave caps slightly loosened). Place the agar plate upside down in the 37°C incubator			
13. Clean equipment and return to proper storage			
14. Clean work area with surface disinfectant			
15. Wash hands with hand disinfectant			

You must:	S	U	Comments
16. Check the broth, slant, and agar plate for bacterial growth after overnight incubation. The broth should be cloudy, indicating growth of organisms. The slant should have a zigzag formation of bacterial growth on the surface. The agar plate should have bacteria growing in all four quadrants with some isolated colonies in the third and fourth quadrants. (On solid media, growth should appear only along streak lines.)			

Comments:

Student/Instructor:

Date:_____ Instructor:_____

LESSON 6–5

Collection and Handling of Bacteriological Specimens

LESSON OBJECTIVES

After studying this lesson, you should be able to:
- List the most frequently cultured sites.
- Collect a throat culture.
- Instruct a patient to collect a urine specimen for bacterial culture.
- Define the glossary terms.

GLOSSARY

flora / organisms adapted for living in a specific environment

transport medium / a medium into which a specimen is placed to preserve it during transport to the laboratory

INTRODUCTION

The correct collection and handling of the specimens to be used in the various bacteriological procedures is absolutely essential if the results are to be of any value in diagnosis and treatment. Improper collection may result in not obtaining the organisms responsible for the illness. An improperly handled specimen may become contaminated or may contaminate the environment. If a sample is not processed properly the organisms collected may die before they can be transferred to growth media. A variety of disposable, sterile supplies and containers are available to meet most specimen collection and transport requirements (Figure 6–16).

MOST FREQUENTLY CULTURED SITES

Two of the most frequently cultured sites are the throat and the genito-urinary tract. The next most frequently performed cultures are of wounds, sputum, and cultures of suspected fungal infections.

Cultures of the throat are collected by using a cotton or polyester-tipped swab. Polyester swabs are preferred since some interfering substances on the cotton fibers may inhibit or kill certain organisms. The urinary tract can be tested for the presence of disease-causing organisms by sampling a clean-catch urine. The procedure for collecting samples from wounds or fungal infections

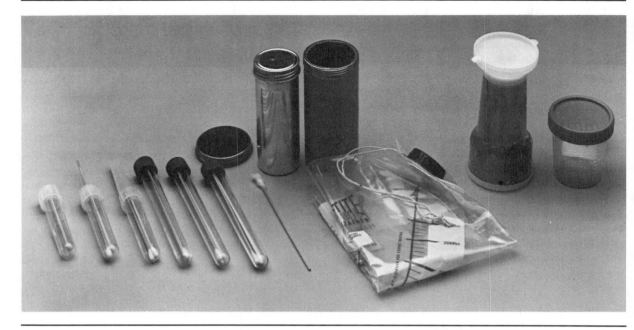

Figure 6–16. Examples of supplies for collection and transport of bacteriological specimens *(Photo courtesy of Becton Dickinson & Co.)*

depends on the particular situation and will not be covered in this lesson.

COLLECTING A THROAT CULTURE

Throat cultures are collected by gently swabbing the back of the throat and the surfaces of the tonsils with a sterile swab. The mouth or tongue surfaces should not be touched. This will prevent contaminating the swab with the normal **flora** of the mouth. The procedure can be accomplished more easily if the patient's tongue is depressed and he/she makes the sound of "ah."

The throat is most often cultured when the physician suspects that the patient has a "strep throat." This disease is caused by organisms called *Streptococci*. The most important group of these is called Group A *Streptococci*. It is essential to identify these organisms if present in the throat and to start antibiotic treatment. Left untreated, this infection can have serious complications such as

rheumatic fever, rheumatic endocarditis, or glomerulonephritis.

PERFORMING A URINE CULTURE

Urine samples for culture must be collected by the clean-catch method (Lesson 5–1) directly into sterile containers. Urine cultures are performed whenever the patient reports symptoms which indicate infection somewhere in the urinary tract. The organism which is most commonly isolated from urine is *Escherichia coli*.

HANDLING THE SPECIMEN AFTER COLLECTION

After the urine sample has been collected into a sterile container, it should have a proper label attached and then be promptly transported to the lab. It should be processed within one to two hours but may be refrigerated if necessary. No

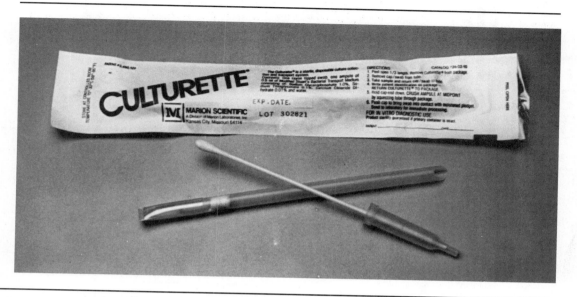

Figure 6–17. Culturette® system for collection and transport of bacteriological specimens *(Photo courtesy of Marion Laboratories, Inc., Marion Scientific Division)*

preservatives should be added since most are toxic to bacteria.

The material on the swab from the throat should be inoculated immediately onto the proper medium. However, that is not always possible and several devices have been marketed which can be used to transport samples to the laboratory. One system widely used is the Culturette® (Figure 6–17). It is a sterile swab in a plastic tube which contains an ampule of modified Stuart's **transport medium** to preserve the organism during transport to the laboratory.

Precautions

■ Materials for laboratory culture should be transported to the laboratory and transferred to growth media as soon as possible.
■ Correct collection procedures must be followed to avoid loss of the organism responsible for the illness.
■ Aseptic techniques must be observed to prevent introduction of a contaminating organism into the culture.

LESSON REVIEW

1. Why is it important to process the bacteriological specimens promptly?
2. What are the most frequently cultured sites?
3. When performing a throat culture, why is it important not to swab the mouth and tongue?
4. What is the usual reason for performing a throat culture?
5. What group of bacteria is usually looked for in a throat culture?
6. What is the organism most commonly isolated from urines?
7. When is the urine culture requested?
8. Define flora and transport medium.

STUDENT ACTIVITIES

1. Re-read the information on the collection and handling of bacteriological specimens.
2. Review the glossary terms.
3. Practice the procedure for the collection and handling of bacteriological specimens as outlined on the Student Performance Guide.

Student Performance Guide

NAME _____

DATE _____

LESSON 6–5
COLLECTION AND HANDLING OF BACTERIOLOGICAL SPECIMENS

Instructions

1. Practice the procedure for the collection and handling of throat and urine specimens.
2. Demonstrate the procedure for collection and handling of the urine and throat specimens satisfactorily for the instructor. All steps must be completed as listed on the instructor's Performance Check Sheet.
3. Complete a written examination successfully.

Materials and Equipment

- gloves
- hand disinfectant
- sterile swabs (or Culturettes®, if available)
- sterile culture tubes with caps (for transporting swabs)
- sterile urine containers
- materials for clean-catch urine collection
- tongue depressors
- labels
- pen, pencil
- surface disinfectant
- biohazard container

Procedure			S = Satisfactory U = Unsatisfactory
You must:	**S**	**U**	**Comments**
1. Wash hands with hand disinfectant and put on gloves			
2. Assemble equipment and materials			

3. Collect a throat culture
   a. Explain the procedure to the patient
   b. Remove the swab from the package or Culturette®tube carefully to avoid contamination of the swab tip			

You must:	S	U	Comments
c. Have the patient open mouth wide			
d. Depress the patient's tongue with a tongue depressor and have the patient say "ah"			
e. Swab the back of the throat and the surfaces of the tonsils gently. Avoid touching the surfaces of the mouth and tongue			
f. Replace swab into Culturette® tube or sterile tube. When using Culturette®, crush the enclosed ampule according to package instructions			
g. Label the tube with the patient's name, the date, time, and patient's ID number if hospitalized			
h. Transport specimen to the laboratory promptly			
4. Collect a urine specimen for culture:			
a. Explain to the patient the procedure for clean-catch urine collection (Lesson 5–1)			
b. Emphasize the necessity of avoiding contamination of the container or the specimen			
c. Label the sterile container with the patient's name, ID number (if hospitalized), time, and date			
d. Transport specimen to the laboratory promptly			
5. Clean equipment and return to proper storage			
6. Dispose of used materials in proper receptacles			
7. Clean work area with surface disinfectant			
8. Remove gloves and discard appropriately			
9. Wash hands with hand disinfectant			

Comments:

Student/Instructor:

Date:_____ Instructor:_____

LESSON 6–6

Performing a Throat Culture and a Rapid Test for Group A *Streptococcus*

LESSON OBJECTIVES

After studying this lesson, you should be able to:
- Collect a throat culture and transfer it to growth media.
- List the different types of media and their uses.
- Discuss the Group A *Streptococci* and their importance.
- List the two main types of rapid diagnostic tests for *Streptococcus* and discuss each.
- Define the glossary terms.

GLOSSARY

antigen / a substance which causes antibody formation and which reacts with that antibody

antibody / a protein that reacts specifically with an antigen

hemolysis / the destruction of red blood cells, with the liberation of hemoglobin

nonselective media / media which will support the growth of most common bacteria

pathogen / any agent capable of causing disease, especially microorganisms

pharyngeal / having to do with the pharynx; the back of the throat

primary plating medium / the initial growth medium upon which the bacterial specimen is placed

selective medium / medium which supports the growth of certain bacteria while inhibiting the growth of others

substrate / a substance upon which an enzyme acts

INTRODUCTION

A throat culture (pharyngeal swab) is a frequently performed test, especially in children and young adults. The test is performed whenever the patient reports clinical symptoms of strep throat. This infection is caused by Group A *Streptococci*. Infection with this group of *Streptococcus* can be dangerous for children and teenagers because of complications that may arise. An untreated tonsilitis caused by the Group A *Streptococcus* can result in conditions such as scarlet fever, rheumatic fever, rheumatic endocarditis or glomerulonephritis. Confirmation of the diagnosis of streptococcal infection can be made either by identifying the organisms in culture or by a positive rapid test result. Correct and rapid identification means that the proper antibiotic can be prescribed and complications avoided.

The throat culture is collected as in Lesson 6–5. It is important that the requested procedure be performed without delay to prevent drying of the swab, which reduces viability of any organisms present.

TYPES OF MEDIA

Once the proper collection of a specimen has been accomplished, it is equally important that it be promptly transferred to an appropriate growth medium. A great variety of growth media is available, and it is imperative that the chosen medium will support optimum growth of the organism.

Liquid, Semi-Solid, and Solid Media

Growth media may be liquid, semi-solid, or solid. One liquid medium suitable for general purposes is tryptic soy broth (TSB). Liquid media, including TSB, can be solidified by the addition of specified amounts of agar. A semi-solid state can be achieved by adding lesser amounts of agar. The broth containing the powdered agar is brought to a boil, allowed to cool slightly, and then poured into tubes or plates where it gels.

Agar slants are made by pouring the still-warm agar medium into tubes placed in a slanted position. For medical work, the agar is more commonly poured into sterile petri dishes and allowed to solidify; these are called agar plates. For observation of bacterial colony characteristics, the bacteria should be grown on solid media.

Selective and Nonselective Media

Media can be further divided into **selective** and **nonselective** types. The selective media allow the growth of certain bacteria while inhibiting the growth of others. The nonselective media are those which support the growth of most common bacteria. An example of a selective medium is MacConkey's, which supports the growth of certain gram-negative bacteria and inhibits the growth of gram positives. Another selective medium is Thayer-Martin, which is used to grow cultures of *Neisseria gonorrhoeae*. Examples of nonselective media include trytose agar (TA) and blood agar (BA).

Primary Plating Media

Most bacteriology departments have a chart of **primary plating media** from which the initial growth media can be selected. This selection is based mainly on the origin of the sample. For example, material from a throat swab is placed on blood agar, which is a good medium for most of the **pathogens** in the throat. Pathogens are agents capable of causing disease. Blood agar supports the growth of the *Streptococci* and also can demonstrate the phenomenon of hemolysis of blood cells. **Hemolysis** is the destruction of red blood cells. A green appearance surrounding colonies on a blood agar plate signifies alpha (α) hemolysis. Complete clearing of the blood in the areas surrounding the colonies is called beta (β) hemolysis. The occurrence of hemolysis can be important in the diagnosis of infection by aiding in the identification of the organism responsible.

CULTURING THE THROAT SPECIMEN

To perform the throat culture, the organisms obtained from a throat swab are transferred to a blood agar plate. This is accomplished by gently rolling the swab across the surface of one quadrant of the plate (Figure 6–18). The inoculating loop is then used to streak the plate to obtain isolated colonies as described in Lesson 6–4. The plate is then incubated upside-down overnight at 37°C. (This procedure should produce isolated individual colonies which can be picked up with the loop and transferred for further study and identification.)

To detect Group A *Streptococci,* a special disk containing the antibiotic bacitracin is placed on the newly streaked plate before it is put into the incubator. The next morning the plate is observed for growth around the disk. No growth in the zone around the bacitracin disk indicates the presence of Group A *Streptococcus.* (See Color Plate 29 for example of zone of inhibition.) If Group A *Streptococcus* is indicated, it must be confirmed by heavily streaking an isolated β hemolytic colony onto a fresh blood agar plate. A bacitracin disk is placed in the center of the streak area and the plate is incubated as above.

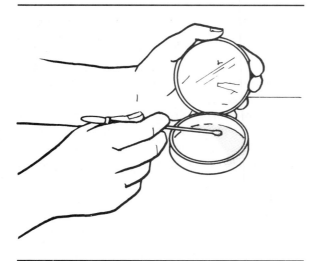

Figure 6–18. Transferring throat culture swab to an agar plate

Growth of some strains of streptococci is enhanced by incubation in an environment of increased CO_2. Special incubators are available for this; alternatively, the plate can be placed in a candle jar or in a special commercial pack into which chemical pellets release high concentrations of CO_2.

If these measures are not sufficient for identification of the organism, one of several identification strips on the market may be used (Color Plate 30). These strips contain small pockets of different biochemical tests into which a solution of an isolated colony is inserted. After incubation, the results of the biochemical tests are used to make an identification.

PERFORMING RAPID TESTS FOR GROUP A *STREPTOCOCCUS*

Although the throat culture is still performed, there are rapid tests available to detect Group A *Streptococcus.* Most of these give results in about five minutes. There are two major types of rapid strep tests on the market. One type of kit utilizes latex agglutination. In this type the **antigen** is the organism itself and latex beads in the kit are coated with antibodies to Group A *Streptococcus.* A throat swab is performed in the usual way. The material from the throat swab is mixed with the antibody-coated beads on a special cardboard slide. The reaction of the antigen and antibody produces agglutination. The appearance of agglutination indicates a positive test for Group A *Streptococcus.* Any test which shows no visible agglutination should be observed microscopically. This will insure that a weak positive reaction will not be reported as a negative.

A second rapid-test method based on the principle of enzyme immunoassay (EIA) is being produced by several manufacturers (Figure 6–19). Because the test is very sensitive, this method supposedly eliminates the problems of reading weak reactions. An example of a kit using the EIA method is the TANDEM® ICON® Strep A test, manufactured by Hybritech. The procedure

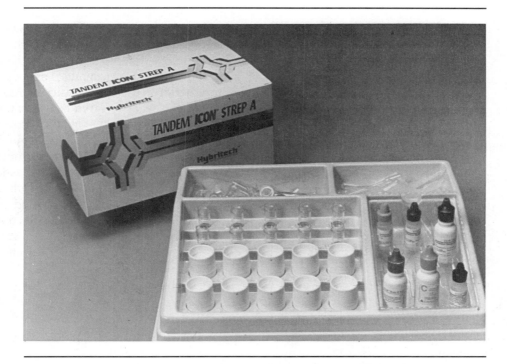

Figure 6–19. EIA test for strep. Components of an enzyme immunoassay rapid test for Group A *Streptococcus*. *(Photo courtesy of Hybritech, Incorporated)*

described is for this test and is given in detail in the Performance Guide. (Inclusion of this test method does not constitute endorsement by the authors.)

The test procedure involves making an extract of bacteria which have been collected on the throat swab, usually by immersing the swab in an acidic reagent. The extract is mixed in a special reagent bottle or tube, and the mixture is expelled onto a filter which is coated with antibody to Group A *Streptococcus*, as well as positive and negative controls. Enzyme-labeled antibody is then added from the kit. The combination of the antibody on the filter, the antigen in the extract mixture, and the enzyme-labeled antibody results in what is called an antibody "sandwich" on the filter. A wash solution is added to the filter membrane to wash off any unbound antibody. An enzyme substrate, a substance upon which an enzyme acts, is then added to the membrane and allowed to incubate, and the filter is observed for color reaction.

Interpreting the Results

If Group A *Streptococcal* antigen (strep) is present, color development will occur. This spot of color will appear in the center of the filter, adjacent to the positive control spot. The reactions of the positive and negative controls included in the filter indicate whether the reagents performed properly and also whether the procedure was executed in the correct manner. The appearance of a positive test with controls is shown in Figure 6–20.

Occasionally, the physician orders both a culture and a rapid test for *Streptococcus*. The swab must be used to inoculate the culture plate before using it in the rapid test. The rapid tests contain chemicals which kill the organisms and the swab would be contaminated if it touched any

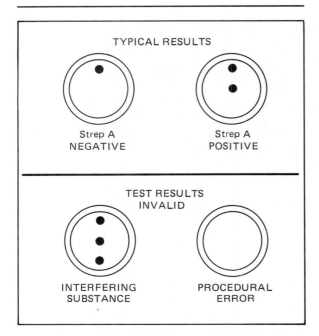

Figure 6–20. Results of a rapid strep test. Illustration of typical results obtained with the TANDEM® ICON® rapid test for Group A *Streptococcus*. When patient is negative for Group A *Streptococcus*, only one spot of color appears. Two spots of color indicate a positive test for patient and positive control. Three spots of color or no color spots indicate problems; the test must be repeated. *(Courtesy of Hybritech, Incorporated)*

surface before inoculating the plate. Some manufacturers recommend the use of two swabs, one for culture and one for the rapid test.

Precautions and Limits

In the performance of either of the methods, certain precautions must be observed. Probably one of the most important points is to use great care in the choice of the swabs used for collecting the sample. In general, cotton-tipped swabs are not recommended, nor any type of tips impregnated with chemicals. The streptococci are sensitive organisms and certain fibers or chemicals may decrease their viability. This is a very important

consideration and the specific instructions for each kit must be followed when choosing swabs for use with these test kits.

If the rapid test is negative and the patient's symptoms persist, the test must be repeated and a culture performed. Some physicians recommend confirming a negative rapid test with throat culture tests. This insures that no one who is infected with strep will go untreated. All guidelines for handling microbiological hazards should be observed. The worker should wear plastic gloves while performing the assay. After completion of the test procedure, all contaminated materials should be disposed of in a biohazard container to be autoclaved or incinerated. The work space should be wiped with surface disinfectant.

LESSON REVIEW

1. Describe how the bacteria on the swab are transferred to the growth media.
2. What is the difference between selective and nonselective media?
3. How is the primary plating medium chosen?
4. Discuss the two types of rapid tests for Group A *Streptococcus*.
5. Define antibody, antigen, hemolysis, nonselective, pathogen, pharyngeal, primary plating medium, and selective media.

STUDENT ACTIVITIES

1. Re-read the information on transferring the throat culture to growth media and rapid tests for Group A *Streptococcus*.
2. Review the glossary terms.
3. Practice the procedures for culturing the throat specimen.
4. Practice the procedures for performing a rapid test for detection of Group A *Streptococcus*.
5. Survey the community to find out which rapid tests are being used.

Student Performance Guide

NAME _____

DATE _____

LESSON 6–6
PERFORMING A THROAT CULTURE AND A RAPID TEST FOR GROUP A *STREPTOCOCCUS*

Instructions

1. Practice transferring the throat culture to growth media and performing a rapid test for Group A *Streptococcus*.
2. Demonstrate the procedure for performing a throat culture and a rapid test for Group A *Streptococcus* satisfactorily for the instructor. All steps must be completed as listed on the instructor's Performance Check Sheet.
3. Complete a written examination successfully.

Materials and Equipment

- gloves
- appropriate swabs
- blood agar plate
- bacterial loop, either wire or sterile plastic
- Bunsen burner or electric loop sterilizer
- incubator set at 37°C with increased CO_2 environment (candle jar* or commercial gas pack may be used)
- kit for performing enzyme immunoassay rapid test for Group A *Streptococcus*
- biohazard container
- surface disinfectant
- hand disinfectant
- bacitracin sensitivity disks

Note: The instructions given are for the Hybritech TANDEM® ICON® Group A *Streptococcus* test. Manufacturer's instructions for the kit being used must be followed. Inclusion of this method does not constitute endorsement by the authors.

*To make a candle jar, place the culture plate and a lighted utility candle in a large glass jar with a metal lid. When the lid is tightened, the candle uses up O_2, leaving increased CO_2 in the jar.

Procedure			S = Satisfactory U = Unsatisfactory
You must:	**S**	**U**	**Comments**
1. Assemble equipment and materials			
2. Wash hands with disinfectant and put on gloves			
3. Collect throat specimen. *Note:* The same swab can often be used for the culture plate and the rapid test. However, some test kits recommend collecting two swabs.			
4. Transfer the bacteria to the properly labeled blood agar plate: a. Roll the swab gently on the surface of one quadrant of the agar plate. Save the swab for rapid test or discard in biohazard container, if two were collected b. Flame a loop for streaking the plate or use sterile disposable plastic loop c. Streak the plate for isolated colonies as demonstrated in Lesson 6–4. Place bacitracin disks on quadrant two d. Place the plate in the 37°C incubator (with increased CO_2) overnight			
5. Perform rapid test for Group A *Streptococcus*. If another type rapid test is more available follow the instructions on the package insert. These instructions are for Hybritech's enzyme immunoassay method: a. Add one drop of Extraction reagent E1 and one drop of Extraction reagent E2 to the sample cup. The solution will turn from pink to yellow b. Add the sample swab to the extraction cup within one minute of the color change. Rotate the swab to mix the reagents. Incubate for one minute (if necessary the reaction may proceed up to five minutes) c. After one minute, add five drops of Extraction Reagent E3 and mix by twirling the swab in the cup. The solution in the cup should be pale yellow. The extracted antigen may remain in the cup, at room temperature (15–30°C), for up to 60 minutes if necessary d. Add one drop of Conjugate Reagent A and mix again by rolling the swab. After mixing, express all fluid from the swab into the cup and discard the swab e. Place the pre-filter top onto the extraction cup. Be sure the top is firmly seated. Proceed to test procedure within 15 minutes after adding the Conjugate			

You must:	S	U	Comments
f. Squeeze the entire sample through the prefilter onto the center of the ICON® cylinder. Incubate for two minutes. It is important to dispense all of the extracted sample			
g. After two minutes, add Wash Solution to the fill line and allow to drain completely			
h. Add three drops of Substrate Reagent B to the center of the ICON® cylinder. Incubate for two minutes			
i. Add Wash Solution to the fill line to stop color development. Allow to drain completely			
j. With the indicator mark (S) facing you, read the patient's results by looking for a purple spot of any intensity in the center of the membrane adjacent to the positive control spot. (See Figure 6–20 for interpretation of results)			
6. Dispose of all contaminated materials in biohazard container			
7. Return all equipment to proper storage			
8. Wipe work area with surface disinfectant			
9. Remove and discard gloves appropriately			
10. Wash hands with hand disinfectant			
11. Observe the throat culture plate after overnight incubation. Record: growth or no growth, presence or absence of hemolysis, and type. Note the presence or absence of a zone of inhibition around the bacitracin disk. Do not open petri dish unless further work is to be done with culture and gloves are worn			
12. If the culture plate indicates Group A *Streptococcus*, an isolated colony may be picked up on a sterile swab and used in the rapid test to confirm the positive			
13. Discard culture plate into biohazard container when finished			

Comments:

Student/Instructor:

Date:_____   Instructor:_____

LESSON 6–7

Performing a Urine Culture

LESSON OBJECTIVES

After studying this lesson, you should be able to:
- Use proper procedure to transfer urine to growth media.
- Choose the correct primary plating media for urine.
- Streak a plate with urine for a colony count.
- Calculate the bacterial count in a urine culture.
- Discuss the antibiotic susceptibility test.
- Define the glossary terms.

GLOSSARY

antibiotic susceptibility test / a test performed to determine which antibiotic is most effective against a particular organism

colony count / a method of counting the isolated colonies resulting from a streak plate

INTRODUCTION

The urine culture is one of the most frequently requested laboratory tests. Urine collected for a culture must be a clean-catch specimen as described in Lesson 5–1. A culture is performed when a patient has the symptoms of urinary tract infection (UTI). Urinary tract infections occur when bacteria migrate up the urethra to the bladder, or further into the kidneys. The organism most commonly involved is *Escherichia coli (E. coli)*, a natural inhabitant of the intestinal tract. Females are especially prone to the development of bladder and kidney infections because of their anatomy. The physician requests a urinary culture to identify the organism(s) causing the infection and to test those

organisms for susceptibility to antibiotics. This information allows the physician to prescribe the antibiotic which is most effective against that particular organism.

TRANSFERRING THE URINE TO MEDIA

Urine specimens are usually transferred onto blood agar and MacConkey's agar. Special calibrated loops which have capacities of either 0.01 or 0.001 ml are used. The agar plates are inoculated by making one streak down the center of the plate, then making 15 to 20 streaks at right angles to the first over the entire surface of the plate. Finally, a third set of streaks is made at right

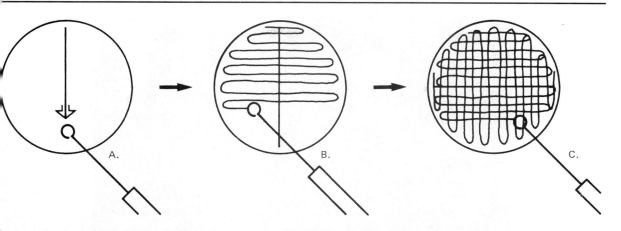

Figure 6–21. Streaking a urine plate. A) Make one streak down the center of the plate using a calibrated loop. B) Make several streaks at right angles to the initial streak, crossing over the original streak several times. C) Make several streaks at right angles to the second set of streaks so that the plate is almost solidly streaked.

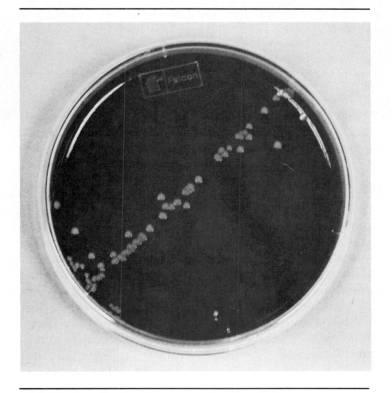

Figure 6–22. Isolated colonies on a blood agar plate *(Photo by John Estridge)*

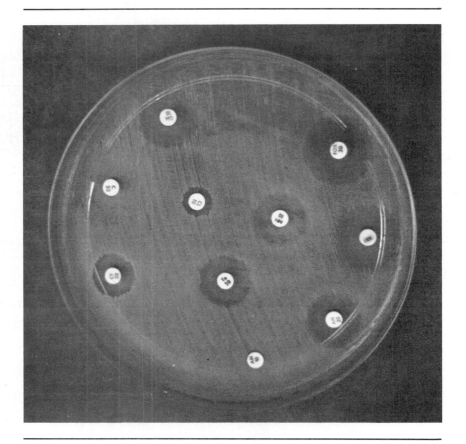

Figure 6–23. Antibiotic susceptibility test plate *(Photo by John Estridge)*

angles to the second so that the plate is almost solidly streaked (Figure 6–21, page 391). The blood agar will support the growth of most bacteria. The MacConkey's agar selects for the growth of gram negatives and also demonstrates the utilization of lactose which is helpful in the identification of the organism. After the plates are streaked in this manner, the MacConkey plate is incubated for 18 to 24 hours at 37°C. The blood agar plate is also incubated for 18 to 24 hours at 37°C, but in an increased CO_2 environment.

Colony Count

The **colony count** of bacteria which grow during the incubation can be used to estimate the number of bacteria in the urine. For example, if 30 colonies are counted on the blood agar plate, and a 0.001 ml loop was used for inoculation, the bacterial count is 30,000 per ml of urine. The number of colonies is multiplied by 1000 since only 1/1000 ml of urine was cultured. An infection is usually indicated when the count is over 100,000 organisms per ml of urine (Figure 6–22, page 391).

IDENTIFICATION OF BACTERIA

After an organism has been isolated from a culture, it may be identified by the use of any one of several identification methods, such as agglutination tests or biochemical strip tests. These strip tests are available for the identification of some of the gram-negative and gram-positive organisms (Color Plate 30).

ANTIBIOTIC SUSCEPTIBILITY

An **antibiotic susceptibility test** is performed on the organisms which grow from the urine culture. This test determines which antibiotics the organism is sensitive to. The physician uses the results to choose the antibiotic which is most effective against the organism causing the urinary tract infection. One method of antibiotic susceptibility is that of Bauer and Kirby. For this method, antibiotic-impregnated disks are placed on a newly inoculated and streaked agar plate. Susceptibility is shown by inhibition of growth in zones around the effective antibiotics (Figure 6–23).

Automated and semi-automated methods are available in which the organism is incubated with a variety of antibiotics in several concentrations. An instrument scans the special test plates for growth. The results are printed out, indicating which antibiotics are most effective against that particular organism.

LESSON REVIEW

1. Explain the proper procedure for transfer of a urine sample to media.
2. How is the primary plating media chosen?
3. Describe how to streak a plate to perform a colony count. What kind of inoculating loop is used?
4. Explain how to estimate the number of bacteria in a urine sample using the colony count.
5. Explain the procedure for the antibiotic susceptibility test.
6. Define antibiotic susceptibility test and colony count.

STUDENT ACTIVITIES

1. Re-read the information on performing a urine culture.
2. Review the glossary terms.
3. Practice performing the urine culture.

Student Performance Guide

NAME _____

DATE _____

**LESSON 6–7
PERFORMING A
URINE CULTURE**

Instructions

1. Practice performing the urine culture.
2. Demonstrate the procedure for urine culture satisfactorily for the instructor. All steps must be completed as listed on the instructor's Performance Check Sheet.
3. Complete a written examination successfully.

Materials and Equipment

- gloves
- clean-catch urine specimen
- blood agar plates
- MacConkey's agar plates
- special calibrated loop (0.01 or 0.001 ml)
- Bunsen burner or electric loop sterilizer
- matches or flint-type lighter
- 37°C incubator
- method for providing increased CO_2 environment
- wax pencil or marking pen
- surface disinfectant
- hand disinfectant
- biohazard container

Procedure

S = Satisfactory
U = Unsatisfactory

You must:	S	U	Comments
1. Assemble equipment and materials			
2. Light the Bunsen burner			
3. Wash hands with disinfectant and put on gloves			
4. Perform the procedure for urine culture using a clean-catch specimen (Lesson 5–1)			
a. Label bottom of blood agar and MacConkey's plates with proper patient identification			
b. Carefully remove lid from specimen container to avoid splashes			
c. Flame the calibrated transfer loop			
d. Insert the loop into the well mixed urine sample			
e. Remove the loop from the urine and check to see that the loop is filled with urine			
f. Transfer the loopful of urine to the surface of the blood agar by making a single streak down the center of the plate			
g. Spread the urine over the plate by making 20 to 25 streaks at right angles to the original streak, crossing the original streak each time			
h. Turn the petri dish one half turn and streak 20 to 25 times at right angles to the first set of streaks, crossing all of them each time			
i. Replace the lid on the petri dish			
j. Repeat steps b–i, using MacConkey's agar			
k. Flame the loop and return it to the holder			
5. Turn off Bunsen burner			
6. Return equipment to proper storage			
7. Place agar plates upside down in 37°C incubator. (Blood agar plate should be placed into increased CO_2 environment)			
8. Dispose of contaminated materials in biohazard container			
9. Wipe the work area with surface disinfectant			
10. Remove gloves and discard appropriately			
11. Wash hands with hand disinfectant			

You must:	S	U	Comments
12. Examine the plates after overnight incubation (18 to 24 hours). If bacterial infection is present, the urine plates should have isolated colonies spread over the entire surface			
13. Count the number of colonies on the blood agar plate			
14. Calculate the number of organisms per ml of urine by multiplying the number of colonies by 1,000 if 0.001 ml loop was used, or by 100 if the 0.01 ml loop was used			
15. Record the results			
16. Dispose of plates as directed by instructor			
17. Wash hands with hand disinfectant			

Comments:

Student/Instructor:

Date:_____ Instructor:_____

UNIT 7
Basic Clinical Chemistry

UNIT OBJECTIVES

After studying this unit, you should be able to:
- Discuss the importance of clinical chemistry.
- Identify the chemistry tests most frequently performed in small laboratories and explain the significance of each.
- Discuss quality control and its importance in the laboratory.
- Use a spectrophotometer.
- Describe the principles of several analyzers used in small laboratories.
- Explain the principles of the clinical chemistry tests for cholesterol.
- Explain the principles of the clinical chemistry tests for glucose.

OVERVIEW

Clinical chemistry is that branch of laboratory medicine which uses chemical analysis to study the level of various body constituents during health and disease. These chemical tests are usually performed on blood samples, but urine and other body fluids are also commonly analyzed. The results from these tests are used by the physician to diagnose disease, institute treatment, and follow the progress of disease. The physician may also use the results to counsel the patient in ways to prevent disease.

The study of body chemistry has a long history; as far back as Hippocrates, certain physicians emphasized chemical analysis in patient care. Early testing was performed on urine and feces samples because of the ease of collection of these specimens. These early tests were qualitative in nature in that they could only detect whether or not a constituent was present. As chemical analytical methods improved it became possible to quantitate substances or measure how much of a substance was present. The results of analyses of some constituents performed by crude methods over 100 years ago compare very well with results obtained today using sophisticated methods.

This unit is an introduction to some basic theories and principles of clinical chemistry. The relationships between the values of certain components and the state of health or disease in the individual are examined in lessons dealing with specific tests, such as glucose and cholesterol, and in the lesson introducing clinical chemistry. In addition, the concept of assuring the reliability and accuracy of a method of analysis is presented in a lesson on basic quality control.

Many laboratory tests which had been performed in the hospital laboratory are now being performed in the physician's office. These laboratories are often referred to as physician's office laboratories (POLs). The increase in testing in POLs has resulted largely from the development of smaller, more diverse instruments which are affordable but still have the ability to perform a variety of tests. A lesson presenting the basic theory and operation of a few of these is included. The inclusion of specific instruments and methods in this unit does not imply endorsement by the authors. These instruments and methods were selected for inclusion because of the basic principles illustrated.

Since blood glucose (sugar) is the most frequently requested chemistry test, one lesson presents information about glucose metabolism and methods of analysis. A lesson is also included on cholesterol. The measurement of serum cholesterol levels has become more important with the release of information linking elevated cholesterol to heart and blood vessel disease. A lesson on the principles and use of the spectrophotometer is placed just before the lessons on glucose and cholesterol; therefore, the worker will become familiar with the spectrophotometer before using it for these two analyses.

The information obtained from a chemical analysis of blood or one of the body fluids may be used to diagnose a disease, prescribe treatment, or monitor progress of the patient. Therefore, it is vital that the laboratory worker be dedicated to insuring that tests are performed and results are reported accurately and precisely, according to accepted procedure.

LESSON 7–1
Introduction to Clinical Chemistry

LESSON OBJECTIVES

After studying this lesson, you should be able to:

- List six body fluids which are frequently tested in clinical chemistry.
- Discuss the proper collection and handling of blood specimens for chemical analysis.
- Discuss five problems associated with blood collection which may cause interference with testing.
- Explain how the blood level of some chemical substances varies according to the time of day.
- Explain the significance or function of each of the constituents commonly included in a chemistry profile.
- List normal or expected values for each of the constituents usually measured in a chemistry profile.
- Define the glossary terms.

GLOSSARY

acidosis / abnormal condition in which blood pH falls below 7.35

alanine aminotransferase / enzyme present in high concentration in liver tissue and which is measured to assess liver function; ALT

albumins / a homogeneous group of serum proteins which are made in the liver and help maintain osmotic balance

alkaline phosphatase / enzyme widely distributed in the body, especially in the liver and bone; ALP or AP

alkalosis / abnormal condition in which blood pH rises above 7.45

aspartate aminotransferase / enzyme present in many tissues, including cardiac, muscle, and liver, and which is measured to assess liver function; AST

bilirubin / product formed in the liver from the breakdown of hemoglobin

BUN / blood urea nitrogen; measurement of urea in blood

creatine kinase / enzyme present in large amounts in brain tissue and in heart and other muscle, and which is measured to aid in the diagnosis of heart attack; CK

creatinine / breakdown product of creatine phosphate, a high energy compound stored in muscle

diurnal / having a daily cycle

electrolytes / the cations and anions which are important in maintaining fluid and acid-base balance

gamma glutamyl transferase / enzyme present in kidney, pancreas, liver and prostate, and measured to assess liver function; GGT

globulins / a heterogeneous group of serum proteins having varied functions

gout / painful condition in which blood uric acid is elevated and urates precipitate in joints

homeostasis / condition in which steady state or equilibrium is maintained

hypercalcemia / blood calcium levels above normal

hyperkalemia / blood potassium levels above normal

hypernatremia / blood sodium levels above normal

hypoalbuminemia / marked decrease in serum albumin concentration

hypocalcemia / blood calcium levels below normal

hypokalemia / blood potassium levels below normal

hyponatremia / blood sodium levels below normal

lactate dehydrogenase / enzyme widely distributed in the body, and measured to assess liver function; LD or LDH

lipemic / having a cloudy appearance due to excess lipid content

uric acid / breakdown product of nucleic acids

INTRODUCTION

In the healthy body, the chemical constituents are in a delicate balance or equilibrium and are influenced by both internal and external factors. This equilibrium or steady state is referred to as **homeostasis.** Changes in the concentration of a chemical constituent will usually trigger a reaction to bring the concentration back to the equilibrium state. For example, when blood glucose levels rise after a meal, the pancreas releases insulin to bring the glucose concentration down to normal levels.

In the clinical chemistry laboratory, tests are performed on blood and other body fluids. These fluids are analyzed for the presence or absence of certain substances or for the level or amount of the substances. The results of the tests are then compared with normal or expected values, the values found in health. Physicians use the results of clinical chemistry tests to aid in the diagnosis, treatment and prevention of disease. The interpretation of test results is based on understanding the physiologic and biochemical processes occurring in health and in disease.

It is important that test results be reliable. The physician must have confidence in test results if patient diagnosis or treatment is to be based on test findings. Reliability is assured when the specimens are collected, handled and stored properly until tests can be performed; when specimens are analyzed using correct procedures and appropriate quality control measures; and when results are calculated and reported properly.

This lesson contains some basics of clinical chemistry including the proper collection and handling of specimens and the significance and expected values of some commonly measured constituents. In order to understand the basis of the chemical tests discussed and the significance of the test results, it is necessary that the student or technologist have at least a basic knowledge of human biology. A short review of organ systems and functions may be appropriate before continuing with the lesson.

TYPES OF SPECIMENS ANALYZED

Fluids which may be submitted for chemical testing include blood, urine, cerebral spinal fluid (CSF), and less commonly, synovial, pleural, or pericardial fluids. Since the most common fluid tested in chemistry is blood, this lesson explains the proper methods of collection and handling of blood for routine chemical analysis. Specimens for most tests require only routine handling, but some require special attention. It is important to know what tests will be performed on a specimen before collection so that the specimen will be collected and stored appropriately.

Urine is also commonly tested in the laboratory. The routine collection, handling and chemical testing of urine is covered in Lessons 5–1 and 5–3. Special collections of urine are beyond the scope of this lesson.

Other fluids, such as synovial, CSF, or pericardial fluids are collected by the physician. The laboratory worker must always be aware that the handling and storage of these specimens are dictated by the test that is to be performed.

COLLECTION AND HANDLING OF BLOOD SPECIMENS FOR CHEMICAL ANALYSIS

Serum, Plasma, and Whole Blood

Chemical tests may be performed on whole blood, plasma, or serum. Whole blood may either be used immediately following a capillary puncture or, if testing is to be delayed, be collected in an anticoagulant such as heparin or EDTA to prevent clotting. (Detailed procedure for venipuncture may be found in Lesson 3–1.) The whole blood sample must be well mixed immediately before testing.

Plasma, the fluid portion of blood, is obtained by removing the liquid portion of anticoagulated blood following centrifugation. Serum is the fluid portion which remains after blood has been allowed to clot. It is obtained by collecting blood in a tube without anticoagulant, allowing the blood to clot, centrifuging the clotted sample, and removing the liquid (serum). If plasma or serum is to be used for testing, it is important to remove the liquid from the cellular portion of the blood as soon as possible after collection to prevent the exchange of substances between the cellular and liquid portions. Serum is the specimen used for most clinical chemistry tests (see Appendix L).

Storage of Specimen

For most routine tests which are to be performed quickly, such as within one hour, it is permissible to allow the specimen to remain at room temperature until testing. If testing is to be delayed, samples should be refrigerated at 4°C in the interim. For some tests, such as those involving certain enzymes, specimens must be frozen until tested to prevent the loss of enzyme activity.

Most specimens may be stored in test tubes or collection tubes until testing. However, certain tests require special handling. For example, since **bilirubin** is degraded by light, the samples should be protected by storage in a dark container until tested.

Effect of Time of Collection on Chemical Constituents

Most blood constituents do not change significantly after eating, so blood for the analysis of these may be collected at any time. However, concentrations of constituents such as glucose, triglycerides, and cholesterol *will* change after eating and specimens are usually collected in a fasting state in the morning before breakfast.

In disease, some blood constituents follow certain patterns of increase or decrease in disease which make the time of collection very important. For example, **creatine kinase,** an enzyme which is measured to detect heart attacks or myocardial infarcts, will rise rapidly and fall back to normal levels in the three to four days immediately following a heart attack. If this enzyme is not measured during this critical period, an infarct may go undiagnosed.

Diurnal variation, or changes with the time of day, can occur with certain blood constituents such as iron and corticosteroids. It is important, therefore, to note the time of collection of specimens for these tests and to consider this when interpreting test results.

Specimens collected shortly after a patient has eaten may appear **lipemic,** having a milky or cloudy serum or plasma. Lipemia may also be seen in some patients with disorders of lipid metabolism. Lipemia may interfere with certain tests, particularly those which use colorimetry or spectrophotometry.

PROBLEMS ASSOCIATED WITH SPECIMEN COLLECTION AND HANDLING

Reliable test results can only be obtained if the technologist has a properly collected specimen to work with. Each test procedure performed in a laboratory will have instructions for proper specimen collection; these should be strictly adhered to. Improperly handled specimens may interfere with tests or cause erroneous test results. Some problems commonly encountered are:

1. **Hemolysis.** Blood that is hemolyzed during collection (or handling) cannot be used for most analyses. The destroyed RBCs will release substances such as lactate dehydrogenase (LD) or potassium (K) and cause a misleading rise of these constituents in the serum. Hemolysis may be caused by overcentrifugation, excessive turbulence of the sample (shaking, etc.), freezing of cells, and forcing blood through the venipuncture needle, as well as by an improperly performed venipuncture.

2. **Hemoconcentration.** If the tourniquet is left on too long during venipuncture, stasis may occur in the vein and the blood constituents may be more concentrated than in properly flowing blood. (See Lesson 3–1.)

3. **Overcentrifugation.** Blood collected to obtain serum should be centrifuged only after it has remained undisturbed for 20–30 minutes to allow clotting to occur. Centrifugation should be gentle to avoid cell damage, and serum should be separated as soon as possible from the cells. To obtain plasma, the anticoagulated specimen may be centrifuged immediately after collection. Cells must be separated from the liquid portion before freezing, since freezing will cause cell lysis.

4. **Evaporation.** Specimens should remain capped until the time of testing. Evaporation will occur in uncapped specimens, with resulting concentration of some constituents, and gas escape or exchange which may alter other values such as pH or HCO_3^- concentration.

5. **Contamination.** Clean pipets or pipet tips should be used for the transfer of each sample. If reusable sample cups are used, they must be clean and dry to avoid contaminating or diluting the samples. Bacterial contamination of specimens must be avoided.

UNITS OF MEASURE

The results of clinical chemistry tests are usually reported in metric units using the International System of Nomenclature, or SI units. (For review, see Lessons 1–7 and 1–8.) Commonly used units are milligrams or micrograms per deciliter or per 100 ml (mg/dl or μg/dl), millimoles per liter (mmol/L), or, in the case of enzymes, enzyme activity units per liter (U/L).

COMMONLY PERFORMED CLINICAL CHEMISTRY TESTS

Chemistry tests can be grouped into two basic categories—tests that are frequently ordered (routine) and special tests. Routine tests, such as glucose or creatinine, are useful in giving an overall view of the state of health (especially when used in combination with other tests). Because they can be performed quickly, in batches, the cost can be kept low. Special chemistry tests, such as those monitoring drug levels or measuring hormone levels, are usually required when a particular diagnosis is suspected or treatment must be monitored. These tests are usually more expensive, take longer to perform, and require special instruments or techniques. Clinical chemistry tests may also be grouped according to the biological system being studied. For example, laboratories may offer a liver profile, which is a group of tests designed to enable the physician to assess liver function, or a cardiac profile, which aids in determining whether or not heart disease is present.

CHEMISTRY PROFILE

Most laboratories have a chemistry analyzer capable of performing chemistry profiles. A chemistry profile is a group of any of twelve to twenty tests performed at one time on one patient sample. The profile is composed of a combination of tests designed to assess the patient's general condition. (An example of a laboratory requisition form for a chemistry profile is in Appendix M.) Tests usually included in the profile reflect the state of carbohydrate and lipid metabolism, and kidney, liver, and cardiac function. Analyzers used for chemistry profiles usually are capable of processing many patient samples per hour. This lesson lists some components commonly included in chemistry profiles, gives the normal or expected serum value for each component, and includes a brief description of the rationale for performing each test.

NORMAL OR EXPECTED VALUES

The normal or expected values of a constituent are determined by measuring the level of the substance in a portion of the general population. For instance, a hospital, when establishing the normal range for a glucose method, may test 100 random samples from the nearby population and calculate the range of values. This range will be used for comparison to patient samples. (See Lesson 7–2 for a more complete explanation of quality control and normal ranges.) The expected ranges of many substances differ according to the age or sex of the patient, the time of day, elapsed time after a meal, or drugs or medications that a person may be taking. Normal ranges may differ slightly for different methods of analysis and geographical areas of the population sample. The normal values given in this lesson are those for an adult male, using commonly accepted testing methodologies. A table of normal values of common chemical tests may be found in Appendix H.

SUBSTANCES TESTED IN CHEMISTRY PROFILES

Proteins

Proteins are essential components of cells and body fluids. They are formed from chains of amino acids; some amino acids are made by the body while others must be provided from dietary protein.

Serum proteins are of two major groups, the **albumins** and the **globulins.** Albumins comprise approximately 60% of total serum proteins, globulins about 40%. The albumins are homogeneous in structure. They transport some insoluble substances and help to maintain fluid balance in the body. The globulins are a heterogeneous group of molecules. Antibodies, blood coagulation proteins, enzymes, and proteins which transport such substances as iron, are all serum globulins.

Protein is most commonly measured in serum, but it can also be measured in urine or CSF where the concentration is normally low. Total serum protein and albumin are usually measured in a sample simultaneously and globulin is computed from the difference (total protein – albumin = globulin). A ratio of albumin to globulin (A/G ratio) may be computed but is of limited value.

Total Serum Protein. The total serum protein concentration is normally 6.0–8.0 g/dl. This represents the sum of many different proteins, all of which may vary independently of each other. Measurement of total protein can provide information about the state of hydration, nutrition, and liver function, since most serum proteins are made in the liver. Total serum protein may be measured chemically or by using a refractometer.

Albumin. The normal serum albumin concentration is 3.5–5.2 g/dl. Albumin is synthesized in the liver. Decreased levels of albumin, or **hypoalbuminemia,** may occur in liver disease, starvation, impaired amino acid absorption, and protein loss through the skin, kidneys, or gastrointestinal tract.

Electrolytes

In clinical chemistry the term **electrolytes** refers to the cations, sodium (Na^+) and potassium (K^+), and the anions, chloride (Cl^-) and bicarbonate (HCO_3^-). These four ions have a great effect on hydration, acid-base balance, and osmotic pressure as well as pH and heart and muscle function.

The electrolytes are distributed unequally between the intracellular (inside the cell) and extracellular (outside the cell) spaces (Figure 7–1). In some illnesses, the normal water and electrolyte balance is altered because of sudden fluid loss due to vomiting, diarrhea, or excessive urination. Such sudden imbalances can be harmful. As shown in Figure 7–1, potassium is the major intracellular cation while sodium is the major extracellular cation. Chloride and bicarbonate are in low concentrations inside the cells and in higher concentrations outside cells.

Sodium. The normal serum sodium concentration is 135–148 mmol/L (meq/L). Sodium has an important influence on osmotic concentration and determines the extracellular fluid volume. Water moves back and forth across membranes to maintain proper sodium balance; rapid shifts in the water volume in cells can damage or destroy cells. Alterations in sodium concentration can influence water intake and excretion.

Sodium is conserved by the kidneys. The sodium concentration is also affected by aldosterone levels. **Hypernatremia,** or increased concentration of sodium, can be seen in dehydration,

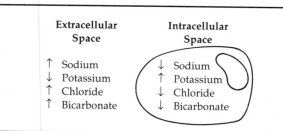

Figure 7–1. Relative intracellular and extracellular electrolyte concentration

hyperadrenalism (Cushing's disease), and diabetes insipidus (a deficiency of antidiuretic hormone). **Hyponatremia,** or decreased concentration of sodium, can be seen in severe diarrhea, acidosis of diabetes mellitus, decreased aldosterone secretion (Addison's disease), or renal disease in which there is poor ion exchange in the tubules.

Potassium. The normal serum potassium is 3.5–5.4 mmol/L (meq/L). Potassium is excreted by the kidney. Abnormally high or low levels of potassium should be reported immediately to the physician because levels outside of normal limits can affect muscle function, particularly heart function. **Hyperkalemia,** increased concentration of serum potassium, can occur when potassium leaves cells rapidly, and may occur in anoxia and acidosis. Increased potassium levels cause a decrease in muscle function, and may occur in circulatory failure (shock) and in renal failure. **Hypokalemia,** decreased concentration of serum potassium, may be due to decreased intake of potassium, increased levels of aldosterone, or increased loss of potassium due to vomiting, diarrhea, or use of diuretics.

Chloride. Chloride is the anion with the highest extracellular concentration; normal serum level is 98–108 mmol/L (meq/L). Its concentration varies inversely with bicarbonate (HCO_3^-). The concentration of chloride will increase in dehydration or in loss of CO_2 by overbreathing (respiratory alkalosis). Decreased chloride concentration may be seen in acidosis caused by uncontrolled diabetes, renal disease and excessive vomiting.

Bicarbonate. The bicarbonate anion is part of the blood buffer system which helps maintain a normal blood pH of 7.4; normal serum concentration is 22–28 mmol/L (meq/L). Carbon dioxide (CO_2) is constantly generated by our metabolic processes. The combination of CO_2 and water (H_2O) creates carbonic acid (H_2CO_3) which is converted to hydrogen ion (H^+) and bicarbonate:

$$H_2O + CO_2 \longrightarrow H_2CO_3 \longrightarrow H^+ + HCO_3^-$$

When the ratio of bicarbonate anion to carbonic acid changes, the pH changes. **Acidosis** occurs when the pH falls below 7.35 and may be caused by decreased HCO_3^- concentrations. **Alkalosis,** caused by increased HCO_3^- concentrations, occurs when the pH is greater than 7.45. The bicarbonate concentration is affected rapidly by changes in respiration, the body's way of eliminating CO_2. Changes in lung function, such as pneumonia, or central nervous system (CNS) depression or stimulation due to drugs will affect HCO_3^- concentrations. Concentration changes may also occur in diabetic ketosis and renal failure.

Mineral Metabolism

Minerals are necessary for good health. Calcium and phosphorus are necessary for proper bone and tooth formation. Calcium, phosphorus (phosphate) and iron are examples of minerals often measured in chemistry profiles. Calcium is also required for blood coagulation. Iron is essential for hemoglobin production and is an integral component of some enzymes.

Calcium. Of all the minerals in the body, calcium is present in the highest concentration. Normal serum calcium is 8.7–10.5 mg/dl (2.18–2.63 mmol/L). Approximately 99% of it is bound in the skeleton in calcium complexes and is not metabolically active. Only unbound calcium ions are metabolically active. Calcium is required for proper blood coagulation and for normal neuromuscular excitability. The calcium balance is influenced by vitamin D_3, and parathyroid hormone and calcitonin. These hormones control dietary absorption of calcium as well as its excretion by kidneys and movement in and out of bone. **Hypercalcemia,** an increased level of calcium, occurs in parathyroidism, bone malignancies, hormone disorders, excessive vitamin D_3, and acidosis. It may cause deposits of calcium in soft organs leading to complications such as kidney stones. Decreased levels of calcium, or **hypocalcemia,** may be life threatening and should be reported to the physician immediately. Extremely low levels may bring on increased muscle contraction leading to tetany. Low calcium levels may be due to hypoparathyroidism, vitamin D_3 deficiency, poor absorption due to intestinal disease, and kidney disease.

Phosphorus. Normal serum phosphorus concentration is 3.0–4.5 mg/dl (0.96–1.44 mmol/L). Most phosphorus in the body is in the form of inorganic phosphate. Approximately 80% is in bone and the rest is mostly in high energy compounds such as adenosine triphosphate (ATP). Phosphorus levels are influenced by calcium and hormones. Children have higher levels than adults because they have higher levels of growth hormone.

Iron. Iron is essential for hemoglobin synthesis and synthesis of heme proteins. Iron is absorbed from dietary sources and is highly conserved by the body. In blood, iron is transported by *transferrin*, a serum protein. Measurement of transferrin levels along with iron levels is helpful. Iron levels differ with age, sex, and time of day, being higher in the A.M. than in the P.M. Serum iron is normally 65–165 µg/dl (11.6–29.5 µmol/L). Iron deficiency may lead to anemia. The deficiency may be due to insufficient iron in diet, poor absorption of iron, impaired release of stored iron or increased loss of iron due to bleeding. Serum iron levels may be increased in hemolytic anemias, increased intake of iron or blocked synthesis of iron-containing compounds, such as occurs in lead poisoning.

Kidney Function

Proper kidney function is important to water and electrolyte balance. The kidneys eliminate waste products, help maintain water and pH balance, and produce certain hormones. Substances are excreted into and reabsorbed from urine to help maintain homeostasis (see Unit 5). The examination of urine may reveal kidney problems; the serum and plasma concentrations of some substances also are altered in certain kidney diseases.

Creatinine. **Creatinine** is a waste product of creatine phosphate, a substance which is stored in muscle and used for energy. Creatinine is excreted by the kidney. When renal function is impaired, blood creatinine levels rise, but more than 50% of kidney function must be lost before this happens. Creatinine levels are not affected by diet or hormone levels. Increases occur when there is impairment of urine formation or excretion, such as occurs in renal disease, shock, water imbalance or blockage of the ureters. Normal serum creatinine is 0.7–1.4 mg/dl (62–125 µmol/L).

BUN. In mammals, surplus amino acids are converted to urea and excreted by the kidney. This surplus is measured as **BUN,** or blood urea nitrogen. The BUN concentration is influenced by the amount of protein degraded, diet, hormones, and kidney function. Therefore, measurement of BUN is not as good an indicator of kidney disease as is creatinine. Normal serum BUN is 8–18 mg/dl (2.9–6.4 mmol/L). BUN levels may be low in starvation, pregnancy, and in persons on a low protein diet. Increased concentration of BUN may be seen during a high protein diet, after administration of steroids, and in kidney disease.

Uric Acid. **Uric acid** is formed from the breakdown of nucleic acids and is excreted by the kidneys. It has low solubility and tends to precipitate as uric acid crystals, or urates. In kidney disease, uric acid concentration changes are similar to changes in BUN and creatinine. However, measurement of uric acid is principally used in the diagnosis and treatment of **gout,** a disease where uric acid precipitates in tissues and joints, causing pain. Uric acid levels may also increase after massive radiation or chemotherapy because of increased cell destruction. Normal serum uric acid is 3.5–7.5 mg/dl (0.210–0.445 mmol/L).

Liver Function

The liver is both a secretory and excretory organ; it has numerous metabolic functions. The liver functions in carbohydrate metabolism, synthesizing glycogen from glucose. Almost all plasma proteins are made in the liver. These include albumin, lipoproteins, blood coagulation proteins such as fibrinogen, and transport proteins. The liver is also important in lipid metabolism. In the liver, cholesterol is formed and degraded into bile acids, which emulsify fats so they can be absorbed. The liver is a storage site for iron, glycogen, vitamins, and other substances. Other functions include destruction of old cells by phagocytosis and the detoxification of many substances. Much liver function must be lost or impaired before some laboratory tests show abnormality. Numerous tests are used to estimate liver function. Most are not specific for a particular disease but only reflect tissue damage.

Total Bilirubin. **Bilirubin,** a waste product from the breakdown of hemoglobin, is formed in the liver and excreted in the bile. Since serum bilirubin levels are normally low, 0.1–1.0 mg/dl (1.7–17.0 µmol/L), only increases are significant. Bilirubin concentration may be increased when there is excessive destruction of hemoglobin such as in hemolytic anemias, impaired bilirubin processing as in hepatitis, or impaired excretion by the liver as in biliary obstruction. Bilirubin measurements are most helpful in diagnosis when both total and direct bilirubin are measured.

Liver Enzymes. A rise in enzymes generally reflects injury to tissue since most enzymes are intracellular. Some enzymes are widely distributed in many body tissues, while others are found in only a few tissues. The measurement of enzyme levels is not always specific for damage to a particular organ, but is most helpful when used with other tests, clinical symptoms, and patient history. Enzymes which may be used to assess liver function or damage include **alkaline phosphatase, lactate dehydrogenase, gamma glutamyl transferase** and the aminotransferases **alanine aminotransferase** and **aspartate aminotransferase.**

Alkaline Phosphatase. Alkaline phosphatase (ALP) is widely distributed in the body, including the bone and the ducts of the liver. Serum ALP levels may greatly increase in liver tumors and lesions, and may show a moderate increase in diseases such as hepatitis. Normal serum ALP is 20–105 U/L.

Aminotransferases. Liver tissue is rich in the aminotransferase enzymes. When liver cells are injured, these enzymes are released. Serum concentrations of these enzymes change with time, rising during acute liver disease and falling as recovery occurs. Generally, only one enzyme need be measured, as levels tend to mirror each other. Alanine aminotransferase (ALT), was formerly called serum glutamic-pyruvic transaminase (GPT or SGPT). Normal serum concentration of ALT is 3–30 U/L. Levels are low in cardiac tissue and high in liver tissue. This enzyme usually rises higher than aspartate aminotransferase in liver disease, with moderate increases (10×) in cirrhosis, infections, or tumors and up to 100× increases in viral or toxic hepatitis. Asparate aminotransferase (AST) was formerly called serum glutamic oxaloacetic transminase (GOT or SGOT). The normal serum concentration of AST is 6–25 U/L. It is present in many tissues, particularly cardiac, muscle, and liver. It is elevated after myocardial infarction as well as in liver disease.

Gamma glutamyl transferase. Gamma glutamyl transferase (GGT) is found in kidney, pancreas, liver and prostate tissue. It may be more helpful than ALP because it is not increased in bone disease, and better than AST because it is not increased in muscle disorders. Measurement of GGT is often used to monitor recovery from hepatitis. Normal serum GGT is 3–35 U/L.

Lactate dehydrogenase. Lactate dehydrogenase (LD or LDH) is widely distributed in tissue. The LDH level increases in the blood following liver disease and myocardial infarction. Hemolysis of a blood sample will cause increased LD levels in the serum because of release of LD from RBCs. Normal serum LD is 125–290 U/L.

Cardiac Function

Creatine kinase. **Creatine kinase** (CK) is an enzyme used to help diagnose myocardial infarction. CK is present in large amounts in muscle and the brain but in small amounts in organs such as the liver and kidneys. Following heart attack, CK is released from the damaged heart muscle. The serum CK level peaks in about 24 hours, reaching 5–8× the upper limit of normal, which is 10–100 U/L. It falls rapidly back to normal levels within three to four days. Serum CK levels also increase following skeletal muscle damage and brain injury.

Lipid Metabolism

Lipids are synthesized in the body from dietary fats and oils that are broken down and reassembled. The most commonly measured lipids are cholesterol and triglycerides.

Cholesterol. Cholesterol is present in all tissues, and serum concentrations tend to increase with age. Elevated cholesterol levels may predispose one to coronary artery disease. It is now generally recommended that serum cholesterol levels be maintained below 200 mg/dl (normal range is 140–250 mg/dl). In Lesson 7–5 in this unit, cholesterol metabolism and methods of analysis of cholesterol are described.

Carbohydrate Metabolism

Glucose. Glucose metabolism is largely regulated by insulin, which is produced by the pancreas, and by other hormones such as growth hormone, glucagon, and cortisol. Glucose is a commonly tested blood constituent. Glucose metabolism and methods of analysis are explained in Lesson 7–6 in this unit. Normal serum glucose is 65–100 mg/dl (3.6-5.6 mmol/L).

LESS COMMONLY ORDERED TESTS

There are dozens of tests available that have not been mentioned here. Many are special tests which measure certain hormones such as insulin, growth hormone, adrenocorticotropic hormone (ACTH),

or follicle stimulating hormone (FSH). Other special tests include the measurement of vitamins or trace minerals such as zinc, measurement of isoenzymes by electrophoresis, or measurement of metabolic products such as methyl malonic acid. Such tests may require special specimen collection as well as special instruments and expertise to perform. A clinical chemistry text should be consulted for more information.

LESSON REVIEW

1. What are the most commonly tested body fluids?
2. Explain how to collect whole blood, serum and plasma for chemical analysis.
3. How may the time a blood sample is collected affect test results?
4. What can cause hemolysis of a specimen? How will test results be affected if hemolysis occurs?
5. What is the cause of lipemia?
6. Give the normal ranges for the constituents included in a chemistry profile. Explain the significance of variations from normal range for each constituent.
7. Name three tests that may be useful in diagnosing kidney disease; liver disease.
8. What enzyme is most useful in diagnosing heart attack?
9. Name the electrolytes and explain their functions. How do intracellular and extracellular concentrations differ?
10. What are the two major types of protein? What are their functions?
11. Define acidosis, alanine aminotransferase, albumins, alkaline phosphatase, alkalosis, aspartate aminotransferase, bilirubin, BUN, creatine kinase, creatinine, diurnal, electrolytes, gamma glutamyl transferase, globulins, gout, homeostasis, hypercalcemia, hyperkalemia, hypernatremia, hypoalbuminemia, hypocalcemia, hypokalemia, hyponatremia, lactate dehydrogenase, lipemic, and uric acid.

STUDENT ACTIVITIES

1. Re-read the information on introduction to clinical chemistry.
2. Review the glossary terms.
3. Ask what tests are included in chemistry profiles in a hospital or laboratory in the nearby area. Find out the laboratory's normal ranges and compare them to those in this lesson.
4. Find out what analyses are performed in special chemistry in a hospital or other large laboratory in the nearby community.

LESSON 7–2
Quality Control

After studying this lesson, you should be able to:
- Explain the importance of quality control in the laboratory.
- Discuss the use of standards and controls in chemistry procedures.
- Determine the mean value for a set of test results.
- Calculate the standard deviation for an analytical method.
- Detect a result which is out of control.
- Explain how to detect the development of a trend in a method.
- Explain coefficient of variation.
- Define the glossary terms.

GLOSSARY

accuracy / a measure of how close a determined value is to the true value

average / the sum of a group of values divided by the number of values; the mean

coefficient of variation / a calculated value to compare the relative variability between different sets of data

control serum / a serum with a known concentration of the same constituents as those being determined in the patient sample

Gaussian curve / a graph plotting the distribution of values around the mean; normal frequency curve

Levey-Jennings chart / quality control chart which demonstrates the precision of a method

mean / the figure obtained when the sum of a set of values is divided by the number of values; the average

population / the entire group of items or individuals from which the samples under consideration are presumed to have come

precision / reproducibility of results; the closeness of obtained values to each other

random error / error whose source cannot be definitely identified

sample / in statistics, a subgroup of a population

standard / a chemical solution whose exact concentration is known and which can be used as a reference or calibration substance

standard deviation / a measure of the spread of a population of values around the mean

statistics / the science of collecting and classifying facts in order to show their significance

systematic error / a variation which may influence results to be consistently higher or lower than the real value

trend / an indication of error in the analysis, detected by an ever increasing or decreasing value in the control sample

Westgard's rules / a set of rules used to determine when a method is out of control

INTRODUCTION

The results obtained from laboratory analyses are often used to diagnose, prescribe treatment, and monitor the progress of the patient. Since such importance may be placed upon the test results, they should be as reliable as possible. It is the ethical and legal responsibility of laboratory workers to insure that the work performed in the laboratory is of the highest quality.

A QUALITY CONTROL PROGRAM

In order to accomplish the goal of producing accurate and reliable results in the laboratory, a regimen of quality control must be instituted. Quality control is a system set up to insure that certain limits for a test result or a product are maintained. In a clinical laboratory, quality control also encompasses the collection and handling of patient samples, and the processing of those samples.

Standards and Controls

The laboratory must also have a program in which standards and controls are run at specified intervals. A **standard** is a substance whose exact concentration is known and which can be used as a reference or calibration solution for a method of analysis. A **control serum** contains the same constituents as those being analyzed in the patient. Most laboratories use commercially produced controls which are made from pooled sera. These controls usually have been assayed for several different constituents; the results of the assays of these controls are included when the laboratories purchase the controls. The control samples must be analyzed along with patient samples using the same methods, reagents and test conditions. Quality control tests should be run once a day, if possible, for each of the procedures performed. Quality control tests should also be run after an instrument has been calibrated and any time patient results seem to be erroneous. The results of these determinations of the control sera are used to construct a quality control chart.

Types of Errors

In general, two basic types of errors can occur during analytical procedures. One of these is **systematic error** (variance) which is defined as a variation that may influence results to be consistently higher or lower than the real value. Examples of factors which may cause this type of error are deteriorated reagents, mechanical change in the instrument, or a peculiarity in worker methodology, such as manner of pipetting. The other basic type of error is random variance, more commonly known as random error. **Random error** is error whose source cannot be identified definitely and causes variations which may occur in both directions. The factors contributing to random error include reagents, the complexity of the analysis, differences in skill levels of workers, and characteristics of the sample.

ACCURACY AND PRECISION

In any discussion of quality control and error, the terms *accuracy* and *precision* must be considered. Although accuracy and precision are sometimes used interchangeably, they do not have the same meaning.

Accuracy refers to the closeness of an analytical result to the actual value. Results which are nearer to the real value are more accurate than ones which are further away from the real value. For example, if the real value for an individual's glucose is 90 mg/dl, analyses which yielded re-

sults of 88, 90, or 92 mg/dl would be more accurate than analyses which yielded values of 80, 75, and 82 mg/dl.

The term **precision** refers to reproducibility of results or the closeness of obtained values to each other. An example of precision would be results of 88, 87, 92, 91, 88, and 90 on the above glucose sample; the results vary little from each other. Another way of thinking about it is to mentally picture a target with all the arrows or bullet holes closely grouped in one area of the target. In like manner, values of 78, 90, and 100 would not represent precision; if places on the imagined target, the "arrows" would be scattered around, not grouped (Figure 7–2). A very important point to remember is that one can have precision without accuracy; in other words, one could produce results that are near in value to each other, but because of an error the values may be inaccurate, not near the real value. The worker's goal should be to achieve both precision and accuracy in the laboratory analyses performed.

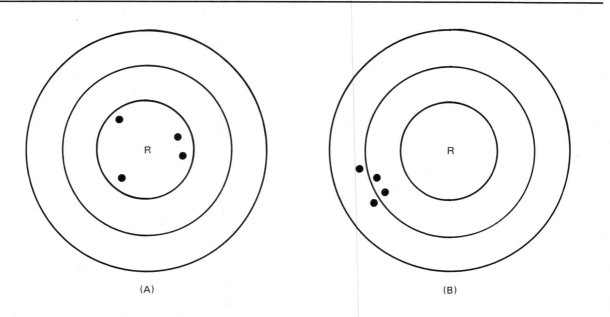

(A)   (B)

Figure 7–2. Accuracy versus precision. Illustrations of (A) accuracy, and (B) precision.

STATISTICS

Quality control involves **statistics,** which is the science of collecting and classifying facts in order to show their significance. The statistics involved in a good quality control program can be very complicated; therefore, only the fundamentals will be covered in this lesson. In practice, laboratories are now able to obtain good quality control programs for computers. The computer interprets the information, makes calculations and provides an evaluation of the precision of the procedure in question. However, the laboratory workers must understand the basics of quality control and statistics to be able to operate the program and correctly interpret the information the computer provides.

In statistics, a collection of observations (results) is called a **population;** a **sample** is a subgroup of values from that population. To make the calculations required for a quality control program, then, a sample or set of values must be obtained to enter into the statistical formulas.

Standard Deviation

One calculation which is always performed in a quality control program is the **standard deviation,** a measure of the scatter of the sample values around the **mean** (average) value. In other words, once the mean value of a sample of values is determined, it is then possible to determine what is the acceptable variation in that method of analysis. When a sample of values is plotted on a graph, the distribution of the values around the mean forms a **Gaussian** curve (Figure 7–3(A)). This curve is also known as a normal frequency or normal distribution curve. In a normal distribution, half of the values are greater than the mean and half are less than the mean. There are also more values close to the mean than values further from the mean.

Calculating the Mean Value. The mean value is the average value of a sample or set of values. The mean is computed by getting the sum of all the values in the sample and dividing this sum by the number of values involved, just as one obtains the **average** of any group of numbers. The formula for calculating the mean is shown here:

$$\overline{X} = \frac{\Sigma X}{n}$$

where $\overline{X}$ is the mean, ΣX is the sum of all the individual values and n is the actual number of determinations involved.

Calculating the Standard Deviation. Once the mean is obtained, the standard deviation of the analysis can be calculated. The standard deviation is a measurement of the variation of any single result (value) from the mean or the spread of any obtained value from the mean. To determine the standard deviation (s) one must first get the variance (s^2) of a sample. The formulas involved are as follows:

(1)
$$s^2 = \frac{\Sigma (\overline{X} - X)^2}{n - 1}$$

where s^2 is the variance, and n is the number of determinations.

(2)
$$s = \sqrt{\frac{\Sigma (\overline{X} - X)^2}{n - 1}}$$

where s is the standard deviation.

Example of Determination of Standard Deviation

The following example illustrates the use of these formulas in the calculation of the standard deviation. For convenience, only 10 values will be included. For more reliable results, one should have a greater number of values in the sample.

Test Value (mg/dl) (X)	Deviation from Mean $(\overline{X} - X)$	Deviation Squared $(\overline{X} - X)^2$
82	−5.4	29.16
85	−2.4	5.76
90	+2.6	6.76
86	−1.4	1.96
91	+3.6	12.96
90	+2.6	6.76
81	−6.4	40.96
86	−1.4	1.96
94	+6.6	43.56
89	+1.6	2.56
sum = 874		sum = 152.4

The first calculation which must be performed is to obtain the mean of the sample of values. This is done by getting the sum of all the values (874). The mean ($\overline{X}$) is then determined:

$$\overline{X} = \frac{\text{sum of X}}{n}$$

$$\overline{X} = \frac{874}{10}$$

$(\overline{X}) = 87.4$.

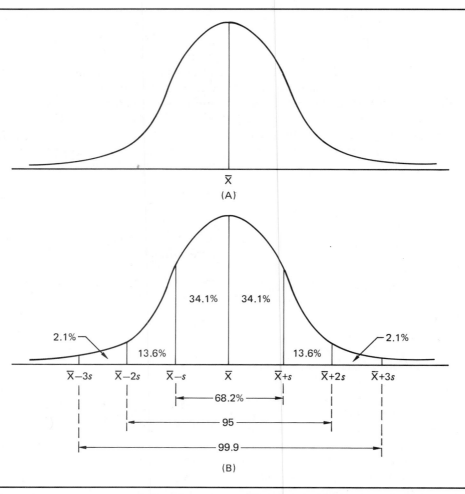

Figure 7–3. Normal distribution curves. (A) Gaussian curve showing normal frequency distribution. (B) Gaussian curve showing the proportion of the population falling between the mean and ±1s, ±2s, and ±3s.

The second calculation is to determine the deviation from the mean for each value. To do this, each individual value is then subtracted from the mean, and the difference, either positive or negative, is entered in column 2. For example, using the first value, 82, and the mean, 87.4, one gets a difference of +5.4, which is squared (or multiplied by itself). The deviation squared (5.4 × 5.4) equals 29.16; therefore 5.4 is entered into column 2 and 29.16 into column 3. These calculations are performed for each of the values in the sample. The squares of all the differences are added together; the sum of the squares in this example equals 152.4.

The standard deviation can then be determined by taking the square root of the sum of the squares divided by the number of samples minus one (n–1).

$$s = \sqrt{\frac{\Sigma\,(\overline{X} - X)^2}{n-1}}$$

$$s = \sqrt{\frac{152.4}{9}}$$

$s = 4.11$ Therefore, the standard deviation is 4.11.

Since the example is an analysis for glucose, which is reported in mg/dl, the standard deviation, s, is equal to 4.11 mg/dl, $2s$ equals 8.22, and $3s$ equals 12.33.

USE OF STANDARD DEVIATION IN THE LABORATORY

Once the standard deviation (s) has been figured, one can then go back to the Gaussian curve and actually make the percent divisions in it as shown in Figure 7–3(B). This shows that in a normally distributed population, 68.2% of all results obtained for this method of glucose analysis will fall between $1s$ below the mean to $1s$ above the mean. In other words, 68.2% of the values will fall between 83.29 (87.4 – 4.11) and 91.51 (87.4 + 4.11) in this particular example, which has a mean of 87.4.

In addition, 95.4% of the values will fall between 2s below the mean to 2s above the mean, or between 79.18 (87.4 – 8.22) and 95.6 (87.4 + 8.22). If 3s is used, 99.6% of the values will be within the range included between 75.07 (87.4 – 12.33) and 99.73 (87.4 + 12.33).

Clinical laboratories establish the allowable standard deviation for each method, basing the decision on the component analyzed and the method used. Two standard deviations (2s) is a common choice. What this signifies is that in this example, using the control which has a mean value of 87.4 mg/dl, the laboratory expects the analysis results of that control serum to be within ±2s (79.18 - 95.62) each time it is analyzed along with patient samples.

QUALITY CONTROL CHARTS

Quality control charts which demonstrate the precision of a method are constructed using the calculated mean and standard deviation results. This chart is called a **Levey-Jennings chart** (Figure 7–4).

The quality control chart shown in Figure 7–4(A) was constructed in the following manner: The mean obtained was 87.4; therefore, the mean line is labeled 87.4. The lines on either side of the mean represent the standard deviation multiplied by two. As the control data are obtained each day they are entered on the chart.

Day	Control Results
1	82
2	85
3	90
4	86
5	91

The process is continued for each day the controls are run.

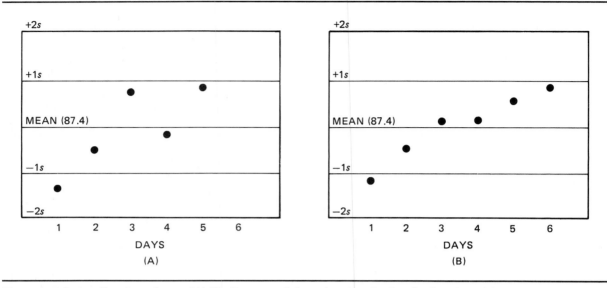

Figure 7–4. Levey-Jennings charts. (A) Quality control chart showing the data for five days. (B) Quality control chart showing a trend.

Trend

Sometimes a control value will consistently increase or decrease during the time which is covered by a quality control chart (a week or a month, etc.). This tendency can be observed after three or four results are either high or low. An uninterrupted rise or decline away from the mean is called a **trend** (Figure 7–4(B)). A trend is a signal that something has gone wrong in the procedure —either in the instrument, the technique, the reagents, or the control substance itself. The laboratory worker must investigate the reason for the trend and change or repair whatever is wrong.

Westgard's Rules

When a laboratory establishes a program of quality control and utilizes it, the workers need guidelines to decide whether or not a method is out of control. One such set of guidelines is called **Westgard's rules.** These rules give specific limits on how much error is allowed in the control values before the results of patient tests are rejected.

In order for these rules to be utilized the laboratory must analyze two control sera of different concentrations in every run of patient samples. The run is out of control and the patient samples are rejected if any of the following are true:

1. both controls are outside the ±2s limit
2. one control (same concentration) is outside the ±2s limit in two successive runs
3. controls in four consecutive runs have values greater than ±1s all in the same direction
4. ten consecutive control values fall either above or below the mean

Coefficient of Variation

Anytime a laboratory changes from one method of analysis to another, the precision of the new method must be compared to the precision of the old one. This can be done by calculating the coefficient of variation (CV) for each method. The **coefficient of variation** is a calculated value which is used to compare the relative variability between two different sets of values. The comparison can be made by expressing each standard deviation as a percentage of the mean.

For example, if the mean glucose for one method was 98.5 mg/dl with a standard deviation (s) of 2.5 mg/dl and 78 mg/dl with a standard deviation of 2.0 mg/dl for the second method, the CV could be calculated as shown below.

1st method $\quad CV = \frac{s}{X} \times 100$

$$CV = \frac{2.5 \text{ mg/dl}}{98.5 \text{ mg/dl}} \times 100$$

$$CV = 2.5\%$$

2nd method $\quad CV = \frac{s}{X} \times 100$

$$CV = \frac{2.0 \text{ mg/dl}}{78 \text{ mg/dl}} \times 100$$

$$CV = 2.6\%$$

In this case the variations are about the same, so the precision of the methods is similar. However, if a third method had a mean of 50 mg/dl and s of 3.0 mg/dl the CV would be calculated:

3rd method $\quad CV = \frac{s}{X} \times 100$

$$CV = \frac{3.0 \text{ mg/dl}}{50 \text{ mg/dl}} \times 100$$

$$CV = 6.0\%$$

Therefore, there is more variation between method three and both methods one and two than there is between methods one and two.

CONCLUSION

In conclusion, quality control in the laboratory is a very necessary procedure if the laboratory is to perform work which has reliable results. In addition, more and more governmental regulations require labs to have programs of quality control and to display Levey-Jennings charts for each procedure. In hospital and other large clinical laboratories, these rules have been in effect for a long time. Compliance has been necessary to receive federal money. At the present time new regulations are being proposed for POLs as a prerequisite to receiving payment from Medicare and Medicaid. However, maintaining a high standard of quality need not be a burden. Almost all instrument manufacturers now furnish some type of controls and standards for their analyzers. In addition, some of the larger, more expensive instruments have programs for quality control built into their computer systems. As an alternative, the laboratory can purchase separate software for quality control.

Precautions

■ Wear gloves when working with blood or blood products.
■ Remember that control sera from human sources carry the potential to cause disease.
■ Be certain that the manufacturer's instructions for instruments are followed carefully.
■ Use care to correctly insert values in the various formulas.
■ Remember that statistics are only as reliable as the analysis values used in the various formulas.
■ Include a sufficient number of results in the calculations to ensure reliability.

LESSON REVIEW

1. What is the importance of a quality control program?

2. Explain the use of standards and controls in chemistry procedures.
3. How is the mean of a sample determined?
4. Explain how to calculate the standard deviation.
5. How can an out-of-control result be detected?
6. Explain how to detect a trend.
7. How is coefficient of variation used?
8. Define accuracy, average, coefficient of variation, control serum, Gaussian curve, Levey-Jennings chart, mean, population, precision, random error, sample, standard, standard deviation, statistics, systematic error, trend, and Westgard's rules.

STUDENT ACTIVITIES

1. Re-read the information on quality control.
2. Practice calculating the standard deviation, using this group of numbers: 10, 9, 15, 10, 12, 11, 10, 12, 14, 12.
3. Using the results of the calculations from above, construct a quality control chart showing the mean, +1s, +2s, +3s, -1s, -2s, and -3s.

Student Performance Guide

NAME _____

DATE _____

LESSON 7–2
QUALITY CONTROL

Instructions

1. Practice gathering data and calculating the mean and the standard deviation for those values.
2. Calculate the mean and standard deviation satisfactorily for the instructor. All steps must be completed as listed on the instructor's Performance Check Sheet.
3. Complete a written examination successfully.

Materials and Equipment

- paper
- pencil
- calculator (optional)

Procedure			S = Satisfactory U = Unsatisfactory
You must:	**S**	**U**	**Comments**
1. Assemble paper, pencil, and calculator			
2. Find the mean of these results from a red cell procedure: 3.2, 3.3, 3.5, 3.2, 3.0, 3.4, 3.8, 3.5, 3.4, and 3.3 a. Give the formula for finding the mean			
b. Substitute the values into the formula			
c. The mean is:			

419

You must:	S	U	Comments
3. Give the formula for determining the standard deviation			
a. Substitute the numbers into the formula			
b. What is the standard deviation?			

4. Construct a Levey-Jennings Chart using the information from #3
   a. Label one line "mean"
   b. Label the lines for +1s and +2s and for -1s and -2s
   c. Plot the following control results: 3.1, 3.4, 3.1, 3.2, 3.5, and 3.8 (days 1–6)			

You must:	S	U	Comments
5. Observe the chart. Do any of the values fall outside the $\pm 2s$ limits?			
6. Put all materials away in their proper places			

Comments:

Student/Instructor:

Date:_____ Instructor:_____

LESSON 7-3
The Spectrophotometer

LESSON OBJECTIVES

After studying this lesson, you should be able to:
- Explain the principle of the spectrophotometer.
- List the parts of the spectrophotometer.
- State Beer's Law.
- Use the spectrophotometer.
- Construct a standard curve.
- List precautions that should be observed when using a spectrophotometer.
- Define the glossary terms.

GLOSSARY

absorbance / the light absorbed by a substance containing colored molecules, designated in formulas by "A"; also called optical density (O.D.)

Beer's Law / a mathematical relationship upon which the basis of analysis by spectrophotometry is formed and which shows that absorbance is related linearly to concentration

cuvette / a tube manufactured to strict standards for clarity and lack of distortion in the glass and used to hold liquids to be examined in the spectrophotometer

diffraction grating / a device which disperses light into a spectrum

galvanometer / instrument which measures electrical current

monochromatic light / light consisting of one color; light which is of one wavelength

monochromator / device which isolates a narrow portion of the light spectrum

percent transmittance / the percentage of light which passes through a substance; %T

photoelectric cell / a device which detects light and converts it into electricity

reagent blank / a solution which contains some or all of the reagents used in the test but does not contain the substance being tested

spectrophotometer / an instrument which measures intensities of light in different parts of the spectrum

standard curve / in spectrophotometry, a graph which shows the relationship between the concentrations and absorbances (or percent transmittances) of a series of standard solutions

INTRODUCTION

The spectrophotometer is a frequently used instrument in the clinical laboratory (Figure 7–5). A spectrophotometer may be a separate instrument used for manual chemical procedures or may be incorporated into an automated chemistry analyzer. Many clinical chemistry methods use the principles of spectrophotometry.

PRINCIPLES OF SPECTROPHOTOMETRY

Spectrophotometers are used to determine the concentrations of colored solutions. This determination is made by passing a narrow beam of light through the solution. The portion of light which passes through the colored solution is the **percent transmittance**. The light which does not pass

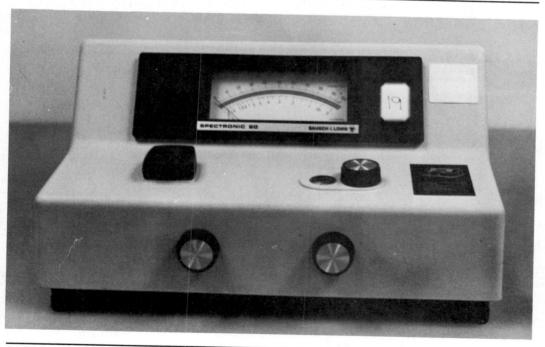

Figure 7–5. An example of a spectrophotometer *(Photo by John Estridge)*

through is absorbed by the solution and is measured as **absorbance.** Concentrated solutions allow less light to pass through than dilute solutions. Thus, it can be said that the more concentrated the solution, the greater its absorbance and the less its transmittance. Either the absorbance or the percent transmittance can be read from most spectrophotometers. For most colored solutions, the absorbance increases with the concentration. These solutions are said to follow **Beer's Law,** a mathematical relationship which shows that the absorbance of a colored solution is directly proportional to its concentration. This relationship is linear. For most colored solutions the percent transmittance decreases as the concentration increases; this relationship is geometric (nonlinear).

PARTS OF THE SPECTROPHOTOMETER

Spectrophotometers vary in external design but have essentially the same internal parts (see Figure 7–6). Each of these parts has a function in the measurement of a solution's concentration. A light source in the spectrophotometer provides a beam of light which passes to a **monochromator.** This monochromator has a **diffraction grating** which disperses the light into a spectrum. It also contains a slit which isolates a narrow beam of **monochromatic light,** light of one wavelength. This monochromatic light is directed toward the sample well in which a cuvette holding the colored solution is placed. The **cuvette** is a special tube manufactured to precise specifications. A portion of the light will be absorbed by the molecules in the solution and a portion of the light will pass through the solution. The light which passes through is detected by a **photoelectric cell** which converts it to electrical current. This current is measured and recorded by a **galvanometer.** The information can be presented as either absorbance (A) units or percent transmittance (%T) on the readout display of the spectrophotometer.

STANDARD CURVE

A **standard curve** can be used to determine the concentrations of colored solutions which follow

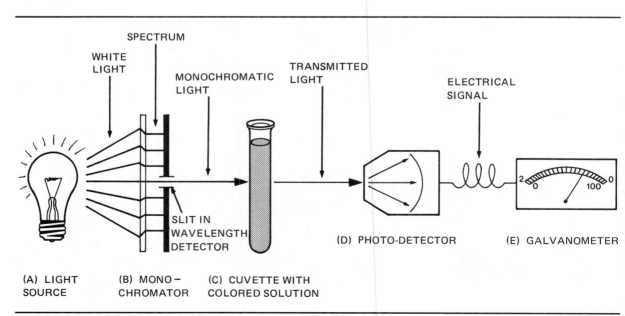

Figure 7–6. Diagram of internal parts of a spectrophotometer

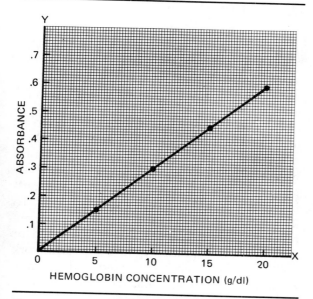

Figure 7–7. Illustration of a standard curve showing absorbance vs concentration

Beer's Law. Dilutions of a standard of known concentration are reacted with a reagent which forms a color whose intensity is proportional to the concentration of the standard substance. The absorbances, or percent transmittances, of the solutions are then determined using the spectrophotometer. The results (A or %T) are plotted against the concentrations of the diluted standards, and a line is drawn through the points (Figure 7–7). Absorbance is plotted using linear graph paper. If percent transmittance is measured, semilog paper must be used to obtain a straight line. This graph, the standard curve, may then be used to find the concentration of unknowns of the same substance. A standard curve must be prepared for each test method and each spectrophotometer.

Example of Preparation of a Standard Curve Using Hemoglobin

A standard curve can be prepared easily using hemoglobin as the standard solution. (Details of hemoglobin analysis are explained in Lesson 2–7.) Hemoglobin, when mixed with Drabkin's reagent, is converted to cyanmethemoglobin, a pigment which absorbs light at 540 nm. A standard curve for hemoglobin can be made using dilutions of a 20 g/dl hemoglobin standard.

Standards are available in various concentrations and manufacturer's instructions should be followed in preparing the dilutions and calculating concentrations. Hemoglobin standards may be purchased as a dry powder to be reconstituted with Drabkin's reagent or in a ready-to-use solution. Drabkin's reagent contains cyanide, must be handled with caution, and must not be mouth pipetted.

Determining the Absorbances of the Standards. Dilutions of the hemoglobin standard are made with Drabkin's reagent, the reagent used in the hemoglobin test. Four tubes consisting of 5, 10, 15, and 20 g/dl hemoglobin are set up. The spectrophotometer wavelength is set to 540 nm and the absorbance is set to zero using Drabkin's reagent as the **reagent blank**. A reagent blank is a solution that contains the reagents of the test but none of the substance being measured. The standard dilutions are transferred to a cuvette and the absorbance of each is determined and recorded.

Plotting the Standard Curve. Using graph paper, the absorbances are plotted on the "Y" axis (ordinate), and the concentrations on the "X" axis (abscissa) as shown in Figure 7–7. A line is drawn through the four points on the graph. If the dilutions were made correctly and the absorbances were measured correctly, a line drawn through the points of the standards should be straight and should pass through the origin (0, 0). If all the points do not fall in a straight line, a ruler can be used to draw a line of "best fit" which connects most of the points. The standard curve is then ready to be used to determine the hemoglobin concentration in a blood sample. The absorbance of the unknown solution is read and the value is matched with an absorbance on the graph. The

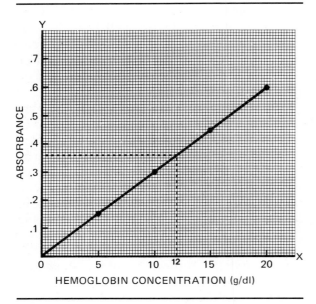

Figure 7–8. Determining the concentration of an unknown using a standard curve. The absorbance of the unknown is .360; the concentration of the unknown is read as 12.0 g/dl from the standard curve.

concentration of the unknown can then be read directly from the graph (Figure 7–8). This method of measurement is valid only when the substance follows Beer's Law. (If %T is read for the standards, the standard curve must be plotted on semi-log graph paper to obtain a straight line.)

If only one standard is used, the concentration of an unknown may be found by using the formula:

$$C_u = \frac{A_u}{A_s} \times C_s$$

Where: C_u = concentration of unknown
C_s = concentration of standard
A_u = absorbance of unknown
A_s = absorbance of standard

Again, this formula may only be used for solutions which are known to follow Beer's Law. A sample calculation using this formula is shown in Figure 2–35.

QUALITY CONTROL

Quality control procedures should be performed on spectrophotometers periodically according to manufacturer's instructions. The spectrophotometer should be checked for stray light before each use. This is done by verifying that the percent transmittance reads zero when the light path is blocked. Wavelength settings may be verified by using a didymium filter or holmium oxide glass, which have maximum absorbance at a particular wavelength. Wavelength verification must be performed routinely, according to manufacturer's instructions, and after any lamp adjustment. To insure that results from a spectrophotometer are reliable, a standard curve must be constructed for each instrument at the beginning of each work day, when new reagents are used, and after any repair or lamp replacement. Controls must also be run with every set of determinations.

CARE OF SPECTROPHOTOMETER AND CUVETTES

The spectrophotometer should be kept covered when not in use to protect it from dust. Jarring the instrument or spilling reagents onto the spectrophotometer should be avoided. The same precautions that are followed when using any electrical instrument should be observed.

Cuvettes should be optically matched and kept free from scratches. They should be washed carefully, avoiding the use of abrasives, rinsed in distilled water, and air-dried. Cuvettes should be inverted when stored to avoid dust. They should be held only by the upper edge, and the outside of the cuvette should be wiped free of fingerprints before using.

Precautions

■ Allow the spectrophotometer to warm up before use.
■ Check the spectrophotometer daily with standards and controls.

■ Use cuvettes which are clean and unscratched.
■ Avoid spilling reagents onto the spectrophotometer.
■ Set the instrument to zero absorbance (100%T) with a water or reagent blank before measuring a sample.
■ Follow test procedures carefully.

What kind of solution is used to set the instrument at 100%T or zero absorbance?
5. Make a simple sketch of a standard curve.
6. List the precautions that should be observed when using a spectrophotometer.
7. Define absorbance, Beer's Law, cuvette, diffraction grating, galvanometer, monochromatic light, monochromator, percent transmittance, photoelectric cell, reagent blank, spectrophotometer, and standard curve.

LESSON REVIEW

1. Explain the principle of operation of the spectrophotometer.
2. Diagram and name the parts of the spectrophotometer.
3 . What is Beer's Law?
4. Explain how a spectrophotometer is used to measure the concentration of a solution.

STUDENT ACTIVITIES

1. Re-read the information on the spectrophotometer.
2. Review the glossary terms.
3. Practice the procedure for using the spectrophotometer to construct a standard curve as outlined on the Student Performance Guide, using the worksheet.

Student Performance Guide

NAME _____

DATE _____

LESSON 7–3
THE SPECTROPHOTOMETER

Instructions

1. Practice the procedure for using the spectrophotometer to prepare a standard curve.
2. Demonstrate the procedure for using the spectrophotometer to prepare a standard curve satisfactorily for the instructor. All steps must be completed as listed on the instructor's Performance Check Sheet.
3. Complete a written examination successfully.

Materials and Equipment

- spectrophotometer
- gloves
- hand disinfectant
- biohazard container
- surface disinfectant
- soft laboratory tissue
- worksheet or graph paper
- pen or pencil
- 5 and 10 ml graduated pipets
- automatic pipetter or safety bulb
- parafilm
- cuvettes (use matched cuvettes for clinical work)
- distilled water
- Drabkin's reagent
- test tubes, 13 × 100 mm
- standard hemoglobin solution (20 g/dl or other available concentration)
- chlorine bleach

Note: The following is a general procedure for use of a spectrophotometer. Consult the instructions in the operating manual for correct procedure for the instrument being used.

Procedure			S = Satisfactory U = Unsatisfactory
You must:	**S**	**U**	**Comments**
1. Wash hands with disinfectant and put on gloves			
2. Turn on spectrophotometer to warm up (use time suggested by manufacturer, usually 10 to 30 minutes)			
3. Set wavelength to 540 nm			
4. Assemble materials			
5. Label five test tubes: 0 (blank), 5, 10, 15, and 20			
6. Reconstitute the hemoglobin standard according to manufacturer's instructions			

7. Make dilutions of the hemoglobin standard as follows:
  a. Pipet Drabkin's reagent into the tubes using a 5 or 10 ml pipet with safety bulb (or automatic pipet):
 	
  Tube
  0 = 6.0 ml
  5 = 4.5 ml
  10 = 3.0 ml
  15 = 1.5 ml
  20 = 0 ml			

b. Pipet the hemoglobin standard solution into the same tubes as follows, using a clean 5 ml pipet:
 	
  Tube
  0 = 0 ml
  5 = 1.5 ml
  10 = 3.0 ml
  15 = 4.5 ml
  20 = 6.0 ml			

8. Observe the tubes to see that each contains the same volume (6.0 ml) and mix each tube well using parafilm to cover top of tube			
9. Transfer contents of the "0" tube to a clean cuvette and place in cuvette well of spectrophotometer. *Note:* Wipe all fingerprints from cuvette with soft tissue before inserting any cuvette into spectrophotometer			

You must:	S	U	Comments
10. Place the cap over the top of the cuvette well and set absorbance to zero using control knob			
11. Remove the "0" cuvette from well			
12. Transfer contents of the "5" tube to a clean cuvette and place in cuvette well			
13. Record absorbance (Do not adjust absorbance control)			
14. Remove cuvette from the sample well			
15. Repeat steps 11–13 for tubes 10, 15, and 20			
16. Record the results on worksheet			
17. Draw the "X" and "Y" axes as shown in Figure 7–7			
18. Label the "X" axis in units of hemoglobin concentration: 0, 5, 10, 15, 20 g/dl			
19. Label the "Y" axis in absorbance (A) units from 0–1.0 using intervals of 0.100			
20. Plot the absorbances of tubes 5, 10, 15, 20			
21. Draw the best straight line through the points, being sure it passes through the origin (0, 0)			
22. Save this graph for use in determining the hemoglobin concentration of a blood sample (Lesson 2–7)			
23. Disinfect and clean the equipment and return to proper storage			
24. Dispose of used reagents and contaminated materials properly			
25. Disinfect working area with surface disinfectant			
26. Remove and discard gloves appropriately and wash hands with hand disinfectant			

Comments:

Student/Instructor:

Date:_____ Instructor:_____

Worksheet

NAME _____ DATE _____

LESSON 7–3 THE SPECTROPHOTOMETER

1. Record results from spectrophotometer:

Concentration of Standard	A (or %T)
0 (blank)	_____
_____	_____
_____	_____
_____	_____
_____	_____

2. Label the "X" and "Y" axes appropriately. Plot A vs. concentration. Draw a line connecting the points. The line should pass through the origin (0, 0). (If %T is used, semi-log paper must be used to obtain a straight line.)

LESSON 7–4
Instrumentation in the Small Laboratory

LESSON OBJECTIVES

After studying this lesson, you should be able to:

- Explain the differences in the types of instruments used in small and large laboratories.
- Discuss the reasons for the increase in testing in small laboratories.
- Discuss the basic differences in continuous flow, discrete, and centrifugal analyzers.
- Explain the principle of solid-phase analyzers.
- Explain the principle of ion selective electrodes.
- Discuss the importance of maintenance and quality control of instruments.
- Define the glossary terms.

GLOSSARY

centrifugal analysis / a type of discrete chemical analysis in which the reagents and sample are mixed together by centrifugal action

continuous flow analysis / a method of analysis in which the reagents and samples are flowing through the instrument all the time

discrete analysis / a method of analysis in which the assay procedure for each sample is performed in its own separate container

ion selective electrode / an electrode which has been manufactured to be responsive to the concentration of a specific ion

POL / physician's office laboratory

reflectance photometry / method of analysis in which the light reflected off a colored reaction product is measured by a light detector

solid-phase chemistry / an analytical method in which the sample is added to a strip or slide containing, in dried form, all the reagents for the procedure

spectrophotometer / an instrument which can be used to measure the amount of light absorbed by a colored solution or light transmitted through such a solution

INTRODUCTION

Automated instruments make it possible for laboratories to perform test procedures with more speed and better precision, in general, than can be obtained in manual methods. However, it must be kept in mind that, for the most part, automation involves adapting the principles of manual methods to instruments. This, of course, is especially important in larger laboratories where several hundred analyses are run daily. However, automation also has a place in smaller laboratories. The initial purchase price, cost per test and ease of operation and maintenance are points to be considered when choosing an instrument, whether for a small or large laboratory.

In the last three to four years, laboratory instrumentation has undergone a sort of revolution. When the main workload of clinical tests was performed in hospital laboratories, the major instrument manufacturers concentrated on developing larger and more diversified instruments capable of performing an ever larger variety and number of tests on one instrument. The emphasis was on reducing the time required to process a specimen and report the results (turn-around time), along with lowering the cost per test. Medicaid and Medicare payment limits set by government regulations have given added importance to cost control in the laboratory. As a result of these restricting regulations, an increased number of physicians have begun to perform laboratory tests in their offices.

Increase in Physician's Office Testing

The number of physician's office laboratories (POLs) is increasing rapidly. The availability of testing in the physician's office can be a benefit, especially to very sick and elderly patients, if the quality of testing is good. The instrument manufacturers have responded to this demand with the development of small, simple to operate instruments which easily fit on a lab bench in the office laboratory. Some are also being used in small hospital laboratories. The rivalry to produce efficient, reliable, and inexpensive instruments is intense among the manufacturers. Updates and improvements of the instruments are constantly being brought to market. One must be careful in selecting an instrument in order to avoid obsolescence after only a short time.

This lesson presents just a few examples of the many instruments available for the POL or other small laboratory. The principles of each instrument are discussed, and examples of the tests each can perform are provided.

The instruments featured in this lesson were chosen because they are in use in laboratories in the surrounding community and it was convenient to see them in operation. The description of an instrument does not constitute an endorsement of the instrument, just as the ommission of an instrument does not mean lack of endorsement.

Three Basic Types of Technology

Automated clinical chemistry can be separated into three major approaches: continuous flow, discrete analysis, and centrifugal analysis. **Continuous flow analysis** means that reagents and samples are flowing through the instrument all the time, with samples introduced one after another at certain time intervals. The result is that the samples are separated from each other by a known amount of reagent and sometimes by air bubbles.

In **discrete analysis** the assay procedure for each sample is performed in its own separate container, usually a tube or packet. In this method, no mixing of individual samples can occur. Most of the instruments suitable for use in small laboratories use the principle of discrete analysis. **Centrifugal analysis** involves discrete analysis carried out in a centrifuge. The centrifugal force causes the reagents to mix with the patient sample in the packet. The final product is read by a spectrophotometer in the instrument. A **spectrophotometer** is an instrument which can measure the amount of light absorbed by a colored solution or light transmitted through such a solution.

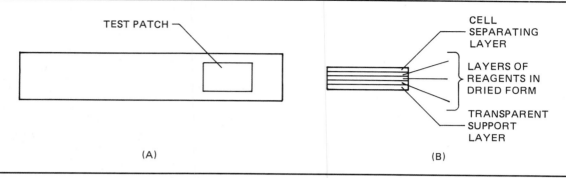

Figure 7–9. Illustration of a solid-phase reagent strip. (A) Top view of a strip, showing reagent test patch. (B) Expanded, side view of a test patch, showing the layers.

Another type of discrete analysis is represented by the **solid-phase chemistry** analyzers. In these analyzers, the sample is added to a strip or slide containing, in dried form, all the reagents used in the test (Figure 7–9). The reagents are in multi-layers, with each layer having a specific function in the reaction. The area where the dried reagents are located is called the *test area* or *reagent pad*. Some reagent pads have the capability to trap the cellular elements of the blood in the top layer and allow only the plasma to proceed down into the pad. The support layer on the bottom is transparent, which makes it possible for the final colored product of the reaction to be read by the instrument after a prescribed incubation time. The instrument calculates and displays the final result. These analyzers use a different strip for each type of test performed: one strip for cholesterol, one for glucose, etc. Each strip also has a magnetic code to tell the machine which test is to be performed. Some test strips come individually wrapped and sealed for the preservation of the reagents and for protection against contamination until the time of use.

EXAMPLES OF AVAILABLE INSTRUMENTS

Discrete Analyzers

Several manufacturers offer discrete analyzers that are very suitable for small laboratories. East-man Kodak Company has on the market several versions of its Ektachem DT system. One which is well suited to small laboratories is the Ektachem DT60. Each test procedure is performed on a slide specific to that analysis. The sample may be from a capillary puncture or a venipuncture, but only plasma or serum can be used for the chemistry tests.

To perform an analysis, the appropriate slide is chosen for the test to be performed—glucose, cholesterol, etc. If the slide has been refrigerated it must be warmed up according to the manufacturer's instructions. The slide is placed into the sample drawer of the instrument which is then closed (Figure 7–10). The instrument reads the magnetic code on the slide to determine which test is to be performed. A pipet which comes with the instrument is used to draw up 10 microliters (μl) of the sample. The tip of this pipet is then placed into a pipet opening in the top of the instrument and the 10 μl are dispensed onto the test slide. The reaction is allowed to proceed and the colored product obtained is measured by a reflectance photometer. A **reflectance photometer** measures the light which a colored product reflects onto a light detector in the instrument. The instrument converts this information into the test result.

New tests are constantly being added, but currently at least 27 different procedures are available. The basic unit is capable of analyzing glucose, BUN/urea, uric acid, total protein,

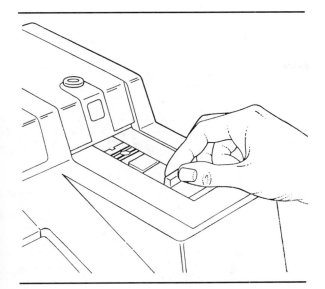

Figure 7–10. Illustration of the insertion of the sample card into the Kodak Ektachem DT60 *(Courtesy of Kodak)*

triglycerides, cholesterol, HDL cholesterol, magnesium, creatinine, ammonia, amylase, total bilirubin, hemoglobin and phosphorous. These can be run at the rate of 65 tests per hour. The instrument will print out all results.

New modules are available for the DT60 which provide additional capabilities. The DTE module permits testing of sodium, potassium, chloride and CO_2 levels. The DTSC module adds the ability to analyze AST, ALT, LDH, CK, CKMB, ALKP, GGT, calcium, theophylline, lipase and creatinine. The DTE module performs tests at a rate of 15 per hour and DTSC module performs 20 tests per hour.

Kodak is currently developing materials for additional tests such as thyroid function, therapeutic drug screening and the fractions of bilirubin. At the present time the DT60 is being used in many POLs, outpatient clinics, intensive care units, and in small hospital laboratories; it is even used on cargo and passenger ships.

The Reflotron® is an instrument manufactured by Boehringer Mannheim Diagnostics. This instrument is also a popular choice for POLs or other small laboratories. Narrow strips called

reagent tabs come with the reagents already applied in dried form to an area designated as the test patch. This test patch is protected by foil until immediately before the sample is applied. The reagent tabs for each of the various individual tests are kept in separate vials. As in the DT60 slides, the layers have distinct functions. Whole blood, serum, or the plasma from EDTA and heparinized blood can be used, depending on which test is being performed. The hemoglobin test utilizes only whole blood.

To perform the test, the sample is drawn up into the Reflotron® pipette and dispensed onto the reagent pad which had been covered by foil. The tab is inserted into the instrument within 15 seconds of sample application. The instrument reads the magnetic code to determine which test to perform. Confirmation of which assay is being performed is shown in the display area. This assures the worker that the correct strip is being used. The time required for the assay is also displayed until the reaction is finished. The result for the procedure is displayed on the read-out screen.

The time required for most reactions is 180 seconds (three minutes). The absorbance of the colored product of the reactions is read by reflectance photometry as in the DT60. The instrument converts the absorbance value into mg/dl for conventional units, or mmol/L for SI units.

Discrete Analyzers, Centrifugal Type

Abbott Laboratories has available on the market an analyzer called the VISION™ System (Figure 7–11). The instrument is a discrete centrifugal analyzer. For this instrument, the reagents are prepackaged in a testpack into which the sample is added. The action of centrifugation mixes the reagents and sample together inside the pack and all reactions take place within that pack. At the end of the reaction time the absorbance of the final product is measured by a spectrophotometer in the instrument.

The VISION™ System testpacks resemble small recording cassettes. Each test procedure, such as

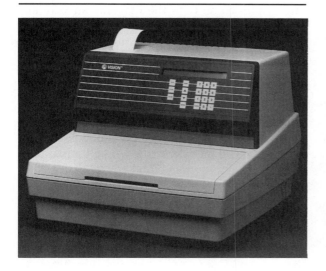

Figure 7–11. The VISION™ System clinical chemistry analyzer *(Photo courtesy of Abbott Laboratories)*

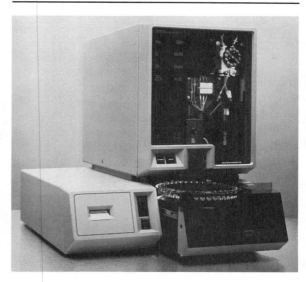

Figure 7–12. The NOVA 12 clinical chemistry analyzer *(Photo courtesy of NOVA Biomedical)*

glucose or cholesterol, is contained in its own individual pack. Only two drops of sample are required for each procedure. The sample of whole blood, plasma or serum is added into the pack through a special opening. If whole blood is used for a clinical chemistry test, the cells are removed from the plasma by a cell-separating chamber in the testpack; the plasma then proceeds through the pack to be analyzed. During the reaction time, the testpack is centrifuged and rotated in various directions to force the sample and reagents together in sequenced chambers. Different portions of the reaction occur in each chamber as the sample travels through the pack. The method allows for an incubation time if one is necessary for a particular test. At the end of the reaction time the absorbance of the final product is measured by a built-in spectrophotomer, using a chamber of the pack as the cuvette.

Presently at least 23 clinical chemistry test procedures are available for the VISION™ including alkaline phosphatase, glucose, cholesterol, creatinine, AST, theophylline, triglycerides, urea nitrogen, ALT, and potassium. Tests for calcium,

HDL-cholesterol, amylase, CK, T_4, LDH, and total bilirubin have recently been added. Additional procedures are constantly being developed. Testpacks for immunochemistry, hematology and coagulation are either available or under development.

Up to ten testpacks can be processed at the same time in the VISION™ System. The average time required for an analysis is about eight minutes.

Ion Selective Electrodes

Another type of technology which is increasing is ion-selective electrodes. The NOVA 12, by NOVA Biomedical (Figure 7–12), has the capability to perform the tests most frequently requested in emergency situations such as in the hospital emergency room, and can also be valuable in a physician's office. Analysis of sodium, potassium, chloride, CO_2, blood urea nitrogen and glucose can be performed. Either serum or plasma can be used in the analysis and the sample volume required is 450 μl.

This analyzer utilizes the technology of **ion selective electrodes** (ISE). Each electrode in the instrument has been manufactured to be responsive to the presence of a specific ion; for example, the Na^+ electrode will measure only the Na^+ ions present in the solution.

Two electrodes are used in an analysis. One electrode contains a known concentration of the substance to be measured and is called the reference electrode. The other electrode, responsive only to the ion being analyzed, is exposed to the unknown solution. The difference in concentration between the two solutions causes an electrical potential to develop across a membrane in the electrode. This potential is measured in voltage and is proportional to the difference in concentrations of the two solutions. A microprocessor converts this voltage into a number representing the concentration of the ion in the unknown sample.

All of the test procedures performed on the instrument use the ISE principle. The patient sample is used undiluted so that no dilutor or dispenser is needed. The need for a spectrophotometer is eliminated since no colorimetric reaction is involved. The use of a single technology reduces the number of things that can go wrong in the instrument. Each type of electrode has an expected period of service and can be individually replaced.

The NOVA 12 has the capacity to process up to 360 samples every hour. A maximum of 40 samples can be loaded at one time. If a stat is ordered, the batch that is running can be interrupted and the stat can be analyzed in less than 90 seconds. This instrument could be used in a physician's office lab which has a steady volume of testing, but would be of optimum value in a small hospital laboratory or in an emergency room laboratory.

An additional instrument which is in use in physicians' office laboratories and which uses ISE technology is the Ionetics Electrolyte Analyzer II. This instrument has miniature electrodes which can measure the concentration of sodium and potassium in an undiluted sample of whole blood, plasma or serum. Many small laboratories combine this instrument with one which has the capability to perform other clinical chemistry tests, but can't perform electrolytes.

MAINTENANCE AND QUALITY CONTROL

All of these analyzers have the capability to provide reliable results for the constituents being examined. However, there are certain maintenance and upkeep procedures which must be performed at regular intervals if the results of the analyses are to remain credible. Although some of these instruments operate on quite similar principles, one must always consult each manufacturer's protocol for that specific instrument. Also, the reagents or strips for one instrument should never be used on another instrument. Another important point is to be certain that as new modules or acessories become available for an instrument, the worker follows the instructions for the operation, care and maintenance of these additions.

The manufacturers of each of the instruments discussed have developed a program of quality control for the laboratory to follow when using one of their analyzers. Each type of instrument has control materials available to be used in the procedures which it performs. These materials may include calibrator solutions, control solutions, and control sera with normal and abnormal values. The specifics for certain instruments are included below.

Solid Phase

The solid-phase analyzers' control solutions are applied to test strips in the same manner as patient samples. The Reflotron® controls are performed using control sera which have known assay values. Control sera for normal levels and abnormal levels of the constituent being analyzed are available. Also available are solutions which are used to calibrate the instrument.

Discrete Analyzers

The VISION™ System supplies quality control materials to help insure that the results obtained on the instrument are reliable. The manufacturer also makes available a Quality Commitment Program in which the purchaser is provided with QCP samples about four times a year. These samples are analyzed by the laboratory and the results sent to Abbott. If the laboratory's results are within two standard deviations of the known value, a certificate verifying the success is sent to the laboratory. If the results are not within two standard deviations, a technical representative will be sent to the laboratory to help review procedures and to check the instrument.

Ion Selective Electrodes

The instruments which utilize ISE technology are checked by the use of calibration standards containing known concentrations of specific ions. Control sera which have known concentrations of ions are analyzed and used for quality control programs. The electrodes used in the ISE type instrument require special care if error is to be kept to a minimum. The electrodes must be rinsed immediately after use to prevent damage caused by serum, plasma or whole blood drying on them. When the blood sample is collected, the manufacturer's instructions regarding the use of anticoagulants must be strictly followed. Most analyzers require heparinized specimens and prohibit the use of any anticoagulant containing potassium salts because they interfere with analysis of potassium ions in patient samples.

CONCLUSION

In conclusion, the worker's responsibility is to be able to run the instruments in the laboratory in a conscientious way. The worker must keep abreast of new developments or any revisions in established methods. Principles and operation of instruments must be understood. Manufacterers' instructions for test procedures must be followed exactly. All maintenance and repair instructions must be adhered to and a logbook should be kept concerning any maintenance and repairs made. If the laboratory worker incorporates these goals into the daily routine, the instruments will perform reliably and produce results in which the physician can have confidence.

LESSON REVIEW

1. Explain why different types of instruments might be used in small and large laboratories.
2. Discuss the reasons for the increase in physician's office testing.
3. What are the basic differences in continuous flow, discrete, and centrifugal analyzers?
4. How do the solid-phase analyzers operate?
5. What is the principle of the ion selective methods?
6. Discuss the importance of a regular maintenance program.

STUDENT ACTIVITIES

1. Re-read the information on instrumentation in the small laboratory.
2. Review the glossary terms.
3. Arrange a tour of a small laboratory to observe some instruments in operation.
4. Select the appropriate worksheet (instrument available or no instrument available) and complete the activities listed.

Instrumentation Worksheet—If No Instrument Is Available

NAME_____ DATE _____

LESSON 7–4 INSTRUMENTATION IN THE SMALL LABORATORY

1. What are the three major technologies of clinical chemistry analyzers?

2. How would the requirements for an instrument used in a POL differ from those for an instrument in a large hospital laboratory?

3. Name an instrument which utilizes each of these technologies: solid-phase, centrifugal, and ISE.

4. What is the major cause of the increase in the amount of testing performed in physicians' office laboratories?

5. List five precautions to be observed when an instrument is being used for an analysis.

6. Why would the information in a maintenance logbook be important when a problem arises with an instrument?

Instrumentation Worksheet—If An Instrument Is Available

NAME_____ DATE _____

LESSON 7–4 INSTRUMENTATION IN THE SMALL LABORATORY

1. What is the name of the available instrument?

2. Is this instrument of the continuous flow, discrete, or ISE type?

3. If the instrument does not fit any of these categories, what type technology is involved?

4. List two test procedures which can be performed using this instrument.

5. How does the worker communicate to the instrument which test procedure is to be performed?

6. How are the control solutions utilized on this instrument?

7. Has a Levey-Jennings chart been constructed for the procedures run on this instrument? Are values plotted daily? Weekly?

8. Is plasma, serum, or whole blood used for the analyses performed on this instrument?

9. Are maintenance and repair records kept in a logbook?

10. List in order the steps for performing an analysis for glucose (or other component) using this instrument.

LESSON 7–5

Measurement of Blood Cholesterol

LESSON OBJECTIVES

After studying this lesson, you should be able to:
- Explain the functions of cholesterol in the body.
- Discuss the dangers of an elevated cholesterol.
- Explain the importance of HDL and LDL cholesterol.
- Give the mean values for total cholesterol for males and females in each age group.
- Give the normal mean values for HDL for males and females in each age group.
- Explain how the risk factor for heart disease can be calculated from the HDL and LDL values.
- Explain the principle of the enzymatic methods of cholesterol measurement.
- Perform a cholesterol determination.
- Define the glossary terms.

GLOSSARY

atherosclerosis / a condition in which a deposit of fatty material narrows the interior of the arteries

endogeneous / produced within; growing from within

enzyme / a complex substance produced in living cells and able to cause or accelerate changes in other substances without being changed itself

exogenous / originating from the outside

HDL / high density lipoprotein; a fraction of total blood cholesterol

LDL / low density lipoprotein; a fraction of total blood cholesterol

myocardial infarction / heart attack caused by the obstruction of the blood supply to the heart or within the heart; abbreviated MI

photometer / any of various instruments for measuring the intensity of light

INTRODUCTION

Cholesterol is an important component of the body. It is used to make many of the different structural parts of all cells in the body. In addition, cholesterol is used in several other essential functions of the body. The cholesterol molecule is the basis for the manufacture of bile acids which enable the body to digest various types of fats and lipids; in fact, about 80% of cholesterol is utilized in this way. A small quantity of cholesterol is used to make certain hormones which are secreted by the adrenal cortex of the kidney, the testes and the ovaries. Some examples of these are adrenocortical hormones, testosterone, and progesterone and estrogen, respectively. Since cholesterol is classified chemically as a sterol these hormones are called steroid hormones.

A relatively large amount of cholesterol is located in the skin where it provides protection by making the skin highly resistant to the absorption of water-soluble substances. It also aids in protection against the action of chemical agents such as acids. Another function of cholesterol in the skin is to prevent excess evaporation of water from the body.

Sources of Cholesterol

Some cholesterol is found in the diet of all persons. This cholesterol from dietary sources is called **exogenous** cholesterol. Sources of cholesterol in the diet include animal fats and egg yolks. People who eat a rich, fatty diet may develop dangerously increased blood cholesterol levels. Certain tissues of the body, especially the liver, have the capability to make cholesterol from other components; this is called **endogenous** cholesterol.

BLOOD CHOLESTEROL

When blood cholesterol levels remain elevated, a condition known as **atherosclerosis** may occur. In this condition, fat accumulates on the inner walls of blood vessels, narrowing the vessel opening. These deposits form especially on any damaged surface of the vessel wall. Although other fats (lipids) are found in these deposits, the major portion is cholesterol. Once these deposits form, their rough edges may cause blood clots to develop. These clots can either damage the area they are in or travel to smaller vessels in vital organs such as the brain, heart, kidneys or liver and cut off the blood supply to these organs. The result may be stroke, heart attack, damage to other organs, or disease of the blood vessels themselves.

Total Cholesterol, HDL, and LDL

Cholesterol testing has become very common and popular in the eighties as diet and its relationship to well-being has become one of the latest health fads. It is not unusual for cholesterol testing booths to be set up in shopping malls; there may be a small fee or no charge at all for the test. However, the cholesterol level is very important to health and well-being and the current interest in the subject should not be regarded lightly.

In the past, blood cholesterol was reported only as total cholesterol. Now it is more meaningful to measure total cholesterol and the fractions of cholesterol. These two fractions are called high density lipoprotein (**HDL**) cholesterol and low density lipoprotein (**LDL**) cholesterol. The HDL is the molecule which transports cholesterol from the tissues to the liver to be broken down, mostly into bile acids. Because of this, HDL is called the "good" cholesterol. The LDL molecule transports cholesterol to the tissues to be deposited as fat. The LDL is sometimes referred to as the "bad" cholesterol. Some experts now believe that the amount of HDL or LDL in a person is genetically determined. If the total cholesterol concentration is elevated in a patient, the physician can use the HDL and LDL values to aid in determining the heart attack risk factor of the elevated cholesterol.

Normal Values for Cholesterol

At birth the serum cholesterol ranges from about 50 mg/dl to 100 mg/dl. At one month the levels approach 100 to 230 mg/dl and remain at those levels until the age of 20 or 21 years. The cholesterol levels for adults are affected by age, diet, and sex of the individual. Estrogen in women seems to have a lowering effect on cholesterol since in postmenopausal women the cholesterol level tends to increase. In some people, diet has a direct effect on the serum cholesterol levels while in others a high cholesterol diet does not seem to affect the serum level; presumably this is because of the HDL and LDL levels. Typical cholesterol values for the various age groups are shown in Table 7–1. Typical values for HDL and LDL are shown in Table 7–2.

Determining the Heart Attack Risk Factor

To determine the risk, the physician uses the ratio of LDL divided by the HDL. The smaller the ratio, the less the risk factor. When the HDL is elevated above the average value, it may reduce the risk of **myocardial infarction** by as much as one third.

As an example, a 45-year-old male (patient one) with an LDL level of 80 mg/dl and an HDL of 59 mg/dl would have a lower risk of heart attack than a second male (patient two) of the same age and identical LDL level, but an HDL of

Table 7–2. Normal ranges for HDL and LDL cholesterol

Age	HDL		LDL
(years)	Male Range mg/dl	Female Range mg/dl	Male and Female mg/dl
0–19	30–65	30–70	50–170
20–29	30–65	36–78	60–170
30–39	30–59	33–77	70–190
40–49	25–61	40–81	80–190
50–75	29–72	38–91	80–210

30 mg/dl. The risk factor (RF) is calculated by dividing the LDL value by the HDL value (RF = LDL/HDL). A low number means the risk of heart attack is decreased.

Patient one: $\dfrac{LDL}{HDL}$ = risk factor

$$\dfrac{80 \text{ mg/dl}}{59 \text{ mg/dl}} = 1.3$$

Patient two: $\dfrac{LDL}{HDL}$ = risk factor

$$\dfrac{80 \text{ mg/dl}}{30 \text{ mg/dl}} = 2.7$$

Therefore, in this comparison of two patients, patient one has a lower risk factor for heart attack than does patient two.

CHOLESTEROL TESTS

The serum cholesterol level can be determined in the laboratory using either chemical or enzyme methods. Techniques for total cholesterol have been in use for decades, but efficient, easy methods for HDL and LDL have been available only since about 1980. The enzymatic methods for testing cholesterol and its fractions are simpler and also use less hazardous chemicals than the non-enzyme (chemical) methods. Several kits for

Table 7–1. Normal levels of blood cholesterol

Age (years)	Range mg/dl	Males mg/dl	Females mg/dl
0–19	120–230	—	—
20–29	120–240	235	220
30–39	140–270	265	240
40–49	150–310	280	265
50–59	160–330	300	320

the enzymatic methods are available commercially. Serum is used as the sample; the volume required ranges from five to 100 μl, depending on which kit is being used. The enzymatic methods have also been adapted to automated instruments.

Manual Methods for Cholesterol

Several enzymatic methods are available for the determination of total cholesterol and the HDL fraction. The principle of the different methods is similar. The reactions described here are in procedure 352 from Sigma Diagnostics®. The method is a modification of one by Allain et al. Cholesterol is separated from the other constituents in the sample by an enzyme, cholesterol esterase. Cholesterol oxidase oxidizes the cholesterol released in the previous reaction, producing a ketone (cholestenone) plus hydrogen peroxide (H_2O_2). The hydrogen peroxide produced is then coupled with the chromagen, 4-aminoantipyrine, and p-hydroxybenzenesulfonate in the presence of peroxidase. A quinoneimine dye whose absorbance can be measured at 500 nm is the end product of the reaction. The intensity of the color of the dye is proportional to the concentration of cholesterol present in the sample. The reactions are as follows:

$$Cholesterol\ esters + H_2O \xrightarrow[\text{Esterase}]{\text{Cholesterol}} cholesterol + fatty\ acids$$

$$Cholesterol + O_2 \xrightarrow[\text{Oxidase}]{\text{Cholesterol}} cholest\text{-}4\text{-}en\text{-}3\text{-}one + H_2O_2$$

$$2\ H_2O_2 + 4\text{-}aminoantipyrine + p\text{-}hydroxybenzenesulfonate$$

$$\xrightarrow[]{\text{Peroxidase}} Quinoneimine\ dye + 4\ H_2O$$

The preferred specimen for this procedure is either serum or heparinized plasma. Anticoagulants such as oxalate, citrate, or EDTA yield slightly lower total cholesterol values.

All of the reactants necessary to perform the test are contained in one reagent called Cholesterol Reagent, which is reconstituted by the addition of deionized water just before use. A series of tubes is set up for Blank, Calibrator, Control and Sample. The reagent is warmed to the assay temperature. One milliliter of reagent is added to each of the tubes in the series. The test specimens—Blank 10 μl of deionized water, Calibrator, Control and Sample—are added to appropriately labeled tubes. The tubes are then mixed by gentle inversion, using parafilm to cover the tops. All the tubes are incubated for the length of time appropriate to the selected temperature of incubation. The absorbance of each tube is read at 500 nm. The readings must be completed within 30 minutes after incubation is finished. The concentration of cholesterol is calculated using the following formula:

$$\text{serum cholesterol (mg/dl)} = \frac{A_{TEST} - A_{BLANK}}{A_{CALIBRATOR} - A_{BLANK}} \times Calibrator\ \text{(mg/dl)}$$

For example, when serum was assayed for total cholesterol concentration by the described procedure, the following absorbance values were obtained:

$$A_{BLANK} = 0.022$$
$$A_{TEST} = 0.325$$
$$A_{CALIBRATOR} = 0.310$$

$$\text{serum cholesterol (mg/dl)} = \frac{A_{TEST} - A_{BLANK}}{A_{CAL} - A_{BLANK}} \times Cal\ mg/dl$$

$$\text{serum cholesterol (mg/dl)} = \frac{0.325 - 0.022}{0.310 - 0.022} \times 200^* = 210$$

*Concentration (mg/dl) of cholesterol in calibrator

The serum total cholesterol of this sample = 210 mg/dl.

The instructions are accompanied by a list of materials required, calibration facts and quality control information. It is important to always read the procedure bulletin which accompanied the assay kit being used, since procedures are periodically modified.

Determination of HDL Cholesterol

Some kits allow for the assay of the HDL fraction of cholesterol using the same kit used for total cholesterol. To determine the HDL level in serum, other lipoproteins are precipitated out with a precipitating reagent, and the sample is centrifuged. The liquid portion (supernatant) contains the HDL fraction of cholesterol. The supernatant is used as the sample in the reactions for cholesterol. In this case, the color of the dye is proportional to the amount of HDL cholesterol in the serum.

Automated Methods for Cholesterol

The most popular automated methods for cholesterol are based on the same principles as the enzymatic manual methods. However, many of these automated methods are simple to perform and take much less time to complete than the manual methods. The majority of the automated methods for use in small laboratories utilize what are called *solid-phase reagent strips.* These strips resemble the strips used for urinalysis. All of the reagents needed for the test reactions are embedded in a reagent pad on the plastic strip. As in the manual method, the reaction is enzymatic, and uses the same enzymes. The worker selects the appropriate strip for cholesterol. A drop of whole blood, serum or plasma from the patient is placed directly on the test area (reagent pad). If whole blood is being used, the cellular elements of the blood are removed by a special layer in the pad. The plasma then proceeds down into the pad and mixes with the reagents. The strip must be placed into the reading instrument within a short specified time after application of the sample. A magnetic code on the back of the strip signals to the instrument which test is being performed. The instrument then displays this information in the read-out area and the worker can confirm that the correct test strip is being used.

The reading instrument is a reflectance photometer which detects color changes in the reagent pad. The reaction is allowed to proceed for the required time, usually about three minutes. The instrument then displays the result in the read-out area. The simplicity, the short time requirement, and the option of using a drop of whole blood from a fingerstick make this a very desirable test method for physicians' office laboratories.

Quality Control

Quality control materials are available from the manufacturers of automated and manual methods. For the manual methods, a standard solution of known concentration is available. If the measured value of the controls is not within the limits defined by the manufacturer, the cause of the error must be discovered before any patient results can be released. The manufacturers of the automated solid-phase strip methods also offer controls to be applied to the strips to check reliability. If the control assay value is not within acceptable limits, no patient results can be released until the problem is identified. These control strip results can indicate whether or not the instrument is working properly or if the strips are reacting correctly.

LESSON REVIEW

1. What are the functions of cholesterol in the body?
2. What are the dangers of an elevated serum cholesterol value?
3. What is the importance of the HDL and LDL levels?
4. What is the average normal value for total cholesterol for males and females in the age groups 20–29 and 40–49?
5. Give the normal mean values for HDL for males and for females in the 40–49-year-old age range.

6. How is the risk factor for heart disease calculated using the HDL and LDL values?
7. Explain the principles of the enzymatic methods of cholesterol measurement.
8. Explain how to perform a manual cholesterol determination.
9. Define atherosclerosis, endogenous, exogenous, HDL, LDL, and myocardial infarction.

STUDENT ACTIVITIES

1. Re-read the information on cholesterol.
2. Review the glossary terms.
3. If cholesterol screening is offered in the community, ask which method is being used.
4. If possible, determine which instruments are in use in some physician's office laboratories in the community.
5. Review the general instructions for performing an automated cholesterol test.
6. Practice performing a cholesterol determination as outlined in the Student Performance Guide, using whatever method is available to you.

NAME _____

DATE _____

LESSON 7–5
MEASUREMENT OF
BLOOD CHOLESTEROL

Instructions

1. Practice the procedure for determination of cholesterol.
2. Demonstrate the cholesterol procedure(s) satisfactorily for the instructor. All steps must be completed as listed on the instructor's Performance Check Sheet.
3. Complete a written examination successfully.

Materials and Equipment

- gloves
- blood collecting equipment
- hand disinfectant
- spectrophotometer
- chlorine bleach
- commercial kit for manual determination of cholesterol
- necessary controls and standards
- marking pencil
- test tubes (13 × 100)
- test tube rack
- cuvettes for spectrophotometer
- laboratory tissue
- calculator (optional)
- pipetter with disposable tips
- water bath at 30°C or 37°C (optional)
- surface disinfectant
- biohazard container
- instrument for performing cholesterol determination
- materials to accompany the instrument
- necessary controls and standards
- Levey-Jennings chart

Note: The following is a general procedure for measuring cholesterol using Sigma Diagnostics® procedure no. 352. Consult the manufacturer's instructions for the specific method being used.

Procedure			S = Satisfactory U = Unsatisfactory
You must:	**S**	**U**	**Comments**
1. Assemble equipment and materials			
2. Wash hands with disinfectant and put on gloves			
3. Obtain blood sample from the patient, either by finger-stick or venipuncture, depending on the type of sample required			

4. Perform either method A or B:
  A. Manual Method
      1. Prepare Cholesterol Reagent according to instructions			

2. Set spectrophotometer wavelength to 500 nm			
3. Set the absorbance reading to zero using water as the blank (reference)			
4. If using spectrophotometer with temperature-controlled cuvette compartment, set temperature to 37° C If the instrument in step 4, above, is not available, the assay may be performed at ambient (room) temperature, or using a water bath at 30° or 37° C			
5. Label cuvettes or test tubes for Blank, Calibrator, Control and Sample			
6. Warm reagent to the temperature being used for the assay			
7. Pipet 1.0 ml of reagent into each of the prepared tubes			
8. Add 0.01 ml (10 µl) deionized water to the Blank			
9. Add 10 µl of Calibrator, Control, or Sample to the appropriately labeled tubes. Mix tubes by gentle inversion			
10. Incubate tubes or cuvettes for 10 minutes at 37°C (If assay temperature is ambient, incubate 18 minutes and if 30°C, incubate for 15 minutes)			
11. Read and record absorbances of all tubes at 500 nm. Complete the readings within 30 minutes after the end of incubation time			
12. Calculate total cholesterol in sample and control, using the absorbance formula (p. 444). Record the results			

You must:	S	U	Comments
B. Automated Method (general)			
1. Turn on the instrument			
2. Wash hands with disinfectant and put on gloves			
3. Prepare any control or calibrator reagents			
4. Run appropriate controls and/or calibrator samples			
5. Obtain correct patient specimen			
6. Choose appropriate test strip or pack for cholesterol determination			
7. Add patient sample to test system			
8. Insert strip or pack into instrument			
9. Insure that correct test is being performed			
10. Wait for results to be displayed or printed out			
11. Record results			
5. For whichever method is used, add the control values to a Levey-Jennings chart			
6. If the method is in control, report patient values			
7. Disinfect and clean reusable equipment			
8. Dispose of contaminated materials in biohazard container			
9. Wipe work area with surface disinfectant			
10. Turn instrument "OFF" (or leave as manual instructs)			
11. Remove gloves and discard properly			
12. Wash hands with hand disinfectant			
Comments:			
Student/Instructor:			

Date:_____   Instructor:_____

LESSON 7–6

Measurement of Blood Glucose

After studying this lesson, you should be able to:
- Explain the function of glucose in the body.
- Describe factors which affect blood glucose levels.
- Name two disorders of glucose metabolism.
- Explain how blood specimens for glucose measurement should be collected.
- Explain the purpose of a post-prandial glucose test.
- Explain how a glucose tolerance test is performed.
- Give the normal values for fasting blood glucose, two-hour post-prandial glucose, and glucose tolerance test.
- Explain the principles of the glucose oxidase and hexokinase methods of glucose analysis.
- Discuss the importance of performing quality control tests when using a glucose analyzer and performing a manual glucose procedure.
- Perform a blood glucose measurement using either a manual or automated method.
- Define the glossary terms.

GLOSSARY

chromogen / a substance which becomes colored when it undergoes a chemical change

diabetes mellitus / a disorder of carbohydrate metabolism characterized by a state of hyperglycemia due to insulin deficiency

glucagon / hormone produced in the pancreas, and which increases blood glucose concentration by promoting the conversion of glycogen to glucose

glucose oxidase / enzyme which converts glucose to gluconic acid and which is used in many glucose analytical methods

glucose tolerance test / testing of blood glucose at timed intervals following the ingestion of a standard glucose dose; oral glucose tolerance test; GTT

glycogen / storage form of glucose which is found in high concentration in the liver

glycolysis / energy production as a result of the conversion of glucose to pyruvate

hexokinase / enzyme which converts glucose to glucose-6-phosphate and which is used in glucose analytical methods

hyperglycemia / blood glucose concentration above normal

hypoglycemia / blood glucose concentration below normal

insulin / pancreatic hormone which lowers blood glucose concentration

peroxidase / enzyme which converts hydrogen peroxide to water and oxygen

post-prandial / after eating

renal threshold / the blood concentration above which a substance which is not normally excreted by the kidneys appears in the urine

INTRODUCTION

Glucose is the major carbohydrate in the blood. It is used for energy by the body's cells. Excess carbohydrates are stored for reserve energy. The short-term storage form of glucose is **glycogen,** which is stored primarily in the liver. Long-term storage is in fat.

Although the body has many enzymatic pathways which use glucose, the concentration of blood glucose is normally constant within a fairly narrow range, due to the controlling action of hormones. One such hormone is **insulin,** which is produced by the pancreas. Insulin lowers the concentration of glucose by increasing cells' glucose intake and increasing the rate of glycogen formation. Insulin also increases the rate of **glycolysis,** the process in cell cytoplasm by which glucose is enzymatically converted to pyruvate or lactic acid. Hormones such as growth hormone, epinephrine, cortisol and **glucagon** act in a variety of ways to increase blood glucose concentration.

The two major types of disorders involving glucose metabolism are 1) those such as **diabetes mellitus** in which there is an increased blood glucose level, or **hyperglycemia;** and 2) those

having a decreased blood glucose level, or **hypoglycemia,** as may be seen in deficiencies of ACTH or growth hormone.

Measurement of blood glucose is a commonly performed chemistry test. The test is most often used to aid in the diagnosis and management of diabetes, but can also be used in the management of hypoglycemia, a less common condition.

SPECIMENS FOR GLUCOSE ANALYSIS

Glucose quantitation may be made on whole blood, plasma, serum, urine or cerebral spinal fluid. If serum or plasma is to be used, it must be separated from cells as soon as possible after collection. The cells contain glycolytic enzymes which can rapidly lower the concentration of plasma or serum glucose. If whole blood glucose is to be measured, the test should be performed immediately following capillary puncture or on blood collected in an anticoagulant. A mixture of sodium fluoride and potassium oxalate, an anticoagulant which inhibits the enzymes of glycolysis, is sometimes used. However, this anticoagulant interferes with some automated glucose methods, such as the glucometer method, and cannot be used. In those instances, an alternate anticoagulant such as EDTA or heparin must be used.

TIME OF SPECIMEN COLLECTION

The time of specimen collection is important, since blood glucose concentration rises rapidly after eating and then falls. The rate of increase depends on the rate of digestion, absorption, and clearance or removal from blood. Usually, fasting (10–12 hours after last meal) or two-hour **post-prandial** (after eating) specimens are tested. Post-prandial tests are most reliable if the patient is given a standard dose of carbohydrate or glucose for breakfast.

GLUCOSE TOLERANCE TEST

In the diagnosis of diabetes mellitus it is often helpful to perform a **glucose tolerance test** (GTT). In this test, the patient's fasting glucose level is measured. The patient is then given a standard dose of glucose (usually a drink) to ingest. The blood glucose is then measured at set intervals for three hours following the ingestion of the glucose. A typical GTT would include the fasting assay and testing at 30 minutes, 1 hour, 2 hours, and 3 hours after the glucose dose. (It is important that the patient be on a 300 g/day carbohydrate diet for the three days preceding the GTT.)

Urine samples may be collected and tested for glucose at the same times as blood for the GTT. Glucose is reabsorbed from the blood by the kidney tubules, so the blood glucose level must be elevated before it exceeds the kidney's capacity to reabsorb. The blood glucose concentration above which glucose can be detected in urine is called the **renal threshold** for glucose, and is normally approximately 160–180 mg/dl.

NORMAL OR EXPECTED GLUCOSE VALUES

Normal Fasting and Two-Hour Post-Prandial Values

The normal or expected value for serum or plasma glucose following an overnight fast is 65–100 mg/dl. Whole blood levels are slightly lower. Fasting levels above 120 mg/dl indicate hyperglycemia. The normal blood glucose level should be less than 109 mg/dl two hours post-prandial. Patients with two-hour post-prandial glucose levels above 110 mg/dl should be tested further.

Generally, a patient is considered to be hypoglycemic if the blood glucose level falls below 50 mg/dl. Abnormally low glucose levels must be reported immediately so appropriate action can be taken. Hypoglycemic patients may experience faintness, weakness, confusion, and incoordination, and may lapse into unconsciousness and coma if left untreated.

Normal GTT Values

In a glucose tolerance test, a person with normal glucose metabolism would have a normal fasting glucose level (65–100 mg/dl), a one-hour level of 120–150 mg/dl and a two- and three-hour level at or below the fasting level. Values outside of these ranges may indicate a problem with carbohydrate metabolism.

PRINCIPLES OF GLUCOSE ANALYSIS

Until about ten years ago, glucose was measured by a complicated oxidation-reduction test which used hot alkaline potassium ferricyanide or copper solutions. This method has since been replaced by simpler, quicker, and more specific methods which use the enzymes **glucose oxidase** or **hexokinase.** In general, tests which use hexokinase are more specific and have less interferences than those using glucose oxidase.

Glucose Oxidase Method

The glucose oxidase method of analysis is a two-step reaction. In the first part of the reaction, glucose is converted to gluconic acid and hydrogen peroxide (H_2O_2) in the presence of glucose oxidase and oxygen. The resulting concentrations of gluconic acid and H_2O_2 are proprotional to the amount of glucose originally present. In the second part of the reaction, in the presence of the **peroxidase** enzyme and a **chromogen,** H_2O_2 is converted to water (H_2O) and the chromogen becomes colored or changes colors:

1) $\text{glucose} + H_2O + O_2 \xrightarrow[\text{Oxidase}]{\text{Glucose}} \text{gluconic acid} + H_2O_2$

2) $H_2O_2 + \text{chromogen} \xrightarrow{\text{Peroxidase}} 2\,H_2O + \text{color formation}$

The color intensity is proportional to the amount of H_2O_2 (and thus the amount of glucose) and can be measured using a spectrophotometer (see Lesson 7–3, The Spectrophotometer).

Hexokinase Method

The hexokinase method is also a two-step reaction. This method has advantages over the glucose oxidase method, primarily because it has less interfering substances and uses safer reagents. In the first step, hexokinase, in the presence of adenosine triphosphate (ATP), adds a phosphate to glucose to form glucose-6-phosphate (G6P). In the second step, G6P in the presence of NADP and the enzyme glucose-6-phosphate dehydrogenase (G6PD) is converted to 6-phosphogluconate (6PG) with the production of NADPH:

1) $\text{Glucose} + \text{ATP} \xrightarrow{\text{Hexokinase}} \text{G6P} + \text{ADP}$

2) $\text{G6P} + \text{NADP} \xrightarrow{\text{G6PD}} \text{6PG} + \text{NADPH}$

NADPH absorbs ultraviolet light at 340 nm. This absorbance can be measured using a spectrophotometer. The increase in absorbance in the solution is proportional to the glucose concentration in the original reaction.

GLUCOSE ANALYZERS

There are several types of glucose analyzers on the market today. Most analyzers which are suitable for small laboratories use enzymatic methods for analysis. This lesson describes both a manual method of glucose analysis and the use of a simple, inexpensive glucose analyzer, the Ames Glucometer® II (Figure 7–13), which can be used in physicians' offices, as well as at home by patients.

MANUAL METHOD OF GLUCOSE ANALYSIS

Many companies have kits available for glucose measurement by enzymatic methods. The method given is from Sigma Diagnostics® Procedure No. 315, which is a modification of the Trinder method of glucose analysis. The procedure requires only one reagent which contains chromogens and the enzymes glucose oxidase and peroxidase. When the reagent is added to a serum sample, the glucose oxidase and peroxidase enzymes generate hydrogen peroxide from the glucose, which then reacts with the chromogens to form a color:

$\text{Glucose} + H_2O + O_2 \xrightarrow{\text{Glucose Oxidase}} \text{Gluconic acid} + H_2O_2$

$H_2O_2 + 4\text{-Aminoantipyrene} \atop + \text{p-Hydroxybenzene Sulfonate} \xrightarrow{\text{Peroxidase}} \text{Quinoneimine dye} + \atop H_2O$

With this procedure, glucose may be measured in serum or plasma. To perform the test, 10 μl of

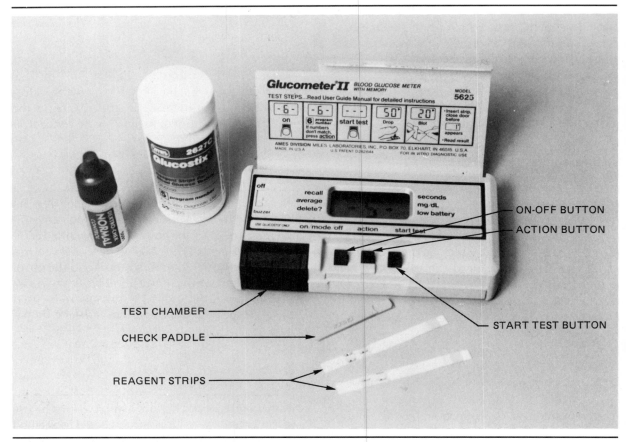

Figure 7–13. Glucometer® II with parts labeled

serum or plasma is mixed with 3 ml of the Trinder reagent and is allowed to react for 18 minutes at room temperature, 15 minutes at 30°C, or 10 minutes at 37°C. Standards and controls are set up in the same manner. A reagent blank is made from 3.0 ml of the Trinder reagent and 10 µl of distilled water. At the end of the incubation period, the absorbances of the tubes are read at 505 nm using a water blank. The change in absorbance (ΔA) due to glucose (in the samples) is calculated by subtracting the reagent blank absorbance from the absorbance of each tube. The glucose concentrations may then be determined by reading from a standard curve or using the absorbance formula:

$$\text{glucose (mg/dl) conc.} = \frac{A_U - A_{BK}}{A_{STD} - A_{BK}} \times \text{conc. (mg/dl) gluc. std.}$$

Lesson 7–3 in this unit describes the use of the spectrophotometer and the above formula. Detailed instructions for the manual glucose method are given in the Student Performance Guide at the end of this lesson.

GLUCOSE ANALYSIS USING THE GLUCOMETER® II

The Glucometer® II is a small, hand-held reflectance photometer. It measures glucose levels from 25–399 mg/dl. It has buttons for on-off and for programming test and check modes. The instrument also has a small memory program. The test chamber contains a lamp and a slot into which the reagent strip is placed. A display screen shows the glucose value and is also used as a timer and for display of the program modes. Figure 7–13 shows the parts of the glucometer.

Principles of Analysis

The Glucometer® II uses Glucostix® reagent strips which contain two reagent pads: a high range and low range. Both pads contain the enzymes glucose oxidase and peroxidase. The low range pad also contains o-tolidine, which, in the presence of H_2O_2, forms a green color, the intensity of which is proportional to the glucose concentration. On the high range pad, the chemicals aminoantipyrine and dichlorohydroxybenzene sulfonate are present. These chemicals are oxidized by H_2O_2 to form an orange color; the color intensity is proprotional to the glucose concentration. The chemical reactions are similar to those described earlier in "Principles of Glucose Analysis."

To use the glucometer, a blood sample is placed on the reagent strip pads. The glucose in the sample reacts with the reagents in the pads causing a color to form. The more glucose present in the sample, the darker the color. At the appropriate time, the strip is blotted and placed into the glucometer test chamber where light is directed onto the pads. The amount of light reflected from the pads is measured by the photometer and converted to a digital read-out showing the glucose concentration in mg/dl or mmol/L.

If a glucometer is not available, the strips may be read visually using the color blocks on the label of the Glucostix® container. The color of the pads is compared to the color chart after the appropriate time interval. However, this gives only a semi-quantitative measurement. The timing differs for visual reading and glucometer reading. *Instructions included with the strips must be carefully followed for reliable test results.*

Glucometer® II Procedure

A general procedure for performing the check test, control test, and patient blood glucose test is given. However, the package inserts and glucometer instruction manual should be consulted and followed.

Performing the Check Test. The check test is a test of the electronics of the glucometer. This test should be performed daily and anytime results are questionable.

The glucometer is turned on; the "action" button is pressed until the number 5 appears. The check test must be performed in mode 5. With the test door closed, the "start" button is pressed; the instrument will count down from 50 seconds to 0, with the seconds displayed on the screen. At the 20 second beep, the check paddle is inserted into the guide (the word "check" should be facing away from the instrument). The door is closed immediately. After the last beep (time 0) a value will be displayed. This value should be compared to the range given with the check paddle. It should fall within the range listed. If the value falls within the given range, the control test should be run. If not, the paddle and test chamber should be cleaned and the test rerun. If it is still out of range, the instrument should be checked by a service technician before it is used to test patient samples.

Performing the Control Test. A control test should be performed daily and anytime results are questionable. A control test lets you know that the strips and instrument are working properly and that technique is adequate. A control test requires Glucostix® reagent strips and Dextro-Chek® controls. These controls are solutions of known concentrations of glucose which will react similarly to blood when used with Glucostix® strips. The controls are available in normal, low and high concentrations.

To perform the control test, the program number is set to match the program on the reagent strip bottle using the "action" button. *The program* mode must match the number on the Glucostix® bottle. A clean reagent strip is removed from the bottle and the cap is replaced tightly. The "start" button is pressed; at the 50 second beep, a large drop of control solution should be applied to the test pads. At the 20 second beep, the strip is blotted two times with soft tissue, immediately inserted into the test chamber, and the door is closed. (This must be done before the number "1" appears on the display.) The control results on the display screen are recorded and compared to the values printed on the control bottle or package insert. If the results are within the given range, the patient test may be run. If not, the control test should be repeated using a new strip and being certain that correct technique is used. If the test is still out of the given range, the strips may be defective and a new lot should be tested. Patient samples must not be tested until the instrument and strips are working properly as indicated by the check and control tests. A log of check and control test results should be kept. In this way, any deterioration of the test system may be noted early and corrective action taken.

Performing the Test. *The program mode is set to match the number on the Glucostix® bottle.* A clean strip is removed from the bottle, and blotting tissue is prepared. A capillary puncture is performed using proper technique and a large drop of blood is allowed to form. The "start" button is pressed; at the 50 second beep, a large drop of blood is applied to cover both pads on the strip. At the 20 second beep, the pads are immediately blotted by folding thick tissue over the pads and pressing on a firm surface. The blotting is quickly repeated with a clean part of the tissue (pads must be blotted, not wiped). Before the display reaches "1", the strip is inserted into the test chamber and the door is closed (the pad on the strip should be facing toward the instrument). The glucose value from the display screen is recorded, and the strip and capillary puncture materials are discarded into a biohazard container. The glucometer is turned off and the test chamber is cleaned with a moist, soft cloth.

Precautions

■ *When Using the Glucometer:*
- Observe proper safety precautions.
- Have all materials ready before beginning.
- Follow the manufacturer's instructions for the use of the glucometer, reagents and reagent strips.
- Do not use the Glucometer® II to test blood that contains a fluoride anticoagulant.
- Use fresh reagent strips.
- Cover the surface of both reagent pads with blood.
- Blot pads thoroughly—do not rub.
- Observe carefully the time intervals for each step.
- Compare results with normal values for whole blood; serum or plasma normal values will be 10–15% higher.
- Be certain test chamber is clean before use and before storing instrument.

■ *When Measuring Glucose Manually:*
- Observe proper safety precautions.
- Follow manufacturer's instructions carefully.
- Pipet reagents accurately.
- Observe carefully the time intervals for each step.
- Make mathematical calculations correctly.
- Compare results with normal values for the type sample tested (whole blood glucose values are lower than serum and plasma glucose).

LESSON REVIEW

1. How are glucose levels in the body controlled?
2. What are the storage forms of glucose?
3. What are two major types of disorders of glucose metabolism?
4. Why must serum or plasma be separated from cells immediately following collection if the specimen is to be tested for glucose?

5. What is a two-hour post-prandial glucose test?

6. What are the normal values for glucose?

7. Explain how a glucose tolerance test is performed. What results would be expected if the patient is normal?

8. Explain the glucose oxidase and hexokinase methods of analyzing glucose. What end product is measured in the glucose oxidase method—in the hexokinase method?

9. What is the difference in the check test and control test for the glucometer? What function does each serve?

10. Define chromogen, diabetes mellitus, glucagon, glucose oxidase, glucose tolerance test, glycogen, glycolysis, hexokinase, hyperglycemia, hypoglycemia, insulin, peroxidase, post-prandial, and renal threshold.

STUDENT ACTIVITIES

1. Re-read the information on glucose measurement.

2. Review the glossary terms.

3. Practice performing a manual glucose measurement as outlined on the Student Performance Guide, using the worksheet.

4. Practice performing a glucose measurement using the Glucometer® II as outlined on the Student Performance Guide, using the worksheet.

Student Performance Guide

NAME _____

DATE _____

LESSON 7–6
MEASUREMENT OF GLUCOSE — MANUAL METHOD

Instructions

1. Practice performing a manual glucose measurement.
2. Perform the manual glucose procedure satisfactorily for the instructor. All steps must be completed as listed on the instructor's Performance Check Sheet.
3. Complete a written examination successfully.

Materials and Equipment

- gloves
- spectrophotometer
- cuvettes
- timer
- chlorine bleach
- serum controls
- serum unknowns
- glucose standard, 500 mg/dl
- pipets, 10 µl and 3 ml
- safety bulb or automatic pipetter
- hand disinfectant
- surface disinfectant
- biohazard container
- test tubes, 13 × 75 or 13 × 100
- worksheet or graph paper
- glucose reagent (Trinder)
- parafilm

Note: The following is a general procedure for measuring glucose using Sigma Diagnostics® Trinder reagent (Procedure No. 315). Consult the procedure outlined in the package insert for specific instructions.

Procedure	S	U	S = Satisfactory U = Unsatisfactory
You must:	**S**	**U**	**Comments**
1. Wash hands with disinfectant and put on gloves			
2. Assemble materials and supplies			
3. Reconstitute the glucose (Trinder) reagent as directed on package insert			
4. Turn on the spectrophotometer and set the wavelength to 505 nm			
5. Label 8 test tubes: H_2O blank, reagent blank, control, patient sample, and standards—100, 200, 300, and 400 mg/dl. (*Note:* Prepare standards by diluting 500 mg/dl standard with distilled water to make a series of glucose solutions of 100, 200, 300, and 400 mg/dl)			
6. Pipet 3.0 ml of distilled water into the H_2O blank			
7. Pipet 3.0 ml of reagent into each of the remaining seven tubes			
8. Pipet 10 µl of distilled water into the reagent blank			
9. Pipet 10 µl each of control, patient serum, and the 100, 200, 300, and 400 mg/dl standards into appropriate tubes at 30 second to one minute intervals. Start the timer when the first sample is pipetted			
10. Mix each tube well by inversion, using parafilm to cover top of tube			
11. Incubate the tubes at room temperature (18–26°C) for 18 minutes. (Alternatively, tubes may be incubated 15 minutes at 30°C or 10 minutes at 37°C)			
12. Pour the water blank into a cuvette, place it into the spectrophotometer cuvette well, and set the absorbance to zero			
13. Read the absorbances of the reagent blank, standards, control and patient tubes at the same time intervals used for pipetting samples			
14. Record the absorbances for each tube on the worksheet			
15. Subtract the absorbance of the reagent blank tube from the absorbances of the other six tubes to get the ΔA for each			

You must:	S	U	Comments
16. Record the ΔA for each tube on the worksheet			
17. Construct a standard curve using the ΔA of the four standard solutions			
18. Determine the concentrations of the control and patient sample using the standard curve			
19. Disinfect and clean reusable equipment			
20. Dispose of all samples and used reagents properly			
21. Disinfect work area with surface disinfectant			
22. Turn off spectrophotometer			
23. Remove gloves and discard into biohazard container			
24. Wash hands with hand disinfectant			

Comments:

Student/Instructor:

Date:_____ Instructor:_____

Worksheet

NAME_____ DATE _____

LESSON 7–6 MEASUREMENT OF BLOOD GLUCOSE—MANUAL METHOD

1. Record spectrophotometer wavelength _____

2. Record absorbances (A) and calculate the change in absorbance (ΔA) by subtracting the blank A from the A of each tube.

	Observed A	−	Blank A	=	ΔA
Reagent Blank	_____				
100 mg Std	_____	−	_____	=	_____
200 mg Std	_____	−	_____	=	_____
300 mg Std	_____	−	_____	=	_____
400 mg Std	_____	−	_____	=	_____
Control	_____	−	_____	=	_____
Patient Sample	_____	−	_____	=	_____

3. Use the ΔA of the standard solutions to construct a standard curve using the graph below.

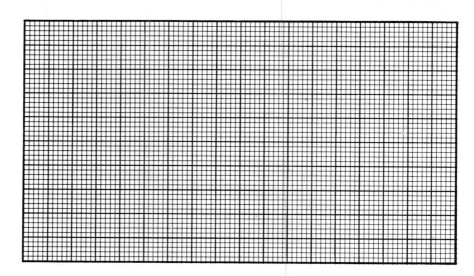

4. Determine the concentration of the control and patient samples using the standard curve. Record results below.

Control results   _____

Patient results   _____

Student Performance Guide

NAME _____

DATE _____

LESSON 7–6
MEASUREMENT OF GLUCOSE—
GLUCOMETER® II METHOD

Instructions

1. Practice performing a glucose measurement.
2. Using the Glucometer® II, perform the measurement of glucose satisfactorily for the instructor. All steps must be completed as listed on the instructor's Performance Check Sheet.
3. Complete a written examination successfully.

Materials and Equipment

- gloves
- Glucometer® II
- Check paddle
- Dextro-Chek® controls
- soft laboratory tissue
- sterile lancet
- hand disinfectant
- surface disinfectant
- biohazard container
- Glucostix® reagent strips and bottle with color chart
- worksheet
- 70% alcohol and cotton balls, or alcohol swabs

Note: The following is a general procedure for the use of the Glucometer II® and Glucostix® reagent strips. Consult the procedure manual and package inserts for specific instructions.

Procedure			S = Satisfactory U = Unsatisfactory
You must:	**S**	**U**	**Comments**
1. Wash hands with disinfectant and put on gloves			
2. Assemble materials and supplies			
3. Record check paddle range, control ranges and lot #, and Glucostix® lot # on the worksheet			
4. Perform the check test: a. Turn on the glucometer			
b. Set mode to 5 by pressing "action"			
c. Press "start"			
d. Insert check paddle into test chamber at 20 second beep and close the chamber door			
e. Read the check value and record on worksheet			
f. Compare the value to the range given with the check paddle			
g. Proceed to step 5, control test, if the value is within range, or			
h. Repeat the check test (steps c–f) after cleaning the test chamber and the check paddle if the check test is out of range			
5. Perform the control test: a. Set mode to match the number on the Glucostix® bottle by pressing "action"			
b. Remove a clean reagent strip from the bottle and replace lid			
c. Press "start"			
d. Apply a large drop of control solution to the reagent pads at the 50 second beep			
e. Blot the reagent strip with tissue two times at the 20 second beep			
f. Insert the reagent strip into the test chamber immediately and close the door (this must be done before the display reads "1")			
g. Read the control value and record on worksheet. Discard the reagent strip appropriately			
h. Compare the control value to the range on the control bottle			
i. Proceed to step 6, glucose test, if the control value is within range, or			

You must:	S	U	Comments
j. Repeat the control test (steps a–h), being careful to use correct technique, if the control value is out of range			
6. Perform glucose test:			
a. Set the program mode to match the number on the Glucostix® bottle by pressing "action"			
b. Remove a clean reagent strip from the bottle and replace lid			
c. Perform a capillary puncture			
d. Press "start"			
e. Apply a large drop of blood to the strip at the 50 second beep, covering both pads			
f. Blot the reagent strip with tissue two times at the 20 second beep			
g. Insert the reagent strip into the test chamber immediately and close the door (this must be done before the display reads "1")			
h. Read the glucose concentration and record on the worksheet			
7. Discard the used reagent strip into a biohazard container			
8. Turn off the glucometer			
9. Clean the test chamber			
10. Discard used lancet and tissues into biohazard container			
11. Disinfect work area with surface disinfectant			
12. Remove and discard gloves appropriately and wash hands with hand disinfectant			

Comments:

Student/Instructor:

Date:_____   Instructor:_____

Worksheet

NAME_____ DATE _____

LESSON 7–6 MEASUREMENT OF BLOOD GLUCOSE— GLUCOMETER® II METHOD

1. Check test: Record the accepted check test range from the check paddle container and the check test results. If test is within range, mark acceptable (A); if not, mark unacceptable (U).

Accepted Check Test Range	Test Results	A	U
_____	_____	___	___
_____	_____	___	___

   Action taken if test is unacceptable: _____

   _____

2. Control test: Record lot numbers and accepted ranges of Dextro-Chek® controls and Glucostix® strips. Record results of control test(s). If test(s) is within range, mark acceptable (A); if not, mark unacceptable (U).

   Glucostix® Lot # _____

   Dextro-Chek® Controls

	Lot No.	Accepted Range	Control Results	A	U
Normal	_____	_____	_____	___	___
Low	_____	_____	_____	___	___
High	_____	_____	_____	___	___

Action taken if control test is unacceptable: _____

_____

_____

3. Patient Test: Record the results below and compare with the normal range given.

Patient Test Result	Normal Range (whole blood)
_____	65–95 mg/dl

References and Suggested Readings

Anderson, Shauna C. *Introductory Laboratory Exercises for Medical Technologists*. St. Louis: C. V. Mosby, 1978.

Barrett, James T. *Basic Immunology and Its Medical Applications*. 2nd ed. St. Louis: C. V. Mosby, 1980.

Bauer, John D., Ackerman, Phillip G., and Toro, Gelson. *Clinical Laboratory Methods*. 8th ed. St. Louis: C. V. Mosby, 1974.

Brock, Thomas D. et al. *Basic Microbiology with Applications*. 3rd ed. Englewood, N.J.: Prentice-Hall, Inc., 1986.

Brown, Barbara A. *Hematology: Principles and Procedures*. 5th ed. Philadelphia: Lea & Febiger, 1988.

Bryant, Neville J. *An Introduction to Immunohematology*. 2nd ed. Philadelphia: W. B. Saunders, 1982.

Bryant, Neville J. *Laboratory Immunology and Serology*. 2nd ed. Philadelphia: W. B. Saunders, 1986.

Clansky, K. B., ed. *Chemical Guide to the OSHA Hazard Communication Standard*. 3rd ed. Burlingame, CA: Roytech Public., Inc., 1988.

Coltey, Roger W. *Survey of Medical Technology*. St. Louis: C. V. Mosby, 1978.

Crabtree, Koby T., and Hinsdill, Ronald D. *Fundamental Experiments In Microbiology*. Philadelphia: W. B. Saunders, 1974.

Cronenberger, J. Helen, and Jennette, J. Charles. *Immunology: Basic Concepts, Diseases, and Laboratory Methods*. Norwalk, CT: Appleton & Lange, 1988.

Davidsohn, Israel, and Henry, John Bernard. *Clinical Diagnosis By Laboratory Methods*. 15th ed. Philadelphia: W. B. Saunders, 1974.

Diggs, L. W., Sturm, Dorothy, and Bell, Ann. *The Morphology of Human Blood Cells*. 5th ed. Abbott Park, IL: Abbott Laboratories, 1988.

Dougherty, William M. *Introduction to Hematology*. 2nd ed. St. Louis: C. V. Mosby, 1976.

Finegold, Sydney M., and Baron, E.J. *Bailey and Scott's Diagnostic Microbiology*. 7th ed. St. Louis: C. V. Mosby, 1986.

Fischbach, Frances T. *A Manual of Laboratory Diagnostic Tests*. 3rd ed. Philadelphia: J. B. Lippincott, 1988.

Frosbisher, Martin, and others. *Fundamentals of Microbiology*. 9th ed. Philadelphia: W. B. Saunders, 1974.

Gile, T. J., and Wire, K. K. Hazard-Communication Program for Clinical Laboratories. *Clinical Lab. Sci.* 1988: 1:88-89.

Harmening, D. *Modern Blood Banking and Transfusion Practices*. 2nd ed. Philadelphia: F. A. Davis Co., 1989.

Henry, John B. *Clinical Diagnosis and Management by Laboratory Methods*. 17th ed. Philadelphia: W. B. Saunders, 1984.

Kaplan, Martin, and others. *Clinical Chemistry: Interpretation and Techniques*. 3rd ed. Philadelphia: Lea & Febiger, 1988.

Koneman, Elmer W., and others. *Color Atlas and Textbook of Diagnostic Microbiology*. 3rd ed. Philadelphia: J. B. Lippincott, 1988.

Lamberg, Stanley Lawrence, and Rothstein, Robert. *Laboratory Manual of Hematology and Urinalysis*. Westport, CT: AVI Publishing Co., Inc., 1978.

Lindberg, David S., Britt, Mary Stevenson, and Fisher, Frances W. *Williams' Introduction to the Profession of Medical Technology*. 4th ed. Philadelphia: Lea & Febiger, 1984.

Miale, John B. *Laboratory Medicine—Hematology*. 6th ed. St. Louis: C. V. Mosby, 1982.

Modern Urine Chemistry. 6th printing. Elkhart, Indiana: Ames Division, Miles Laboratories, Inc., 1978.

Nester, Eugene, and others. *Microbiology*. 3rd ed. Philadelphia: Saunders College Publishing, 1983.

Peacock, Julia E., and Tomar, Russel H. *Manual of Labo-*

ratory Immunology. Philadelphia: Lea & Febiger, 1980.

Pittiglio, D. Harmening, ed. *Clinical Hematology and Fundamentals of Hemostasis.* Philadelphia: F. A. Davis Company, 1987.

Raphael, Stanley S. *Lynch's Medical Laboratory Technology.* 4th ed. Vol. I and II. Philadelphia: W. B. Saunders, 1983.

Ross, Doris L., and Neely, Ann E. *Textbook of Urinalysis and Body Fluids.* Norwalk, CT: Appleton-Century-Crofts, 1983.

Scimone, John. *Laboratory Manual of Clinial Bacteriology.* Westport, CT: AVI Publishing Co., Inc., 1978.

Seiverd, Charles E. *Hematology for Medical Technologists.* 5th ed. Philadelphia: Lea & Febiger, 1983.

Simmons, Arthur. *Technical Hematology.* 3rd ed. Philadelphia: J. B. Lippincott, 1980.

Thomas, Clayton L., ed. *Taber's Cyclopedic Medical Dictionary.* 15th ed. Philadelphia: F. A. Davis Company, 1985.

Tietz, Norbert W. *Fundamentals of Clinical Chemistry.* 3rd ed. Philadelphia: W. B. Saunders Co., 1987.

Tietz, Norbert W. *Textbook of Clinical Chemistry.* Philadelphia: W. B. Saunders, 1986.

U. S. Department of Labor, Hazard Communication. Final Rule Part III. *Federal Register,* 1987. (Aug 24): 31852-31886.

Widmann, Frances K. *Technical Manual of the American Association of Blood Banks.* 9th ed. Philadelphia: J. B. Lippincott, 1985.

Williams, Harriet B. *Laboratory Manual of Serology, Immunology and Blood Banking.* Westport, CT: AVI Publishing Co., Inc., 1978.

Wintrobe, Maxwell M. et al. *Clinical Hematology.* 8th ed. Philadelphia: Lea & Febiger, 1981.

Glossary

absorbance the light absorbed by a substance containing colored molecules; designated in formulas by "A"; also called optical density (O.D.)

accuracy a measure of how close a determined value is to the true value

acid a substance which liberates hydrogen ions in solution; turns litmus paper red

acidosis abnormal condition in which blood pH falls below 7.35

acquired immunodeficiency syndrome a form of immune deficiency induced by infection with human immunodeficiency virus; AIDS

aerosol a suspension of fine solid or liquid particles in the air

agar common name for agar-agar; a gelatinous seaweed extract which is added to bacterial media to make it semi-solid and solid

agar plate agar medium dispensed into sterile petri dishes and allowed to solidify

agar slant agar medium dispensed into tubes and allowed to solidify at an angle

agglutination clumping of cells or particles; in serology due to reaction of the particle with antibody

agglutination inhibition interference of agglutination

aggregate total substances making up a mass; a clustering of particles

alanine aminotransferase enzyme with high concentration in the liver, and which is measured to assess liver function; ALT

albumins a homogeneous group of serum proteins which are made in the liver and help maintain osmotic balance

alkaline phosphatase enzyme widely distributed in the body, especially in the liver and bone; ALP or AP

alkalosis abnormal condition in which blood pH rises above 7.45

amorphous without definite shape

anemia decrease below the normal red cell count or in the blood hemoglobin level

anhydrous containing no water

anisocytosis marked variation in the size of erythrocytes

antibiotic susceptibility test a test performed to determine which antibiotic is most effective against a particular organism

antibody serum protein produced in response to a foreign substance (antigen); abbreviated Ab

anticoagulant agent which prevents blood coagulation

antigen a substance which causes the formation of antibodies; abbreviated Ag

antiserum serum containing antibodies

anuria absence of urine production

artery a blood vessel that carries oxygenated blood from the heart to the tissues

aseptic techniques techniques used to maintain sterility or to prevent contamination

aspartate aminotransferase enzyme present in many tissues including cardiac, muscle, and liver, and which is measured to assess liver function; AST

aspiration act of drawing in by suction

atherosclerosis a condition in which a deposit of fatty material narrows the interior of the arteries

autoantibody an antibody which is directed against self

autoclave a device which uses steam pressure for sterilization

average the sum of a group of values divided by the number of values; the mean

bacillus a rod-shaped bacterium (pl. bacilli)

bacteria a group of one-celled microorganisms; germs

bacterial morphology the form or structure of bacteria; color, shape, and size

band cell an immature neutrophil with a nonsegmented nucleus; a stab cell

base a substance which accepts hydrogen ions; turns litmus paper blue

basophil a leukocyte containing basophilic-staining granules

basophilic blue in color; having affinity for the basic stain

Beer's Law a mathematical relationship upon which the basis of analysis by spectrophotometry is formed and which shows that absorbance is related linearly to concentration

bibulous paper a special absorbent paper which is used to dry slides

bilirubin product formed in the liver from the breakdown of hemoglobin

binocular having two oculars or eyepieces

biological safety hood a special cabinet which draws air away from the worker, providing a safe work area for the handling of infectious agents

blank reagent blank; solution which contains some or all of the reagents used in the test but does not contain the substance being measured

blood bank place where blood is typed, tested, and stored until it is needed for transfusion

blood group antibody a serum protein that reacts specifically with a blood group antigen

blood group antigen a substance or structure on the red cell membrane which causes antibody formation and reacts with that antibody

broth liquid nutrient medium in tubes

buffer a substance which prevents changes in the pH of solutions when additional acid or base is added

buffy coat a light-colored layer of leukocytes and platelets which forms on the top of the red cell layer when a sample of blood is centrifuged or allowed to stand

BUN blood urea nitrogen; measurement of urea in blood

capillary a minute blood vessel which connects the smallest arteries to the smallest veins

capillary action the action by which a fluid will enter a tube or pipet because of the attraction between the glass and liquid

capillary tube a glass tube of very small diameter used for laboratory procedures

carcinogen a substance which has the ability to produce or cause cancer

carrier a person who harbors an organism and has no symptoms or signs of disease, but is capable of spreading the organism to others

cast mold; in urinalysis, a protein matrix formed in the tubules that becomes washed into the urine

CBC complete blood count, a commonly performed group of hematological tests

cell diluting fluid diluting solution which will not damage the cells being counted

Celsius temperature scale having the freezing point of water at zero (0°) and the boiling point at one hundred (100°); indicated by ''C''; also called Centigrade

centrifugal analysis a type of discrete chemical analysis in which the reagents and sample are mixed together by centrifugal action

centrifuge an instrument which may be used to spin biological samples at high speeds to separate particulate matter from the liquid portion of the sample

certified medical laboratory technician a professional who has completed a minimum of two years of specific training in an accredited program, consisting of one year of college and one year of clinical training, and has passed a national certifying examination

certified medical technologist a professional who has a bachelor's degree from an accredited college or university, has completed one year of clinical training, and has passed a national certifying examination

chromogen a substance which becomes colored when it undergoes a chemical change

clean-catch urine a mid-stream urine sample collected after the urethral opening and surrounding tissues have been cleansed

coagulation formation of a fibrin clot which aids in stopping bleeding

coagulation factors plasma proteins which interact to form the fibrin clot

coarse adjustment adjusts position of microscope objectives; used to initially bring objects into focus

coccus spherical or oval-shaped bacterium (pl. cocci)

coefficient of variation a calculated value to compare the relative variability between different sets of data

colony a circumscribed mass of bacteria growing in or upon a solid or semi-solid medium; assumed to have grown from a single organism

colony count a method of counting the isolated colonies resulting from a streak plate

condenser apparatus located below the microscope

stage which directs light into the objective

continuous flow analysis a method of analysis in which the reagents and samples are flowing through the instrument all the time

control serum a serum with a known concentration of the same constituents as those being determined in the patient sample

coumarin a class of anticoagulant administered orally to prevent or slow clotting

counterstain a dye which adds a contrasting color

creatine kinase enzyme present in large amounts in brain tissue and in the heart and other muscle, and which is measured to aid in diagnosis of heart attack; CK

creatinine breakdown product of creatine phosphate; a high energy compound stored in muscle

critical measurements measurements made when accuracy of the concentration of a solution is important; measurements made using glassware which is manufactured to strict standards

culture to cultivate bacteria in a nutrient medium; a mass of growing bacteria

cuvette a tube manufactured to strict standards for clarity and lack of distortion in the glass and used to hold liquids to be examined in the spectrophotometer

cyanmethemoglobin a stable compound formed when hemoglobin is combined with Drabkin's reagent

cystinuria the presence of cystine in urine; results in the development of recurrent urinary calculi

cytoplasm the fluid portion of the cell outside the nucleus

deionized water water which has had most of the ions removed

diabetes mellitus a disorder of carbohydrate metabolism characterized by a state of hyperglycemia due to insulin deficiency

differential leukocyte count determination of the relative numbers of each type of leukocyte in a blood smear

diffraction grating a device which disperses light into a spectrum

diplococci round bacteria which occur predominantly in pairs

discrete analysis a method of analysis in which the assay procedure for each sample is performed in its own separate container

distilled water the condensate collected after water has been boiled to remove impurities

diurnal having a daily cycle

Drabkin's reagent a diluting reagent used for hemoglobin determination which contains iron, potassium, cyanide, and sodium bicarbonate

dysfunction impaired or abnormal function

EDTA ethylene diamine tetraacetic acid; commonly used anticoagulant for hematological studies

EIA enzyme immunoassay

electrolytes the cations and anions which are important in maintaining fluid and acid-base balance

embolus a clot that is carried in the bloodstream

endogenous produced within; growing from within

enteric isolation type of isolation used for patients with intestinal infections

enzyme a complex substance produced in living cells, and which is able to cause or accelerate changes in other substances without being changed itself

eosin a dye that produces a red stain

eosinophil a leukocyte containing acid- or eosin-staining granules

eosinophilic having affinity for eosin or acid stain

erythrocyte red blood cell; RBC; cell which transports oxygen to the tissue and carbon dioxide (CO_2) to the lungs

erythrocytosis increase above normal in the number of red cells in circulation

ethics a system of conduct or behavior; professional rules of right and wrong

exogenous originating from the outside

eyepiece ocular

Fahrenheit a temperature scale having the freezing point of water at 32° and the boiling point at 212°; indicated by "F"

fibrin protein filaments formed in the coagulation process resulting from the action of the enzyme, thrombin, on the plasma protein, fibrinogen

fine adjustment adjusts position of microscope objectives; used to sharpen focus

fixative preservative; chemical which prevents deterioration of cells or tissues

flame sterilization of certain materials used in bacteriology by heating or passing through a flame

flora organisms adapted for living in a specific environment

fume hood a device which draws contaminated air out of an area and either cleanses and recirculates it or discharges it to the outside

galvanometer instrument which measures electrical current

gamma glutamyl transferase enzyme present in kidney, pancreas, liver and prostate, and measured to assess liver function; GGT

gauge a measure of the diameter of a needle

Gaussian curve a graph plotting the distribution of values around the mean; normal frequency curve

globin the portion of the hemoglobin molecule composed of protein

globulins a heterogeneous group of serum proteins having varied functions

glomerular pertaining to the glomerulus, the filtering unit of the kidney

glucagon hormone produced in the pancreas, and which increases blood glucose concentration by promoting the conversion of glycogen to glucose

glucose oxidase enzyme which converts glucose to gluconic acid and which is used in many glucose analytical methods

glucose tolerance test testing of blood glucose at timed intervals following the ingestion of a standard glucose dose; oral glucose tolerance test; GTT

glycogen storage form of glucose which is found in high concentration in the liver

glycolysis energy production as a result of the conversion of glucose to pyruvate

glycosuria glucose in the urine; glucosuria

gout painful condition in which blood uric acid is elevated and urates precipitate in joints

graduated flask container used for estimating volumes; has 50 ml to 100 ml increment marks

gram basic metric unit of weight or mass

gram negative refers to bacteria which are decolorized in the Gram stain; pink-red in color after counter-stained

gram positive refers to bacteria which retain the crystal violet dye in the Gram stain; purple-blue in color

Gram stain a stain which differentiates bacteria according to the chemical composition of their cell walls

HCG human chorionic gonadotropin, a hormone found in pregnant women; sometimes called uterine chorionic gonadotropin (UCG)

HDL high density lipoprotein; a fraction of total blood cholesterol

hemacytometer a heavy glass slide made to precise specifications and used to count cells microscopically; a counting chamber

hemacytometer coverglass a special coverglass of uniform thickness used with a hemacytometer

hematocrit the volume of erythrocytes packed by centrifugation of a given volume of blood and expressed as a percentage; abbreviated "crit" or "hct"

hematology the science concerned with the study of blood and blood-forming tissues

hematoma the swelling of tissue around a vessel due to leakage of blood from the vessel into the tissue

hematuria presence of red blood cells in urine

heme the portion of the hemoglobin molecule containing iron

hemoglobin a red blood cell constituent which is composed of heme and globin and which carries oxygen to the tissues of the body; abbreviated "Hb" or "Hgb"

hemolysis the destruction of red blood cells resulting in the liberation of hemoglobin from the cells

hemolytic disease of the newborn (HDN) a disease in which antibody from the mother destroys the red cells of the fetus

hemorrhage excessive or uncontrolled bleeding

hemostasis process of stopping blood flow

heparin an anticoagulant used in certain laboratory procedures

heterophile antibody antibody which is increased in infectious mononucleosis

hexokinase enzyme which converts glucose to glucose-6-phosphate, which is used in glucose analytical methods

homeostasis condition in which steady state or equilibrium is maintained

human immunodeficiency virus a retrovirus which has been identified as the cause of AIDS; HIV

hyaline transparent, pale

hypercalcemia blood calcium levels above normal

hyperglycemia blood glucose concentration above normal

hyperkalemia blood potassium levels above normal

hypernatremia blood sodium levels above normal

hypoalbuminemia marked decrease in serum albumin concentration

hypocalcemia blood calcium levels below normal

hypochromia a condition in which the red cell has a hemoglobin content below normal for its size

hypochromic having reduced color or hemoglobin content

hypodermic needle a hollow needle used for injections or for obtaining fluid specimens

hypoglycemia blood glucose concentration below normal

hypokalemia blood potassium levels below normal

hyponatremia blood sodium levels below normal

immunity resistance to disease or infection

immunization process by which an antibody is produced in response to an antigen

immunoglobulins serum proteins produced in response to antigens; antibodies; abbreviated Ig

immunohematology blood banking; the study of blood group antigens and antibodies

incubator temperature-controlled chamber into which inoculated media is placed so that bacterial growth will occur

indices plural of index; indexes; erythrocyte indices are values which compare a blood sample to standard values

infection the condition in which the body or tissue is invaded by a pathogenic organism

inflammation a tissue reaction to injury

inoculating loop a nichrome or platinum wire fashioned into a loop on one end and having a handle on the other end; used to transfer bacterial growth

inoculation the introduction of organisms into media

inoculum the portion of culture organisms which is being introduced into a medium

insulin pancreatic hormone which lowers blood glucose concentration

intravasuclar inside the blood vessels

ion selective electrode an electrode which has been manufactured to be responsive to the concentration of a specific ion

iris diaphragm regulates the amount of light which strikes the object being viewed through the microscope

isolation the practice of limiting the movement and social contact of a patient who is potentially infectious or who must be protected from exposure to infectious agents

isotonic solution a solution which has the same concentration of dissolved particles as that solution with which it is compared

ketones substances produced during increased metabolism of fat; sometimes called ketone bodies

ketonuria ketones in the urine

lactate dehydrogenase enzyme widely distributed in the body and measured to assess liver function; LD or LDH

lancet a sterile, sharp, pointed blade which can be used to perform a capillary puncture

lateral toward the side

LDL low density lipoprotein; a fraction of total blood cholesterol

lens a transparent material, curved on one or both sides, which spreads or focuses light

lens paper a special nonabrasive material used to clean optical lenses

leukocyte white blood cell; WBC; cell which provides protection from disease

leukocytosis increase above normal in the number of leukocytes in the blood

leukopenia decrease below the normal number of leukocytes in the blood

Levey-Jennings chart quality control chart which demonstrates the precision of a method

lipemic having a cloudy appearance due to excess lipid content

liter basic metric unit of volume

lumen the open space within a tubular organ or tissue

lymphocyte a small basophilic staining leukocyte having a round or oval nucleus and which is important in the immune process

lymphocytosis an increase above normal in the number of lymphocytes in the blood

macrocytic having a larger than normal cell size

mean the figure obtained when the sum of a set of values is divided by the number of values; the average

mean corpuscular hemoglobin MCH; average red cell hemoglobin concentration; an estimate of the hemoglobin concentration in a red cell in a blood specimen; measured in picograms (pg)

mean corpuscular hemoglobin concentration MCHC; compares the weight of hemoglobin in a red cell to the size of the cell; reported in percentage or g/dl

mean corpuscular volume MCV; average red cell volume; an estimate of the volume of a red cell in a blood specimen; measured in femtoliters (fl) or cubic microns (μ^3)

median cephalic vein a vein located in the bend of the elbow and frequently used for venipuncture

medical technology the health profession concerned with the performance of laboratory analyses used in the diagnosis and treatment of disease as well as in health maintenance

medium   a nutritive substance, either solid or liquid, in or upon which microorganisms are grown for study (pl. media)

megakaryocyte   a large bone marrow cell which releases platelets into the blood stream

melanin   a dark pigment

meniscus   the curved surface of a liquid in a container

meter   basic metric unit of distance or length

Methylene Blue   a dye that produces a blue stain

microbe   a microscopic single-celled organism

microbiology   the scientific study of microorganisms such as bacteria

microcytic   having a smaller than normal cell size

microhematocrit   a hematocrit performed on a small sample of blood

microhematocrit centrifuge   a machine which spins capillary tubes at a high speed to cause rapid separation of liquid from solid components

micron   a unit of measurement, 1×10^{-6} meter or one micrometer

micropipet   pipet which holds a very small volume

microscope arm   the portion of the microscope which connects the lenses to the base

microscope base   the portion of the microscope which rests on the table and supports the instrument

mid-stream urine   a urine sample collected in the middle of voiding

monochromatic light   light consisting of one color; light which is of one wavelength

monochromator   device which isolates a narrow portion of the light spectrum

monocular   having one ocular

monocyte   a large leukocyte which usually has a convoluted or horseshoe-shaped nucleus

mordant   a substance which fixes a dye or stain to an object

morphology   study of form and structure of cells, tissues, organs

myocardial infarction   heart attack caused by the obstruction of the blood supply to the heart or within the heart; abbreviated MI

myoglobin   protein found in muscle tissue

neutrophil   a neutral staining leukocyte; first line of defense against infection

nocturia   excessive urination at night

noncritical measurements   measurements which are estimated; measurements made in containers (such as the Erlenmeyer flask) which estimate volume

nonpathogenic   unable to cause disease in a normal individual

nonselective media   media which will support the growth of most bacteria

normochromic   having normal color

normocytic   having a normal cell size and shape

nosepiece   revolving unit to which microscope objectives are attached

nosocomial infection   infection acquired in a hospital or health-care facility

nucleus   the central structure of a cell which contains DNA and controls cell growth and function (pl. nuclei)

objective   magnifying lens which is closest to the object being viewed with a microscope

ocular   eyepiece of a microscope; contains a magnifying lens

oliguria   decreased production of urine

opalescent   reflecting an iridescent light

pathogen   a microorganism or substance which causes disease

pathologist   a physician specially trained in the nature and cause of disease

percent transmittance   the percentage of light which passes through a liquid sample; "%T"

peroxidase   enzyme which converts hydrogen peroxide to water and oxygen

petri dish   a shallow covered dish made of plastic or glass

pH   an expression of the degree of acidity or alkalinity of a solution; a measure of the hydrogen ion (H+) concentration of a substance

pharyngeal   having to do with the pharynx, the back of the throat

phlebotomist   one trained to draw blood; venipuncturist

phlebotomy   venipuncture; entry of a vein with a needle

photoelectric cell   a device which detects light and converts it into electricity

photometer   any of various instruments for measuring the intensity of light

picogram   micromicrogram; 1×10^{-12} gram; pg

plasma   the liquid part of the blood in which the cellular elements are suspended

platelet a small disk-shaped fragment of cytoplasm from a megakaryocyte which plays an important role in blood coagulation; a thrombocyte

poikilocytosis significant variation in the shape of erythrocytes

POL physician's office laboratory

polychromatic multicolored

polyuria excessive production of urine

population the entire group of items or individuals from which the samples under consideration are presumed to have come

porphyrins a group of pigments which are intermediates in the production of hemoglobin

post-prandial after eating

precision reproducibility of results; the closeness of obtained values to each other

prefix modifying word or syllable(s) placed at the beginning of a word

primary plating medium the initial growth medium upon which the bacterial specimen is placed

protective isolation reverse isolation

proteinuria protein in the urine, usually albumin

prothrombin one of the plasma coagulation factors

prothrombin time a test used as a screening test in coagulation; used to monitor oral anticoagulation therapy

quadrant one fourth; one quarter of an agar plate

random error error whose source cannot be definitely identified

ratio relationship in degree or number between two things

reagent blank a solution which contains some or all of the reagents used in the test but does not contain the substance being tested

reagents substances or solutions which are used in laboratory analyses

reciprocal inverse; one of a pair of numbers which has a product of one

red cell diluting pipet pipet used to dilute blood for a red cell count; RBC pipet

reference laboratory an independent regional laboratory which offers routine as well as specialized testing for hospitals and physicians

reflectance photometry method of analysis in which the light reflected off a colored reaction product is measured by a light detector

refractometer an instrument for measuring refraction

renal threshold the blood concentration above which a substance which is not normally excreted by the kidneys appears in the urine

respiratory isolation type of isolation for patients infected with organisms easily transmitted through the air

reticulocyte an immature erythrocyte which has retained basophilic substance in the cytoplasm

reticulocytopenia decrease below the normal number of reticulocytes

reticulocytosis an increase above the normal number of reticulocytes in the circulating blood

reticulum a network

reverse isolation a type of isolation designed to protect highly susceptible patients from exposure to infectious agents; protective isolation

Rh (D) immune globulin a concentrated purified solution of human anti-D used for injection; RhIG

rheumatoid arthritis an inflammatory disease characterized by inflammation of the joints

rheumatoid factors autoantibodies against human IgG which are often present in the serum of patients with rheumatoid arthritis

rotor the part of the centrifuge which holds the samples and rotates during the operation of the centrifuge

rouleau a group of red cells arranged like a roll of coins (pl. rouleaux)

Sahli pipet a pipet with a volume of 0.02 ml which was formerly widely used for manual hemoglobin determinations

saline an isotonic solution of sodium chloride and distilled water; normal saline; physiological saline; usually made in 0.85 or 0.9% concentration for use in medical laboratory procedures

sample in statistics, a subgroup of a population

sediment solid substances which settle to the bottom of a liquid

sedimentation the process of solid particles settling at the bottom of a liquid

selective media media which support the growth of certain bacteria while inhibiting the growth of others

serofuge a centrifuge which spins small tubes

serology laboratory study of serum and the reactions between antigens and antibodies

serum the liquid portion of blood which has been allowed to clot

SI units standardized units of measure; international units

solid-phase chemistry an analytical method in which the sample is added to a strip or slide containing, in dried form, all the reagents for the procedure

solute a liquid, gas, or solid which is dissolved in a liquid to make a solution

solvent that liquid into which the solute is dissolved

specific gravity ratio of weight of a given volume of a solution to the weight of the same volume of water; a measurement of density

spectrophotometer an instrument which measures intensities of light in different parts of the spectrum

spirochete a slender, spiral microorganism

stage platform on which object to be viewed microscopically is placed

standard a chemical solution whose exact concentration is known and which can be used as a reference or calibration substance

standard curve in spectrophotometry, a graph which shows the relationship between the concentrations and the absorbances (or percent transmittances) of a series of standard solutions

standard deviation a measure of the spread of a population of values around the mean

stat test a test that should be performed immediately

statistics the science of collecting and classifying facts in order to show their significance

stem main part of a word; root word

strict isolation type of isolation for patients with highly contagious diseases

substrate a substance upon which an enzyme acts

suffix modifying word or syllable(s) placed at the end of a word

supernatant clear liquid remaining at the top after centrifugation or settling of precipitate in a solution

supravital stain a stain which will color living cells or tissues

synthesis the combination of parts or elements into a whole

syringe a hollow, tube-like container with a plunger used for injecting or withdrawing fluids

systematic error a variation which may influence results to be consistently higher or lower than the real value

TC to contain

TD to deliver

terminology special terms used in any specialized field

thrombocyte platelet

thrombocytopenia a decrease below the normal number of platelets in the blood

thrombocytosis an increase above the normal number of platelets in the blood

thrombus a clot which forms in a blood vessel or in the heart

titer reciprocal of the highest dilution which gives the desired reaction

tourniquet a band used to constrict the blood flow in the vein from which blood is to be drawn

transport medium a medium into which a specimen is placed to preserve it during transport to the laboratory

trend an indication of error in the analysis, detected by ever increasing or decreasing values in the control sample

turbid having a cloudy appearance

universal precautions precautions to be used in the handling of all patients and biological specimens in order to prevent exposure of health care workers to infectious or harmful agents

uric acid breakdown product of nucleic acids

urinometer a float with a calibrated stem used to measure specific gravity

urobilinogen a derivative of bilirubin formed by the action of intestinal bacteria

urochrome yellow pigment which gives color to urine

vacuole a clear space in cytoplasm filled with fluid or air

vasoconstriction a contracting or narrowing of a vessel

vein a blood vessel that carries deoxygenated blood to the heart

venipuncture entry of a vein with a needle; a phlebotomy

Westgard's rules a set of rules used to determine when a method is out of control

white cell diluting pipet pipet used to dilute blood for white cell count; WBC pipet

Wintrobe tube a slender thick-walled tube marked from 0–100 mm; used in Wintrobe method of macrohematocrit and erythrocyte sedimentation rate

working distance distance between the microscope objective and the slide when the object is in sharp focus

wound or skin isolation type of isolation for patients with skin infections or open wounds

Appendix A
Safety Agreement Form

Although there are certain hazards present in the medical laboratory, it is possible to make the laboratory a safe working environment. Each laboratory worker must agree to observe all safety rules posted or unposted which are required by the instructor or employer. No set of rules can cover all of the hazards that may be present. However, several general rules are listed below:

1. Refrain from horseplay.
2. Avoid eating, drinking, smoking, gum chewing or applying makeup in the work area.
3. Wear a laboratory jacket or coat and closed-toe shoes.
4. Pin long hair away from face and neck to avoid contact with chemicals, equipment, or flames.
5. Avoid wearing chains, bracelets, rings, or other loose hanging jewelry.
6. Use gloves when handling blood, biological specimens, and hazardous chemicals or reagents.
7. Use universal barrier precautions in handling patients and biological specimens, including human blood and diagnostic products made from human blood.
8. Disinfect work area before and after laboratory procedures and at any other time necessary.
9. Wash hands before and after laboratory procedures, before putting on and after removing gloves, and any other time necessary.
10. Discard all contaminated materials into an appropriate, labeled biohazard container. (A rigid, puncture-proof container must be used for disposal of sharp objects such as needles and lancets.)
11. Wear safety goggles when working with strong chemicals and when splashes are likely to occur.
12. Wipe up spills promptly and appropriately for the type of spill.
13. Avoid tasting, smelling, or breathing the dust of any chemicals.
14. Follow the manufacturer's instructions for operating equipment.
15. Handle equipment with care and store it properly.
16. Report any broken or frayed electrical cords, exposed electrical wires, or damaged equipment.
17. Discard any broken glassware into a safe container.
18. Allow visitors only in the nonworking area of the laboratory.
19. Report any accident to the supervisor immediately.

Please initial the items listed below:

Initial

_____   I agree to follow all set rules and regulations as required by the instructor or supervisor, including those listed above.

_____   I have been informed that biological specimens and blood products may possess the potential of transmitting diseases such as hepatitis and acquired immunodeficiency syndrome (AIDS).

_____   I understand that even though diagnostic products are tested for HIV antibodies and Hepatitis B surface antigen (HBsAg), no known test can offer 100% assurance that products derived from human blood will not transmit disease.

Student Name (please print) _____

Student Signature _____   Date _____

Parent Signature (if student under 18) _____   Date _____

Appendix B
Abbreviations, Prefixes, Suffixes, and Stems

ABBREVIATIONS COMMONLY USED IN A MEDICAL LABORATORY

A	absorbance
AIDS	acquired immunodeficiency syndrome
ALP, AP	alkaline phosphatase
ALT	alanine aminotransferase
AST	aspartate aminotransferase
BP	blood pressure
BUN	blood urea nitrogen
C	Centigrade, Celsius
CBC	complete blood count
cc, ccm	cubic centimeter
CK	creatine kinase
Cl	chloride
cm	centimeter
CNS	central nervous system
CO	carbon monoxide
CO$_2$	carbon dioxide
crit	hematocrit
CSF	cerebral spinal fluid
cu mm	cubic millimeter, mm^3
E.U.	Ehrlich units
F	Fahrenheit
FUO	fever of unknown origin
g, gm	gram
GGT	gamma glutamyl transferase
GI	gastrointestinal
GTT	glucose tolerance test
GU	genitourinary
Hb, Hgb	hemoglobin
HCl	hydrochloric acid
HCO$_3$	bicarbonate
Hct	hematocrit
HDL Chol	high density lipoprotein cholesterol
HIV	human immunodeficiency virus

H_2O	water
HPF	high power field
IM	infectious mononucleosis
IU	international unit
IV	intravenous
K	potassium
L	liter
LD, LDH	lactate dehydrogenase
LDL Chol	low density lipoprotein cholesterol
LPF	low power field
MCH	mean corpuscular hemoglobin
MCHC	mean corpuscular hemoglobin concentration
MCV	mean corpuscular volume
meq	milliequivalent
mg	milligram
MI	myocardial infarction
mL, ml	milliliter
MLT	medical laboratory technician
mm	millimeter
mmol	millimole
MT	medical technologist
Na	sodium
NaCl	sodium chloride, saline
nm	nanometer
O.D.	optical density
pH	a number indicating the relative acidity of a solution
PP	post-prandial
RA	rheumatoid arthritis
RBC	red blood cell
RF	rheumatoid factors
SI	Le Systeme International d'Unites (International System of Units)
sp. gr.	specific gravity
Staph	*Staphylococcus*
stat	immediately
Strep	*Streptococcus*
UA	urinalysis
μl	microliter
μmol	micromole
WBC	white blood cell

SELECTED PREFIXES COMMONLY USED IN MEDICAL TERMINOLOGY

Prefix	Definition	Example of term
a, an	absent, deficient	anemia
ab	away from	absent
ad	toward	adrenal
ambi	both	ambidextrous
aniso	unequal	anisocytosis
ante	before	antenatal
ant(i)	against	antibiotic
auto	self	autograft
baso	blue	basophil
bi	two	binuclear
bio	life	biology
brady	slow	bradycardia
circum	around	circumnuclear
co, com, con	with, together	concentrate
contra	against	contraception
de	down, from	decay
di	two	dimorphic
dia	through	dialysis
dipl	double	diplococcus
dis	apart, away from	disease
dys	bad, difficult, improper	dysphagia
e, ecto, ex	out from	ectoparasite
end(o)	inside, within	endoparasite
enter(o)	intestine	enterotoxin
epi	upon, after	epidermis
equi	equal	equilibrium
hemi	half	hemisphere
hyper	above, excessive	hyperglycemia
hypo	under, deficient	hypoventilation
infra	beneath	infracostal
inter	among	intercostal
intra	within	intracranial
iso	equal	isotonic
macr(o)	large	macrocyte
mal	bad, abnormal	malformation
medi	middle	median
mega	huge, great	megaloblast
melan	black	melanoma

Prefix	Definition	Example of term
meta	after, next	metamorphosis
micro	small	microscope
mon(o)	one, single	monoxide
morph	shape	morphology
necro	dead	necropsy
neo	new	neoplasm
neutro	neutral	neutrophil
olig	few	oliguria
orth	straight, normal	orthopedic
pan	all	pandemic
para	beside	paraplegic
per	through	percolate
peri	around	pericardium
phago	to eat	phagocyte
poly	many	polyuria
post	after	post-op
pre, pro	before	prenatal
pseudo	false	pseudoappendicitis
psych(o)	mind	psychology
py(o)	pus	pyuria
quad(r)	four	quadrant
retro	backward	retroactive
semi	half	semiconscious
steno	narrow	stenosis
sub	under	subcutaneous
super, supra	above	superinfection
syn	together	synergistic
tachy	swift	tachycardia
tetra	four	tetramer
therm	heat	thermometer
trans	through	transport
tri	three	trimester
uni	one	unicellular

SELECTED SUFFIXES COMMONLY USED IN MEDICAL TERMINOLOGY

Suffix	Definition	Example of term
algia	pain	neuralgia
blast	primitive, germ	erythroblast
centesis	puncture, aspiration	amniocentesis
cide	death, killer	bacteriocide
ectomy	excision, cut out	gastrectomy
emesis	vomiting	hematemesis
emia	in the or of the blood	bilirubinemia
ferent	carry	afferent
genic	origin, producing	pyogenic
ia, iasis	state, condition	iatrogenic
iole	small	bronchiole
itis	inflammation	pharyngitis
lysis	free, breaking down	hemolysis
oid	resembling, similar to	blastoid
(o)logy	study of	pathology
oma	tumor	hepatoma
opathy, pathia	disease	adenopathy
osis	state or condition, increase	leukocytosis
ostomy	create an opening	ileostomy
otomy	cut into	phlebotomy
penia	lack of	leukopenia
phil	affinity for; liking	eosinophil
phyte	plant	dermatophyte
plastic, plasia	to form or mold	hyperplasia
pnea	breathing	apnea
poiesis	to make	hemopoiesis
rrhage	excessive flow	hemorrhage
rrhea	flow	diarrhea
scope, scopy	view	arthroscope
stasis	same, standing still	hemostasis
troph(y)	nourishment	hypertrophy

SELECTED STEMS COMMONLY USED IN MEDICAL TERMINOLOGY

Stem	Definition	Example of term
adeno	gland	lymphadenitis
alg	pain	analgesic
arter	artery	arteriogram
arthr	joint	arthritis
audio	hearing	auditory
brachi	arm	brachial
bronch(i)	air tube in lungs	bronchitis
calc	stone	calcify
carcin	cancer	carcinogen
cardi	heart	myocardium
caud	tail	caudate
ceph(al)	head	encephalitis
chol	bile, gall bladder	cholesterol
chondr	cartilage	chrondroplasia
chrom	color	chromogen
cran	skull	craniotomy
cut	skin	subcutaneous
cyan	blue	cyanosis
cyst	bladder, bag	cystocele
cyt(o)	cell	monocyte
dactyl	finger	arachnodactyly
dent, dont	teeth	orthodontist
derm	skin	dermatitis
edema	swelling	edematous
erythro	red	erythrocyte
febr	fever	afebrile
gastr(o)	stomach	gastritis
genito	reproductive	genital
gloss	tongue	glossitis
glyco	sweet	glycosuria
gran	grain	granulocyte
hem(a), haem	blood	hematology
hepat(o)	liver	hepatitis
histo	tissue	histology
hydro	water	hydrocephalic
hystero	uterus	hysterectomy
iatro	physician	podiatrist

Stem	Definition	Example of term
leuk	white	leukocyte
lip	fat	lipoma
lith	stone	cholelithiasis
mening	membrane covering brain	meningitis
myel	marrow	myelogram
myo	muscle	myositis
nephro	kidney	nephron
neur	nerve	neurectomy
noct	night	nocturia
onc	tumor	oncology
oo	egg	oogenesis
ophthal	eye	ophthalmologist
os, osteo	bone	osteosarcoma
oto	ear	otitis
path	disease	pathogen
ped	child	pediatrician
phleb	vein	phlebitis
phob	fear	phobia
phot	light	photosensitive
pneum	air	pneumonitis
pod	foot	pseudopod
pulm	lung	pulmonary
ren	kidney	adrenal
rhin	nose	rhinoplasty
scler	hard	sclerosis
sep	poison	septic
soma(t)	body	somatic
sperm	seed	spermatogenesis
stoma	mouth, opening	stomatitis
therm	temperature	thermometer
thorac	chest	thoracotomy
thromb	clot	thrombocyte
tome	knife	microtome
tox	poison	toxin
ur(o)	urine	urochrome
vas	vessel	intravascular
ven	vein	intravenous

Appendix C
Metric Conversions

COMMONLY USED PREFIXES IN THE METRIC SYSTEM

Abbreviation	Prefix		Meaning	Multiple of basic unit	Weight gram (g)	Length meter (m)	Volume Liter (L)
k	kilo	=	1000	10^3	kg	km	kl
h	hecto	=	100	10^2	hg*	hm*	hl*
da	deca	=	10	10^1	dag*	dam*	dal*
d	deci	=	.1	10^{-1}	dg*	dm*	dl
c	centi	=	.01	10^{-2}	cg*	cm	cl*
m	milli	=	.001	10^{-3}	mg	mm	ml
μ	micro	=	.000001	10^{-6}	μg	μm	μl
n	nano	=		10^{-9}	ng	nm	nl*
p	pico	=		10^{-12}	pg	pm*	pl*

*units not commonly used in the laboratory

COMMON METRIC EQUIVALENTS

Mass							
	10^{-3} kg	=	1 gram	=	10^3 mg	=	10^6 μg
	10^{-3} g	=	1 mg	=	10^3 μg	=	10^6 ng
	10^{-9} g	=	1 ng	=	10^3 pg		
Volume	10^{-3} kl	=	1 liter	=	10^3 ml	=	10^6 μl
	10^{-3} l	=	1 ml	=	10^3 μl	=	10^6 nl
	10^{-1} l	=	1 dl	=	10^2 ml		
Length	10^{-3} km	=	1 meter	=	10^3 mm	=	10^6 μm
	10^{-3} m	=	1 mm	=	10^3 μm	=	10^6 nm
	10^{-2} m	=	1 cm	=	10 mm	=	10^4 μm
	10^{-3} mm	=	1 nm	=	10 Å		

CONVERSION OF ENGLISH UNITS TO METRIC UNITS

	English unit	English abbreviation		Multiply by	To get metric unit	Metric abbreviation
Distance	1 mile	mi	=	1.6	kilometers	km
	1 yard	yd	=	0.9	meters	m
	1 inch	in	=	2.54	centimeters	cm
Mass	1 pound	lb	=	0.454	kilograms	kg
	1 pound	lb	=	454	grams	g
	1 ounce	oz	=	28	grams	g
Volume	1 quart	qt	=	0.95	liters	l
	1 fluid ounce	fl. oz.	=	30	milliliters	ml
	1 teaspoon	tsp	=	5	milliliters	ml

CONVERSION OF METRIC UNITS TO ENGLISH UNITS

	Metric unit	Metric abbreviation		Multiply by	To find English unit	English abbreviation
Distance	1 kilometer	km	=	0.6	miles	mi
	1 meter	m	=	3.3	feet	ft
	1 meter	m	=	39.37	inches	in
	1 centimeter	cm	=	0.4	inches	in
	1 millimeter	mm	=	.04	inches	in
Mass	1 gram	g	=	.0022	pounds	lb
	1 kilogram	kg	=	2.2	pounds	lb
Volume	1 liter	l	=	1.06	quarts	qt
	1 milliliter	ml	=	.03	fluid ounces	fl. oz.

INTERNATIONAL SYSTEM OF UNITS (SI UNITS)

Common Usage	SI Equivalents
micron (μ)	micrometer (μm; 10^{-6} meter)
cubic micron (μ^3)	femtoliter (fl; 10^{-15} liter)
micromicrogram ($\mu\mu$g)	picogram (pg; 10^{-12} gram)
microgram (mcg or μg)	microgram (μg; 10^{-6} gram)
Angstrom (Å)	nm $\times 10^{-1}$
millimicron (mμ)	nanometer (nm; 10^{-9} meter)
lambda (λ)	microliter (μl; 10^{-6} liter)

Test	Old Unit	SI Unit
Cell counts	cells/mm^3 or cells/cumm	cells/μl or cells/liter
Hematocrit	% (Ex. 41%)	decimal (Ex. 0.41)
Hemoglobin	g/dl	g/liter
MCV	μ^3	fl
MCH	$\mu\mu$g	pg
MCHC	%	g/dl (or g/l)

Appendix D
Temperature Conversions

Temperatures may be converted from Fahrenheit to Celsius (or Celsius to Fahrenheit) by using the conversion chart below.

F	C	F	C	F	C
23	−5	101	38.3	115	46.1
32	0	102	38.9	116	46.7
70	21.1	103	39.4	117	47.2
75	23.9	104	40	118	47.8
80	26.7	105	40.6	119	48.3
85	29.4	106	41.1	120	48.9
90	32.2	107	41.7	125	51.7
95	35	108	42.2	130	54.4
96	35.6	109	42.8	135	57.2
97	36.1	110	43.3	140	60
98	36.7	111	43.9	150	65.6
98.6	37	112	44.4	212	100
99	37.2	113	45	230	110
100	37.8	114	45.6		

Temperature conversions may also be performed using the formulas below:

Problem: Convert 98.6° F (normal body temperature) to Celsius (C) degrees.

Formula: $C = \dfrac{5}{9}(F-32)$

Solution: $C = \dfrac{5}{9}(98.6-32)$

$C = \dfrac{5}{9}(66.6)$

$C = 36.99 \text{ or } 37$

Answer: 98.6° F is equal to 37° C

Problem: Convert 37° C to Fahrenheit (F) degrees.

Formula: $F = \dfrac{9}{5}(C) + 32$

Solution: $F = \dfrac{9}{5}(37) + 32$

$F = 66.6 + 32$

$F = 98.6$

Answer: 37° C is equal to 98.6° F

Appendix E
Examples of Preparing Solutions and Dilutions

Preparation of a v/v Percentage Solution

Problem: Prepare one liter of 2% acetic acid from concentrated (glacial) acetic acid.

Solution:
1. A 2% solution of acetic acid contains 2 ml of concentrated acetic acid in each 100 ml of solution.
2. Therefore, one liter of 2% acetic acid contains 2 ml × 10, or 20 ml of concentrated acetic acid.
3. To prepare the solution:
   a. Fill a one-liter volumetric flask approximately half full with distilled water.
   b. Add 20 ml of concentrated acetic acid and swirl to mix.
   c. Fill the flask to the line with distilled water.

Preparing a Solution Using Proportions

Problem: A buffer is made by adding 2 parts of "solution A" to 5 parts of "solution B." How much of solution A and solution B would be required to make 70 ml of the buffer?

Formula: $\dfrac{\text{Total volume required}}{\text{parts of ''A'' + parts of ''B''}} = \text{volume of one part}$

Solution: $\dfrac{70 \text{ ml required}}{2 \text{ parts ''A'' + 5 parts ''B''}} = \text{volume of one part}$

$\dfrac{70}{7} = 10 \text{ ml} = \text{volume of one part}$

2 parts of solution "A" = 2 × 10 = 20 ml
5 parts of solution "B" = 5 × 10 = 50 ml

Answer: The buffer would be made by mixing 20 ml of solution A with 50 ml of solution B to give a total volume of 70 ml.

Using the Formula: $C_1V_1 = C_2V_2$ to Prepare a Solution

Problem: Prepare 100 ml of a 2% solution of acetic acid using a 10% acetic acid solution.

Formula: $C_1V_1 = C_2V_2$

Solution: $(2)(100 \text{ ml}) = (10)(V_2)$

$200 \text{ ml} = 10(V_2)$

$\dfrac{200}{10} \text{ ml} = V_2$

$20 \text{ ml} = V_2$

where: $C_1 =$ concentration of first solution
$C_2 =$ concentration of second solution
$V_1 =$ required volume of first solution
$V_2 =$ required volume of second solution

Answer: Twenty ml of 10% acetic acid are added to 80 ml of distilled water to make 100 ml of a 2% solution of acetic acid.

Preparation of a w/v Percentage Solution

Problem: Prepare 500 ml of 0.85% saline.

Solution:
1. A 0.85% solution contains 0.85 g of the solute in every 100 ml of solution.
2. Therefore, to prepare 500 ml, 5×0.85 g or 4.25 g of sodium chloride (NaCl) must be used.
3. To prepare the solution:
   a. Weigh out 4.25 g of NaCl.
   b. Fill a 500 ml volumetric flask approximately half full with distilled water.
   c. Add 4.25 g of NaCl and swirl gently to dissolve.
   d. Fill the flask to the line with distilled water.

Preparation of a 1:10 Dilution

Problem: Prepare 10 ml of a 1:10 dilution of serum using saline as the diluent.

Solution:
1. A 1:10 dilution contains one part of a substance combined with 9 parts of a diluent to give a total of 10 parts.
2. Add 1 ml of serum to 9 ml of saline to form 10 ml of a 1:10 dilution of the serum.
3. If 50 ml were required, 5 ml of serum would be added to 45 ml saline.

Appendix F
Table of Normal Hematological Values

Test	Normal Range	
Hemoglobin:		
Newborn	16.0–23.0 g/dl	
Children	10.0–14.0 g/dl	
Adult males	13.5–17.5 g/dl	
Adult females	12.5–15.5 g/dl	
Microhematocrit:		
Newborn	51–60%	
One year	32–38%	
Six years	34–42%	
Adult males	42–52%	
Adult females	36–48%	
Leukocyte Counts:		
Newborn	$9.0–30.0 \times 10^9/1$	
One year	$6.0–14.0 \times 10^9/1$	
Six years	$4.5–12.0 \times 10^9/1$	
Adult	$4.5–11.0 \times 10^9/1$	
Erythrocyte Counts:		
Adult males	$4.5 \times 6.0 \times 10^{12}/1$	
Adult females	$4.0 \times 5.5 \times 10^{12}/1$	
Erythrocyte Indices:		
Mean Corpuscular Volume (MCV)	80–100 fl	
Mean Corpuscular Hemoglobin (MCH)	27–32 pg	
Mean Corpuscular Hemoglobin Concentration (MCHC)	33–38%	
Platelet Count	$0.15–0.40 \times 10^{12}/1$	
Reticulocyte Percentages:		Upper limit of Normal
Newborn	2.5–6.5%	10%
Adult	0.5–1.5%	3%

Test	Normal Range

Erythrocyte Sedimentation
Rate (ESR), Wintrobe method

Children	0–13 mm/hr
Adult males	0–9 mm/hr
Adult females	0–20 mm/hr

Prothrombin Time 11–13 sec

Bleeding Time:

Ivy method	1–7 minutes
Duke method	1–3 minutes

Capillary Coagulation 2–6 minutes

Differential Leukocyte Count:

White Cell	one month	six-year-old	12-year-old	adult
Neutrophil (seg)	15–35%	45–50%	45–50%	50–65%
Neutrophil (band)	7–13%	0–7%	6–8%	0–7%
Eosinophil	1–3%	1–3%	1–3%	1–3%
Basophil	0–1%	0–1%	0–1%	0–1%
Monocyte	5–8%	4–8%	3–8%	3–9%
Lymphocyte	40–70%	40–45%	35–40%	25–40%

Platelets   An average of 5-15 platelets per oil immersion field is considered normal

Appendix G
Hematology—CBC Report Form

Date _____

Student _____

Specimen No. _____

Normal

WBC/1 _____ $4.5–11.0 \times 10^9/1$

RBC/1 _____ $4.5–6.0 \times 10^{12}/1$ Male
$4.0–5.5 \times 10^{12}/1$ Female

Hgb g/dl _____ 13.5–17.5 g/dl Male
12.5–15.5 g/dl Female

Hct % _____ 42–52% Male
36–48% Female

MCV (fl) _____ 80–100 fl

MCH (pg) _____ 27–32 pg

MCHC (%) _____ 33–38%

Differential count: **Normal**

___% segmented neutrophils   50–65%

___% lymphocytes   25–40%

___% monocytes   3–9%

___% eosinophils   1–3%

___% basophils   0–1%

___% bands   0–7%

___ other

RBC morphology:

Cell size: ☐ normocytic
                ☐ microcytic   normocytic
                ☐ macrocytic

Cell color: ☐ normochromic   normochromic
                ☐ hypochromic

Platelet: ☐ appear adequate   5–15/ oil immersion field

Estimate: ☐ appear decreased   <4/ oil immersion field
                ☐ appear increased   >16/ oil immersion field

Comments: _____

                _____

Appendix H
Table of Normal
Clinical Chemistry Values

Substance Measured	Conventional Units	S.I. Units
Alanine aminotransferase (ALT)	3–30 U/L	
Albumin	3.5–5.2 g/dl	
Alkaline phosphatase (ALP)	20–105 U/L	
Aspartate aminotransferase (AST)	6–25 U/L	
Bicarbonate (HCO_3^-)	22–28 meq/L	22–28 mmol/L
Bilirubin (Total)	0.1–1.0 mg/dl	1.7–17 µmol/L
BUN	8–18 mg/dl	2.9–6.4 mmol/L
Calcium	8.7–10.5 mg/dl	2.18–2.63 mmol/L
Chloride	98–108 meq/L	98–108 mmol/L
Cholesterol	140–250 mg/dl	
Creatine kinase (CK)	10–100 U/L	
Creatinine	0.7–1.4 mg/dl	62–125 µmol/L
Gamma glutamyl transferase (GGT)	3–35 U/L	
Glucose	65–100 mg/dl	3.6–5.6 mmol/L
Lactate dehydrogenase (LD)	125–290 U/L	
Iron	65–165 µg/dl	11.6–29.5 µmol/L
Phosphorus	3.0–4.5 mg/dl	0.96–1.44 mmol/L
Potassium	3.5–5.4 meq/L	3.5–5.4 mmol/L
Sodium	135–148 meq/L	135–148 mmol/L
Total Protein	6.0–8.0 g/dl	
Uric Acid	3.5–7.5 mg/dl	0.21–0.45 mmol/L

Appendix I

Percent Transmittance–Absorbance Conversion Chart

%T	A	%T	A	%T	A	%T	A
1	2.000	1.5	1.824	34	.469	34.5	.462
2	1.699	2.5	1.602	35	.456	35.5	.450
3	1.523	3.5	1.456	36	.444	36.5	.438
4	1.398	4.5	1.347	37	.432	37.5	.426
5	1.301	5.5	1.260	38	.420	38.5	.414
6	1.222	6.5	1.187	39	.409	39.5	.403
7	1.155	7.5	1.126	40	.398	40.5	.392
8	1.097	8.5	1.071	41	.387	41.5	.382
9	1.046	9.5	1.022	42	.377	42.5	.372
10	1.000	10.5	.979	43	.367	43.5	.362
11	.959	11.5	.939	44	.357	44.5	.352
12	.921	12.5	.903	45	.347	45.5	.342
13	.886	13.5	.870	46	.337	46.5	.332
14	.854	14.5	.838	47	.328	47.5	.323
15	.824	15.5	.810	48	.319	48.5	.314
16	.796	16.5	.782	49	.310	49.5	.305
17	.770	17.5	.757	50	.301	50.5	.297
18	.745	18.5	.733	51	.2924	51.5	.2882
19	.721	19.5	.710	52	.2840	52.5	.2798
20	.699	20.5	.688	53	.2756	53.5	.2716
21	.678	21.5	.668	54	.2676	54.5	.2636
22	.658	22.5	.648	55	.2596	55.5	.2557
23	.638	23.5	.629	56	.2518	56.5	.2480
24	.620	24.5	.611	57	.2441	57.5	.2403
25	.602	25.5	.594	58	.2366	58.5	.2328
26	.585	26.5	.577	59	.2291	59.5	.2255
27	.569	27.5	.561	60	.2218	60.5	.2182
28	.553	28.5	.545	61	.2147	61.5	.2111
29	.538	29.5	.530	62	.2076	62.5	.2041
30	.523	30.5	.516	63	.2007	63.5	.1973
31	.509	31.5	.502	64	.1939	64.5	.1905
32	.495	32.5	.488	65	.1871	65.5	.1838
33	.482	33.5	.475	66	.1805	66.5	.1772

%T	A	%T	A	%T	A	%T	A
67	.1739	67.5	.1707	84	.0757	84.5	.0731
68	.1675	68.5	.1643	85	.0706	85.5	.0680
69	.1612	69.5	.1580	86	.0655	86.5	.0630
70	.1549	70.5	.1518	87	.0605	87.5	.0580
71	.1487	71.5	.1457	88	.0555	88.5	.0531
72	.1427	72.5	.1397	89	.0505	89.5	.0482
73	.1367	73.5	.1337	90	.0458	90.5	.0434
74	.1308	74.5	.1278	91	.0410	91.5	.0386
75	.1249	75.5	.1221	92	.0362	92.5	.0339
76	.1192	76.5	.1163	93	.0315	93.5	.0292
77	.1135	77.5	.1107	94	.0269	94.5	.0246
78	.1079	78.5	.1051	95	.0223	95.5	.0200
79	.1024	79.5	.0996	96	.0177	96.5	.0155
80	.0969	80.5	.0942	97	.0132	97.5	.0110
81	.0915	81.5	.0888	98	.0088	98.5	.0066
82	.0862	82.5	.0835	99	.0044	99.5	.0022
83	.0809	83.5	.0783	100	.0000		

Appendix J
Table of Normal Urine Values

Urine Volume:

Age	Volume (ml/24 hours)
Newborn	20–350
One year	300–600
Ten years	750–1500
Adult	750–2000

Physical and Chemical Characteristics of Urine:

	Range	Average/Normal
Color	straw to amber	yellow
Transparency		clear
Specific gravity	1.005–1.030	1.015
pH	5.5–8	6
Protein	negative-trace	negative
Glucose		negative
Ketone		negative
Bilirubin		negative
Blood		negative
Urobilinogen		0.1–1.0 EU/dl
Bacteria (nitrite)		negative
Leukocyte esterase		negative

Components of Urine Sediment:

	Normal
RBC/HPF	rare
WBC/HPF	0–4
Epith/HPF	occasional (may be higher in females)
Casts/LPF	occasional hyaline
Bacteria	negative
Mucus	negative to 2+
Crystals	only crystals such as cystine, leucine, tyrosine, and cholesterol are considered clinically significant

Appendix K
Routine Urinalysis Report Form

ROUTINE URINALYSIS REPORT FORM

Date _____

Student _____

Specimen No. _____

Instructions: Record results as indicated:

1. *Physical Examination*

   <u>Normal Values</u>

   Volume (ml): _____   (only report if 24-hour urine)

   Transparency: _____ clear   clear
   _____ hazy (slightly cloudy)
   _____ cloudy (turbid)

   Color: _____   straw to amber

   Specific gravity: _____   1.005–1.030

2. *Chemical Examination*

   A. Multistix   <u>Normal Values</u>

pH	_____	5.5-8.0
protein	_____	negative, trace
glucose	_____	negative
ketone	_____	negative
bilirubin	_____	negative

blood	_____	negative
urobilinogen	_____	0.1–1.0 e.u./dl urine
bacteria (nitrite)	_____	negative
leukocyte esterase	_____	negative

B. *Confirmatory Test Results* (circle results)

Protein (sulfosalicylic acid):	negative	trace 1+ 2+ 3+ 4+
Reducing substances (Clinitest®):	negative	¼% ½% ¾% 1% 2% or more
Ketones (Acetest®):	negative	positive
Bilirubin (Ictotest®):	negative	positive

3. *Microscopic Examination*

Normal Values

WBCs:	_____/HPF	0–4
RBCs:	_____/HPF	rare
Epithelial cells:	_____/HPF	occasional (higher in females)
Casts:	_____/LPF	occasional, hyaline

Type present: _____

Crystals: _____ none seen

_____ present

(type) _____

Amorphous deposits: _____ none seen

_____ present

Yeasts:	negative 1+ 2+ 3+ 4+	negative
Bacteria:	negative 1+ 2+ 3+ 4+	negative
Mucus:	negative 1+ 2+ 3+ 4+	negative–2+

Other: _____

Appendix L
Guide for Selection of Vacuum Tubes

Stopper Color	Anticoagulant	Examples of Use
red	none	tests which require serum: cross matches, serology tests, electrolytes, glucose, BUN, creatinine, cholesterol, enzymes, bilirubin and most other blood chemistries
lavender	EDTA	blood typing; most hematological tests: cell counts, hematocrit, hemoglobin, differential count
green	heparin	LE test; lymphocyte studies; and some special chemistry tests: cortisol, blood gases
blue	sodium citrate	most coagulation studies: prothrombin time, partial thromboplastin time
gray	sodium fluoride	certain glucose methods

Appendix M
Examples of Laboratory Requisition Forms

HEMATOLOGY

CBC		HEMA LOG #		INSTR. OPER
HGB & HCT				
WBC				X2
PLATELET CT.				

TEST NO.

SA	OP CODES	NORMAL VALUES		
	•	WBC x10³	M F	7.8±3
	•	RBC x10⁶	M 5.4±0.7 F 4.8±0.6	
	•	Hgb g/dl	M 16.0±2 F 14.0±2	
	•	Hct %	M 47±5 F 42±5	
	•	MCV µm³	M 87±7 F 90±9	
	•	MCH pg	M F	29±2
	•	MCHC g/dl	M F	35±2
	•	RDW %	M F	13±1.5
	•	PLT x10³	M F	130-400
	•	MPV µm³	M F	8.9±1.5
	•	LYMPH %	M F	28±13
	•	LYMPH x10⁴	M F	2.0±1

42474

SEGS		NORMAL RBC				
BANDS		MORPH	1	2	3	4
LYMPHS		POLYCHROM				
MONOS		HYPOCHROM				
EOS		POIK				
BASOS		TARGET				
ATYP LYMPHS		SPHERO / ANISO				
META		MICRO				
MYELO		MACRO				
PRO		SICKLE CELLS				
BLAST		BASO STIP				
		TOXIC GRAN				
NRBC/100 WBC		1. SLIGHT				
WBC CT CORRECTED FOR NRBC's		2. MODERATE 3. MOD TO MARKED				
PLATELETS CK'd		4. MARKED				

Ordering Physician

Nurse/Ward Clerk

Date Ordered

To Be Done:
☐ STAT
☐ Routine ____ AM
☐ Time ____ PM

COMMENTS:

REMARKS (For Lab Use Only)

COLLECTED BY TECH/NURSE	REPORTED TECH	CALLED BY
		TO
DATE	DATE	DATE
TIME	TIME	TIME
☐ AM ☐ PM	☐ AM ☐ PM	☐ AM ☐ PM

HEMATOLOGY I

CHEMISTRY II GENERAL CHEMISTRY BLOOD

FORM # 28065 7/87 CAT # 1035

X	Test (Normal Range)	Result
	Acetone (Negative)	
	Acid Phos. (0.0-0.8 IU/L)	
	Albumin (3.4-4.8 g/dl)	
	Alkaline Phos. (25-97 u/L)	
	Ammonia (11-35 µmol/L)	
	Amylase (35-120 u/L)	
	BHcg Preg Test	
	Bilirubin, Total (< 1.5mg/dl)	
	Bilirubin, Direct (0-.4 mg/dl)	
	BUN (7-22 mg/dl)	
	Calcium (8.7-10.2 mg/dl)	
	Cholesterol (140-300 mg/dl)	
	CPK (21-232 u/L)	
	Creatinine (0.6-1.3 mg/dl)	
	Sodium (135-148mEq/L)	
	Potassium (3.5-5.0mEq/L)	
	CO₂ (24-32 mmol/L)	
	Chloride (98-108 mEq/L)	
	GGT (5-85 U/L)	
	Glucose (Fasting)(70-110 mg/dl)	
	Glucose(2hr.P.P.)(70-110mg/dl)	
	Glucose(Random)(70-110mg/dl)	
	IGG (639-1349 mg/dl)	
	IGA (70-312 mg/dl)	
	IGM (56-352 mg/dl)	
	Iron, Total (42-135ug/dl)	
	TIBC (250-350 ug/dl)	
	Lactic Acid (0.5-2.2 mmol/L)	
	LDH (100-190 u/L)	
	Lipase (4-24 U/dl)	
	Liver LDH (0-20 U/dl)	
	Magnesium (1.8-2.4 mg/dl)	
	Osmolality (277-292 mOsm/kg)	
	Phosphorus (2.5-4.9mg/dl)	
	Protein, Total(6.0-7.7 gm/dl)	
	SGOT (22-47 u/L)	
	SGPT (3-36 IU/L)	
	T3 (22-35%)	
	T4 (4.5-12.0 ug/dl)	
	T7 (1.04-3.84)	
	Triglyceride (30-200mg/dl)	
	TSH (0-7 uIU/ml)	
	Uric Acid (2.6-7.1 mg/dl)	

38874

Ordering Physician

Nurse/Ward Clerk

Date Ordered

To Be Done:
☐ STAT
☐ Routine ____ AM
☐ Time ____ PM

COMMENTS:

CHEM LOG #	ATS #

COLLECTED BY TECH/NURSE	REPORTED TECH	CALLED BY
		TO
DATE	DATE	DATE
TIME	TIME	TIME
☐ AM ☐ PM	☐ AM ☐ PM	☐ AM ☐ PM

CHEMISTRY 1 PROFILE

28060 (2-87)

X	PROFILE NAME

PROFILE 1 (GENERAL)

Glucose	Alkaline Phos.
BUN	SGOT
Bilirubin, Total	LDH
Protein, Total	Cholesterol
Albumin	A/G Ratio
Calcium	Globulin
Phosphorus	T4
Uric Acid	

PROFILE 2 (THYROID)

T3 (22%-35%) ____
T4 (4.5-12.0 ug/ml) ____
T7 (1.10-4.55) ____

PROFILE 3 (RENAL)

Sodium (135-148mEq/L.) ____
Potassium (3.5-5.0mEq/L.) ____
CO₂ (24-32mmol/L..) ____
Chloride (98-110mEq/L.) ____
Glucose (70-110mg/dl) ____
BUN (7-22mg/dl) ____
Creatinine (0.6-1.3mg/dl) ____

PROFILE 4 (HEPATIC)

Bilirubin, Total	Alkaline Phosphatase
Bilirubin, Direct	SGOT
Protein, Total	LDH
Albumin	A/G Ratio
	Globulin

SGPT (3-36 U/L) ____
Gamma GT (5-85 U/L) ____
Liver LDH (0-20 U/L) ____

54248

PROFILE 5 (LIPID)

Cholesterol (140-300 mg/dl) ____
Triglyceride (30-200 mg/dl) ____
HDL Cholesterol (32-96 mg/dl) ____

PROFILE 6 (CARDIAC)

SGOT (22-47 U/L) ____
LDH (100-190 U/L) ____
CPK* (21-232 U/L) ____
*CPK isoenzymes done only if CPK is elevated

PROFILE 7 (IRON)

Total Iron
Total Iron Binding Capacity (TIBC)
Unsaturated Iron Binding Capacity (UIBC)

PROFILE 8 (COAGULATION)

Protime PT. ____ sec.
Control ____ sec.
APTT (23-33 sec) ____
Fibrinogen (177-375mg/dl) ____
Antithrombin III ____
Plasminogen ____

PROFILE 9 (DEMENTIA)

PROFILE I (GENERAL)
B12
FOLATE

Ordering Physician

Nurse/Ward Clerk

Date Ordered

TO BE DONE:
☐ STAT
☐ ROUTINE
☐ TIME ____ AM / PM

COMMENTS

CHEM LOG #	ATS #

Collected By Tech/Nurse	Reported Tech
CALLED TO	
CALLED BY	
DATE	
TIME	

Collected By	Reported
Tech/Nurse	Tech
Date	Date
Time	Time
☐ AM ☐ PM	☐ AM ☐ PM

CHEMISTRY 1 PROFILE

Appendix N
Preparation of Reagents

Listed below are recipes for reagents which are needed in some of the procedures in this book. These reagents, and others, may also be obtained from the companies listed in Appendix O, Sources of Laboratory Supplies.

Unit–Lesson	Reagent	
2–1	70% alcohol	For 100 ml: 74 ml 95% ethanol 26 ml dH$_2$O
2–5	RBC diluting fluids	Gower's: 12.5 g anhydrous sodium sulfate 33.3 ml glacial acetic acid q.s. to 200 ml with dH$_2$O
		Dacie's: 5.0 g sodium citrate 3.0 g NaCl 5.0 ml Formalin 490.0 ml dH$_2$O
2–6	WBC diluting fluids	2% acetic acid: 2 ml glacial acetic acid 98 ml dH$_2$O 1% HCl: 1 ml conc. HCl 99 ml dH$_2$O
3–3	New Methylene Blue stain	0.5 g New Methylene Blue 1.6 g potassium oxalate q.s. to 100 ml with saline Filter before use. Store at 4°C
3–4	platelet diluting fluid 1% ammonium oxalate:	1.0 g ammonium oxalate q.s. to 100 ml with dH$_2$O Store at 4°C. Filter before use.
3–5	Drabkin's reagent	1 g sodium bicarbonate 50 mg potassium cyanide 200 mg potassium ferricyanide q.s. to 1 liter with dH$_2$O
4–1	saline	0.85 g NaCl 100 ml dH$_2$O
4–2	2–5% cell suspension	Suspend red cells in saline. Centrifuge and remove supernatant saline. Add 2 to 5 ml of the packed red cells to saline to make 100 ml.

| 5–3 | urine control solution | 0.5 ml 30% Bovine albumin
300 mg glucose
0.5 g NaCl
0.5 g urea
10 µl whole blood
0.2 ml acetone
q.s. to 100 ml with dH$_2$O |
| 5–3 | 20% sulfosalicylic acid | 20 g sulfosalicylic acid
q.s. to 100 ml with dH$_2$O |

Appendix O
Sources of Laboratory Supplies

American Type Culture Collection 12301 Parklawn Drive Rockville, MD 20852-1776	ATCC bacterial cultures
Abbott Laboratories Dept. 383 Abbott Park, IL 60064	*Morphology of Human Blood Cells*, medical terminology booklets, blood chemistry analyzers
Ames, Division of Miles Laboratories Elkhart, IN 46515	Urinalysis reagents, charts, educational aids, Glucometer®
Scientific Products Division of Baxter Healthcare 1430 Waukegan Road McGaw Park, IL 60085	Hematology, chemistry and blood typing reagents, bacteriology and urinalysis supplies, general laboratory equipment, serology kits, chemistry analyzers
BBL Microbiology Systems Division of Becton, Dickinson & Co. P.O. Box 342 Cockeysville, MD 21030	Bacterial culture media, reagents, and supplies
Boehringer Mannheim Diagnostics 9115 Hague Road Indianapolis, IN 46250-0528	Blood chemistry analyzers
Carolina Biological Supply Co. Burlington, NC 27215	Student kits, equipment and supplies, bacteriological media and cultures, prepared hematology slides, blood typing kits
Centers for Disease Control Atlanta, Georgia 30333	Safety guidelines
DIFCO Laboratories P.O. Box 1058 Detroit, MI 48232	Bacterial cultures, media

Fisher Scientific
711 Forbes Avenue
Pittsburg, PA 15219

Standards, controls, supplies and reagents
for chemistry, hematology, urinalysis and
serology, general laboratory supplies,
Glucometer®, laboratory instruments

Hybritech
P.O. Box 269006
San Diego, CA 92126-9006

TANDEM® ICON® Strep A test

Ionetics
3020 Enterprise Street
Costa Mesa, CA 92626

Ion selective electrode analyzers

ISOLAB Inc.
P.O. Box 4350
Akron, Ohio 44321

HbDirect™, Micro-Pipex

Eastman Kodak Company
343 State Street
Rochester, NY 14650

Chemicals, blood chemistry analyzers

NOVA Biomedical
200 Prospect Street
Waltham, MA 02254-9141

Ion selective electrode analyzers for blood
chemistry tests

Ortho Diagnostics
Raritan, NJ 08869

Blood typing reagents, serology kits, pregnancy
kits

Sigma Chemical Company
P.O. Box 14508
St. Louis, MO 63178

Diagnostics kits for chemistry, chemicals, stains,
standards, controls

Index

Abbreviations, medical terminology, 47–49, 481–482
ABO slide typing,
    ABO system, 258–259
    antibodies, 258–259
    antigens, 258
    importance of, 259
    interpretation of results, 260
    performing, 259–260
    precautions for, 260
    principle of, 259
    worksheet for, 263
ABO tube typing,
    direct or forward typing, 264–265
    precautions for, 265
    reverse or indirect typing, 265
    worksheet for, 269
Absorbance, 424
Accuracy, 412
Acidosis, 405
Acquired immunodeficiency syndrome (AIDS), 15
Aerosols, 369
Agar plate, 371
Agar slant, 368, 371–372
Agglutination, 258
Agglutination inhibition, 277–279
Aggregates, 205
Alanine aminotransferase, 407
Albumins, 404
Alkaline phosphatase, 407
Alkalosis, 405
Amorphous urates, 328–329
Anisocytosis, 179
Antibodies, 258–259
Anticoagulants, 194–195
Antigens, 258, 384
Antiobiotic susceptibility test, 393
Antiserum, 259
Anuria, 301
Artery, 191
Aseptic techniques, 351
Aspartate aminotransferase, 407

Aspiration, 96
Aspirin, affect on bleeding time, 244
Atherosclerosis, 442
Autoantibodies, 290–291
Autoclaves, 15, 30–31
Automatic pipets, 29–30
Automation,
    blood cell counts, 123–124, 138
    blood cholesterol measurement, 445
    blood smear staining, 165–166
    differential leukocyte count, 181
    erythrocyte indices, 238
    hematocrit, 88
    hemoglobin levels, 149
    platelet count, 218–219
    prothrombin time, 231

Bacillus, 346
Bacteria,
    appearance of stained, 346–347
    bacillus, 346
    coccus, 345–346
    colony of, 346
    Gram stain for, 346
    identification in urine culture, 392–393
    presence in urine sediment, 326–327
    spirochete, 346
Bacterial morphology, 347
Bacteriological smear, preparation of, 350
    aseptic techniques, 351
    from bacteria growing on media, 351, 355
    direct smear, 351
    precautions for, 355–356
Bacteriological specimens, collection and handling of,
    most frequently cultured sites, 377–378
    precautions for, 379
    specimen handling after collection, 378–379

    throat culture collection, 378
    urine culture collection, 378
Bacteriology,
    bacteriological smear preparation, 350–355
    Gram stain, 361–363
    identification of stained bacteria, 345–347
    inoculation of media, 368–372
    introduction to, 343–344
    performing a throat culture and rapid test for Group A *Streptococcus*, 382–386
    performing a urine culture, 390–393
    specimen handling and collection, 377–379
Balances, 31
Band cell, 174
Basophil, 174
Beakers, 24
Beer's Law, 424
Bibulous paper, 362
Bicarbonate, 405
Bilirubin, 308, 317, 319, 407
Binocular microscope, 34
Biological hazards, 16–18
Biological safety hood, 17
Biological specimens, rules for handling, 17–18
Bladder, 298
Bleeding time,
    Duke bleeding time, 245
    and hemostasis, 243–244
    Ivy bleeding time, 244–245
    methods of measuring, 244–245
    precautions for, 245
Blood, presence in urine, 317
Blood banks, 6, 255–256, 264
Blood cell count, red,
    automated, 123–124
    calculation of, 114, 122
    conditions associated with changes in, 120

diluting fluids (isotonic solution), 120
manual cell count, 120–123
normal values for, 120
precautions for, 122
procedure for, 120–122
RBC counting area, 110
Unopette microcollection system, 123
Blood cell count, white,
automated, 138
calculation of, 114, 137
counting the cells, 135–137
diluting fluids for, 135
diluting the sample, 135
factors influencing, 135
manual, 135–138
normal values for, 134–135
precautions for, 138
Unopette microcollection system, 138
WBC counting area, 110
Blood cells, 325
Blood cells, identification of normal. *See* Normal blood cells, identification of.
Blood cholesterol measurement,
atherosclerosis caused by elevated levels, 442
automated methods for cholesterol, 445
heart attack risk factor, 443
manual methods for cholesterol, 444
normal values for, 443
sources of cholesterol, 442
total cholesterol, HDL, and LDL, 442
Blood-diluting pipets,
calculating dilutions for RBC pipet, 97–98
calculating dilutions for WBC pipet, 98–99
care and cleaning of, 99–100
parts of, 95
precautions for, 99–100
red-cell-diluting pipet, 95–96
self-filling pipets, 100
using, 96–97
white-cell-diluting pipet, 96
Blood glucose, measurement of,
diabetes mellitus caused by increase in blood glucose, 451
Glucometer II method for glucose analysis, 454–456
glucose analysis principles, 452–453

glucose tolerance test, 452
hypoglycemia caused by decrease in blood glucose, 451
manual method of glucose analysis, 453–454
normal or expected glucose values, 452
precautions for, 456
specimens for analysis, 451–452
time of specimen collection, 452
worksheet for Glucometer II method of glucose measurement, 466–467
worksheet for manual method of glucose measurement, 461–462
Blood group antibodies, 258–259
Blood group antigens, 258
Blood smear, 156
cleaning the slides, 157
factors affecting quality, 158
good smear, features of, 157–158
making the smear, 157
precautions for, 158
preserving and staining, 158
Blood smear staining,
automatic stainers, 165–166
evaluating stain quality, 166
precautions for, 166
quick stains, 165
special stains, 164
storage of stained smears, 166
two-step method, 164
types of stains, 163–164
Broth, 368
Buffer, 164
Buffy coat, 86
BUN (blood urea nitrogen), 406

Calcium, 405–406
Capillary, 79
Capillary action, 96
Capillary coagulation, 249
normal values for, 250–251
performing the procedure, 250
precautions for, 251
Capillary puncture, 79
performing the puncture, 80–81
precautions for, 81
puncture sites, 80
types of capillary tubes, 81
Capillary tubes, 80–81
Carbohydrate metabolism, 408
Carcinogen, 16
Cardiac function, 407–408
Carrier, 67

Casts, presence in urine sediment, cellular, 328
granular, 328
hyaline, 328
CBC (complete blood count), 78, 156
Cell count, red blood; white blood. *See* Blood cell count, red; white.
Cell-diluting fluid, 95
Celsius, 58, 59
Centers for Disease Control (CDC), 16–17
Centrifugal analysis, 433
Centrifuges,
clinical, 30
high speed, 30
microcentrifuges, 30
rules for operation of, 30
Chemical hazards, 15–16
Chemistry department, 4
Chemistry profile, 403
Chloride, 405
Cholesterol, 408
endogenous, 442
exogenous, 442
See also Blood cholesterol.
Chromogen, 453
Clean-catch urine sample, 300
Clinical chemistry,
blood cholesterol measurement, 441–445
blood glucose measurement, 450–456
carbohydrate metabolism, 408
cardiac function, 407–408
chemistry profile, 403
collection and handling of specimens, 401–402
commonly performed tests, 403
electrolytes, 404–405
instrumentation in the small laboratory, 432–440
kidney function, 406
less commonly ordered tests, 408
lipid metabolism, 408
liver function, 406–407
mineral metabolism, 405–406
normal or expected values, 403
overview of, 397–398
problems associated with collection and handling of specimens, 402
proteins, 403–404
quality control in laboratory, 410–417
spectrophotometer use in, 422–427
substances tested in chemistry profiles, 403–408

types of specimens analyzed, 401
units of measure, 403
Clothing, laboratory, 18–19
Coagulation, 229, 249
Coagulation factors, 229, 243
Coagulation tests, 6
Coarse adjustment, 37
Coccus, 345–346
Coefficient of variation (CV), 416–417
Colony, bacteria, 346
Colony count, 392
Communications, 6–7
Complete isolation, 69
Compound microscope, 34, 37–38
Condenser, 34
Confirmatory tests, 318–319
Contamination, specimens, 402
Continuous flow analysis, 433
Control serum, 411
Conversions,
metric, 51-53, 488–489
temperature, 54, 490
Coumarin, 229
Counterstain, 361
Creatine kinase (CK), 402, 407–408
Creatinine, 406
Critical measurements, 25
Crystals, presence in urine sediment,
amorphous phosphates, 329
amorphous urates, 328–329
calcium carbonate, 330
calcium oxalate, 329
cholesterol, 331
cystine, 330
leucine, 331
sulfonamide, 331
triple phosphate, 330
tyrosine, 331
uric acid, 329
Culture, 355
Cuvette, 424
Cyanmethemoglobin, 148
Cytoplasm, 166

Deionized water, 31–32
Diabetes mellitus, 451
Differential leukocyte count. See
Leukocyte count, differential.
Diffraction grating, 424
Dilutions, examples for preparing,
491–492
Direct (forward) typing, 258, 264–265
Direct smear, 351
Discrete analysis, 433–434

Discrete analyzers, 434–435
centrifugal type, 435–436
maintenance and quality control, 438
Distilled water, 31–32
Diurnal variation, 402
Double-bagging, 73
Drabkin's reagent, 148
Duke bleeding time, 245
Dysfunction, 244

EDTA (anticoagulant), 86
EIA (enzyme immunoassay), 279
Electrolytes,
acidosis caused by pH decrease, 405
alkalosis caused by pH increase, 405
bicarbonate, 405
chloride, 405
hyperkalemia caused by increase of
serum potassium, 405
hypernatremia caused by increased
sodium, 404–405
hypokalemia caused by decrease in
serum potassium, 405
hyponatremia caused by decrease in
sodium, 405
potassium, 405
sodium, 404–405
Electron microscope, 39
Embolus, 229
Endogenous cholesterol, 442
Enteric isolation, 68-69
Entering patient's room, procedure for,
72
Enzyme, 229
Eosin, 164
Eosinophil, 174
Epithelial cells, presence in urine
sediment, 326
Epstein-Barr virus, 283
Equipment,
autoclaves, 30–31
automatic pipets, 29–30
balances, 31
centrifuges, 30
distilled and deionized water, 31–32
pH meters, 31
Errors, analytical procedures, 411–412
Erythrocyte indices, 236
automation, 238
factors affecting the indices, 238
mean corpuscular hemoglobin,
calculation of, 237
mean corpuscular hemoglobin concentration, calculation of, 237–238

mean corpuscular volume, calculation of, 237
normal values for, 238
precautions for, 238
Erythrocytes, 95, 172
presence in urine sediment, 325
properties of and ESR, 205
Erythrocyte sedimentation rate (ESR),
202
and disease, 204
and erythrocyte properties, 205
and mechanical of technical factors,
205
other methods of measurement, 204
and plasma properties, 205
Wintrobe method of measurement,
203
Ethics, 10
Evaporation, specimens, 402
Exiting patient's room, procedure for, 72
Exogenous cholesterol, 442
Eyepiece, 34

Fahrenheit, 58, 59
Fibrin, 229, 249–251
Fine adjustment, 37
Fixative, 158
Flame, 355
Flasks,
Erlenmeyer, 24
Florence, 24–25
volumetric, 25
Flora, 378
Fluorescent microscope, 38–39
Forward (direct) typing, 258, 264–265
Fume hood, 16

Galvanometer, 424
Gamma glutamyl transferase, 407
Gauge (needle), 191
Gaussian curve, 413
Glassware,
beakers, 24
care and cleaning of, 28
flasks, 24–25
graduated cylinders, 27–28
pipets, 26–27
precautions when using, 28
test tubes, 25–26
Globin, 147
Globulins, 404
Glomerulus, 297
Glove procedure, 71–72
Glucagon, 451

Glucometer II, 454
    performing check test, 455
    performing control test, 455–456
    performing patient blood glucose
        test, 456
    principles of analysis, 455
Glucose, 408
    presence in urine, 317
    See also Blood glucose.
Glucose oxidase, 453
Glucose tolerance test (GTT), 452
Glycogen, 451
Glycolysis, 451
Glycosuria, 317
Gout, 406
Gown procedure, 71
Graduated cylinders, 27–28
Gram, 51
Gram stain,
    appearance of stained bacteria,
        346–347
    gram negative, 346
    gram positive, 346
    observing stained smear, 362–363
    performing, 361–362
    precautions for, 363
Group A Streptococcus, rapid tests for,
    384–385
    interpreting the results, 385–386
    precautions for, 386

Handwashing procedure, 70
Hazards, laboratory,
    biological, 16–18
    chemical, 15–16
    physical, 15
HCG (human chorionic gonadotropin),
    277
HDL (high density lipoprotein)
        cholesterol, 442
    determination of, 445
Hemacytometer,
    calculating cell counts, 114
    care of, 114
    counting pattern, 112, 114
    coverglass for, 107, 110
    precautions for, 114
    RBC counting area, 110
    viewing ruled areas, 110–112
    WBC counting area, 110
Hemacytometer coverglass, 107, 110
Hematocrit, 86
Hematology,
    advanced, overview of, 187–188

basic, overview of, 77–78
bleeding time, 243–246
blood-diluting pipets, 94–103
blood smear preparation, 156–158
capillary coagulation, 249–251
capillary puncture, 79–81
differential leukocyte count, 178–181
erythrocyte indices, 236–238
erythrocyte sedimentation rate,
    202–205
hemacytometer, 107–114
hematology—CBC report form,
    495–496
hemoglobin determination, 146–149
identification of normal blood cells,
    171–174
microhematocrit, 85–88
platelet count, 215–219
prothrombin time, 228–231
RBC count, 119–124
reticulocyte count, 209–211
staining a blood smear, 163–166
venipuncture, 189–197
WBC count, 134–138
Hematology department, 4, 6
Hematoma, 194
Hematuria, 308, 325
Heme, 147
Hemoconcentration, 402
Hemoglobin,
    automated methods, 149
    cyanmethemoglobin, 148
    determining hemoglobin levels,
        147–149
    factors affecting hemoglobin levels,
        147
    manual methods, 148–149
    normal values for, 147
    specific gravity technique, 147–148
Hemolysis, 120, 383, 402
Hemolytic disease of the newborn
    (HDN), 271
Hemorrhage, 244
Hemostasis, 215
    abnormalities in, 229, 243–244
Heterophile antibodies, 283, 284
Hexokinase, 453
Homeostasis, 400
Human immunodeficiency virus (HIV),
    16
Hyaline cast, 328
Hypercalcemia, 405
Hyperglycemia, 451
Hyperkalemia, 405

Hypernatremia, 404–405
Hypoalbuminemia, 404
Hypocalcemia, 405–406
Hypochromia, 238
Hypochromic cell, 179
Hypodermic needle, 191
Hypoglycemia, 451
Hypokalemia, 405
Hyponatremia, 405

Identification of normal blood cells. See
    Normal blood cells, identification
    of.
Immunity, 134
Immunization, 271
Immunoglobulins, 258
Immunohematology, 6, 255
Immunology, 255
Incubator, 369
Indirect (reverse) typing, 259, 265
Infection, 67
Infectious mononucleosis, 283
    hematological test for, 284
    interpretation of results, 285
    precautions for, 286
    serological test for, 284
    slide test for, 284–285
Inflammation, 202
Inoculating loop, 355
Inoculation, 368
Inoculation of media,
    of agar plate, 371
    of agar slant, 371–372
    of broth, 368–371
    precautions for, 372
Inoculum, 369
Instrumentation, small laboratory,
    centrifugal type discrete analyzers,
        435–436
    discrete analyzers, 434–435
    and increase in physician's office
        testing, 433
    instrumentation worksheet (no
        available instrument), 439
    instrumentation worksheet (with
        available instrument), 440
    ion selective electrodes, 436–437
    maintenance and quality control of
        analyzers, 437–438
    three basic types of technology,
        433–434
Insulin, 451
Intravascular clots, 229
Ion selective electrodes (ISE), 436–437

maintenance and quality control, 438
Iris diaphragm, 37
Iron, 406
Isolation techniques, 67
    complete isolation, 69
    double-bagging, 73
    enteric isolation, 68–69
    entering and exiting patient's room, 72
    glove procedures, 71–72
    gown procedures, 71
    handwashing procedure, 70
    mask procedures, 70
    respiratory isolation, 69
    reverse or protective isolation, 69
    universal barrier precautions, 73
    wound or skin isolation, 68
Isotonic solution, 120
Ivy bleeding time, 244–245

Ketones, 308, 317, 319
Ketonuria, 317
Kidney function, 406

Laboratory. See Equipment; Glassware; Math; Medical laboratory.
Laboratory safety, 14
    biological hazards, 16–18
    chemical hazards, 15–16
    general rules for, 19–20
    laboratory clothing, 18–19
    physical hazards, 15
    safety agreement form, 479–480
    safety check worksheet, 21–22
    teacher/supervisor responsibility, 19
Laboratory supply sources, 507–508
Laboratory test, requesting, 6
Lactate dehydrogenase, 407
Lancet, 80
Lateral site, 80
LDL (low density lipoprotein) cholesterol, 442
Lens, 34
Lens paper, 38
Leukocyte count, differential, 178
    automation, 181
    factors affecting platelets, 181
    factors affecting ratios, 180–181
    factors affecting red cells, 181
    normal values, 179–180
    performing, 179
    precautions for, 181
Leukocytes, 95
    basophil, 174

eosinophil, 174
identification guide for, 173
lymphocyte, 174
monocyte, 174
neutrophil, 172, 174
presence in urine, 318
presence in urine sediment, 325
Leukocytosis, 135
Leukopenia, 135
Levey-Jennings chart, 415–416
Licensing, laboratory personnel, 11
Lipemia, 402
Lipid metabolism, 408
Liter, 51
Liver function, 406
    liver enzymes, 407
    total bilirubin, 407
Lumen, 193
Lymphocyte, 174
Lymphocytosis, 284

Macrocytic cell, 179, 238
Mask procedure, 70
Math for laboratory, 58
    percentage solutions, 60–61
    percentage solutions worksheet, 64
    proportion, 59–60
    proportions worksheet, 63
    ratios, 61–62
    ratios worksheet, 65
    temperature conversion, 59
Mean, 413
Mean corpuscular hemoglobin concentration (MCHC), 237–238
Mean corpuscular hemoglobin (MCH), 236–237
Mean corpuscular volume (MCV), 236–237
Mean value, calculating, 413
Media, 351
    liquid, semi-solid, and solid, 383
    primary plating, 383
    selective and nonselective, 383
    See also Inoculation of media.
Median cephalic vein, 191
Medical laboratory, 3
    blood bank, 6
    chemistry department, 4
    communication problems in, 6–7
    glassware and equipment, 23–32
    hematology department, 4, 6
    isolation techniques for workers, 66–73
    laboratory test request, 6

math used in, 58–65
metric system, 50–57
microbiology department, 4
the microscope, 33–39
non-hospital, 7
organization chart of, 5
overview of, 1–2
personnel in, 8–11
requisition form examples, 504
safety in, 14–20
specimen collection and processing, 6
terminology used in, 44–49
Medical laboratory professional, 8
    career information fact sheet, 12
    educational requirements for, 9–10
    employment opportunities for, 11
    ethics and professionalism, 10
    history of medical technology, 9
    interview fact sheet, 13
    licensing requirements, 11
    and patients, 10
    professional organizations for, 11
    qualities of, 10
    responsibilities of, 10–11
    specialization areas, 10
Medical laboratory technician, 9
Medical technologist, 9–10
Medical technology, 9
Medical terminology. See Terminology.
Megakaryocyte, 172
Melanin, 308
Meniscus, 25
Meter, 51
Methylene blue, 164
Metric system, 50–51
    common measurements, 51
    converting units, 51–53, 488–489
    distance worksheet, 55
    importance of measurements, 51
    temperature conversions, 54, 59, 490
    volume worksheet, 57
    weight worksheet, 56
Microbe, 67
Microbiology department, 4
Microcytic cell, 179, 238
Microhematocrit,
    and automation, 88
    normal values, 87–88
    performance of, 86
    precautions for, 88
Microhematocrit centrifuge, 86
Micropipet, 100
Microscope,
    care of, 39

compound, 34, 37–38
electron, 39
fluorescent, 38–39
parts of, 34–37
phase-contrast, 38
precautions for, 39
Microscope arm, 34
Microscope base, 34
Mid-stream urine sample, 300
Mineral metabolism,
    calcium, 405–406
    hypercalcemia caused by increase in
        calcium, 405
    hypocalcemia caused by decrease in
        calcium, 405–406
    iron, 406
    phosphorus, 406
Monochromatic light, 424
Monochromator, 424
Monocular microscope, 34
Monocyte, 174
Mordant, 361
Morphology, 156
Mucus threads, presence in urine
    sediment, 331–332
Myocardial infarction, 443
Myoglobin, 308

Nephron, 297
Neutrophil, 172
    band cell, 174
Nitrite, 318
Nocturia, 301
Noncritical measurements, 24
Non-hospital medical laboratories, 7
Nonpathogenic, 67
Normal blood cells, identification of,
    and erythrocytes, 172
    and leukocytes, 172–174
    and platelets, 172
    precautions for observing, 174
    Wright's stained blood smear for
        observing, 174
Normal values,
    blood glucose after fasting, 452
    cholesterol, 443
    clinical chemistry tests, 403, 497
    differential leukocyte count, 179–180
    erythrocyte indices, 238
    glucose tolerance test, 452
    hematology, 493–494
    hemoglobin, 147
    microhematocrit, 87–88
    prothrombin time, 229

red blood cell counts, 120
reticulocyte count, 211
urine, 318, 500
urine sediment components, 337
white blood cell counts, 134–135
Wintrobe method for ESR, 203
Normochromic cell, 179
Normocytic cell, 179
Nosepiece, 34
Nosocomial infection, 67
Nucleus, 166

Objective, 34
    high power, 37
    low power, 37
    oil immersion, 37–38
Occupational Safety and Health
    Administration (OSHA), 19
Ocular, 34
Oliguria, 301
Organization chart, medical laboratory,
    5
Overcentrifugation, 402

Parasitology laboratory, 4
Pathogens, 67, 383
Pathologist, 4
Percentage solutions, 60–61
Percent transmittance, 423
Percent transmittance-absorbance
    conversion chart, 498–499
Peroxidase, 453
Petri dish, 216
pH, 317
Pharyngeal swab. *See* Throat culture.
Phase-contrast microscope, 38
Phlebotomist, 6
Phlebotomy, 190
pH meters, 31
Phosphorus, 406
Photoelectric cell, 424
Physical hazards, 15
Physician's office laboratories. *See* POLs.
Picogram, 237
Pipets,
    blood-diluting, 95–106
    graduated, 26–27
    micropipets, 27
    volumetric, 26
    See also Automatic pipets.
Plasma, 86, 401
    and ESR, 205
Platelet count, 215
    automation of, 218–219

calculation of, 216–217
counting the platelets, 216
diluting the sample, 216
filling the chamber, 216
precautions for, 219
procedure for, 216–218
Unopette microcollection system, 218
Platelets, 172
    dysfunction of, 244
    factors affecting, 181
Poikilocytosis, 179
POLs (physician's office laboratories), 7,
    433
Polychromatic stains, 163–164
Polyuria, 301
Population, 413
Porphyrins, 308
Post-prandial specimens, 452
Potassium, 405
Precision, 412
Prefixes, medical terminology, 45–46,
    483–484
Primary plating media, 383
Proportion, 59–60
Protective barriers, 17
Protective isolation, 67
Proteins, 403
    albumins, 404
    globulins, 404
    hypoalbuminemia caused by
        decrease in albumin, 404
    presence in urine, 317, 318
    total serum protein, 404
Proteinuria, 317
Prothrombin, 229
Prothrombin time,
    and abnormalities in hemostasis, 229
    automated method, 231
    manual method, 230–231
    normal values for, 229
    performing the assay, 230–231
    precautions for, 231
    specimen collection, 230
    use of, 229–230
Protozoa, presence in urine sediment,
    327

Quadrant, 371
Qualitative procedures, 6
Quality control,
    accuracy and precision, 412
    analyzers, 437–438
    blood cholesterol measurement, 445
    charts for, 415–416

coefficient of variation, calculating, 416–417
precautions for, 417
spectrophotometer, 426
standards and controls, 411
statistics, 413–415
trends, 416
types of errors, 411–412
Westgard's rules, 416
Quantitative procedures, 4, 6
Quick stains, 165

Random error, 412
Ratios, 58, 61–62
RBC pipet, calculating dilutions for, 97–98
Reagent blank, 425
Reagent pads (test area), 434
Reagents, 24
recipes for preparing, 505–506
Reagent strips, 316–318
Reagent tabs, 435
Reciprocal, 292
Red blood cell count. See Blood cell count, red.
Red-cell-diluting pipet, 95–96
Reducing sugars, presence in urine, 318–319
Reference laboratory, 4, 7
Reflectance photometer, 434
Refractometer, 309
Renal threshold, 452
Respiratory isolation, 69
Reticulocyte count, 209
calculating reticulocyte percentage, 210–211
normal values for, 211
performing, 210
precautions for, 211
Reticulocytopenia, 210
Reticulocytosis, 210
Reticulum, 210
Reverse (indirect) typing , 259, 265
Reverse isolation, 69
Rh blood group, 270–271
Rheumatoid arthritis, 290
Rheumatoid factors, 290
interpretation of results, 291–292
principle of slide agglutination test for, 291
qualitative latex agglutination test for, 291
quantitative latex agglutination test for, 292

significance of results, 292
Rh slide typing,
and hemolytic disease of the newborn, 271
importance of, 271–272
interpretation of results, 272–273
nomenclature for Rh antigens, 271
precautions for, 273
procedure for, 272
Rh blood group system, 270–271
weak D antigen, 271
worksheet for, 276
Rotor, 30
Rouleau(x), 205
Routine tests, 403

Safety. See Laboratory safety.
Sahli pipet, 148
Saline, 58, 59
Sample, 413
Sediment, 324
Sedimentation, 202
Sedimentation rate. See Erythrocyte sedimentation rate.
Self-filling blood-diluting micropipet, 100
Serofuge, 264
Serology, 6
ABO slide typing, 257–260
ABO tube typing, 264–265
overview of, 255–256
Rh slide typing, 270–273
slide test for infectious mononucleosis, 283–286
slide test for rheumatoid factors, 290–292
urine pregnancy test, 277–279
Serum, 4, 401
Simplate device, 245
SI units (International System of Nomenclature), 53, 403
Skin isolation, 68
Slide test. See Infectious mononucleosis; Rheumatoid factors.
Small laboratory instrumentation. See Instrumentation, small laboratory.
Sodium, 404–405
Solid-phase chemistry analyzers, 434
maintenance and quality control, 437
Solid-phase reagent strips, 445
Solute, 25
Solutions, examples for preparing, 491–492
Solvent, 25

Special tests, 403
Specific gravity, urine, 309–310, 318
Specific gravity technique, hemoglobin levels, 147–148
Specimen collection, 6
Spectrophotometer, 433
care of spectrophotometer and cuvettes, 426
parts of, 424
precautions for using, 426–427
principles of spectrophotometry, 423–424
and quality control, 426
and standard curve, 424–426
worksheet for, 431
Spermatozoa, presence in urine sediment, 327
Spirochete, 346
Stage, 37
Standard, 411
Standard curve, 424
determining absorbances of the standards, 425
example of preparation of, 425
plotting, 425–426
Standard deviation,
calculating, 413
example for calculating, 413–415
use of in laboratory, 415
Statistics,
calculating mean value, 413
calculating standard deviation, 413
example for calculating standard deviation, 413–415
population, 413
sample, 413
standard deviation, 413
standard deviation, using in laboratory, 415
Stat test, 7
Stems, medical terminology, 46–47, 486–487
Strict isolation, 69
Suffixes, medical terminology, 46, 48, 485
Supernatant urine, 324
Supravital staining, 210
Synthesis, 147
Syringe, 191
Systematic error, 411

TC, 27
TD, 26-27
Temperature conversions, 54, 59, 490

Terminology,
    abbreviations, 47–49, 481–482
    prefixes, 45–46, 483–484
    pronunciation, 46–47
    stems, 46–47, 486–487
    structure of terms, 44–45
    suffixes, 46, 48, 485
Test tubes, 25–26
Throat culture,
    collecting, 378
    liquid, semi-solid, and solid media
        for, 383
    performing, 384
    precautions for, 386
    primary plating media for, 383
    selective and nonselective media for,
        383
Thrombocytopenia, 216, 244
Thrombocytosis, 216
Thrombus, 229
Titer, 292
Total bilirubin, 407
Total serum protein, 404
Tourniquet, 191
Transferin, 406
Transport medium, 379
Trend, 416
Tubule, 297
Turbidity, 309
Typing. See ABO slide typing; ABO tube
    typing; Rh slide typing.

Universal barrier precautions, 16–17, 73
Ureter, 297–298
Urethra, 298
Uric acid, 406
Urinalysis, 6
    chemical examination of urine,
        315–319
    collection and preservation of urine,
        299–301
    identification of urine sediment,
        324–332
    microscopic examination of urine
        sediment, 336–337
    overview of, 297–298
    physical examination of urine,
        307–310
    routine urinalysis report form,
        501–502
Urine, chemical examination of, 315
    and bilirubin, 317

and blood, 317
    confirmatory tests, 318–319
    and glucose, 317
    and ketones, 317
    and leukocytes, 318
    methods of analysis, 316
    and nitrite, 318
    normal values for urine, 318, 500
    and pH, 317
    precautions for, 319
    principles of chemical tests, 317–318
    and protein, 317
    reagent strip technique, 316–317
    and specific gravity, 318
    and urobilinogen, 317–318
    worksheet for, 323
Urine, collection and preservation of,
    299
    clean-catch specimen, 300
    contamination sources, 300–301
    handling and preserving specimens,
        301
    instructions to female for clean-catch
        sample, 300
    instructions to male for clean-catch
        sample, 300
    mid-stream specimen, 300
    urine volume, 301
Urine, physical examination of,
    color of urine, 308
    odor of urine, 308
    performing physical examination,
        310
    precautions for, 310
    specific gravity of, 309–310
    transparency of urine, 309
    worksheet for, 314
Urine culture,
    antibiotic susceptibility test, 393
    bacteria identification, 392–393
    collecting, 378
    colony count, 392
    performing, 390–393
    transferring urine to media, 390–392
Urine pregnancy test,
    general procedure for, 279
    precautions for, 279
    principle of, 277–279
    specimen requirements, 279
Urine sediment, identification of,
    casts in, 328
    cells in, 325–327

components of, 324–332
    crystals and amorphous deposits in,
        328–331
    microorganisms in, 326–327
    other substances in urine, 331–332
    precautions for analysis, 332
Urine sediment, microscopic examina-
    tion of,
    method for counting cells and
        magnification, 337
    obtaining the sediment, 336
    performing the microscopic
        examination, 337
    precautions for, 337
    worksheet for, 342
Urinometer, 309–310
Urobilinogen, 317–318
Urochrome, 308

Vacuoles, 174
Vacuum tubes, 194–195
    guide for selection of, 503
Vasoconstriction, 244
Vein, 190
Venipuncture,
    equipment selection, 191
    patient preparation, 191
    performing the puncture, 193–194
    precautions for, 195–196
    puncture site care, 194
    puncture site preparation, 193
    puncture site selection, 191
    by syringe method, 190–194
    tourniquet application, 191
    vacuum tubes and anticoagulants,
        194–195
    by vacuum tube system, 194

Walk-in medical facility, 7
WBC pipet, calculating dilutions for,
    98–99
Westgard's rules, 416
White blood cell count. See Blood cell
    count, white.
White-cell-diluting pipet, 96
Whole blood, 401
Wintrobe tube, 203
Working distance, 37
Wound isolation, 68

Yeast cells, presence in urine sediment,
    327